ESSENTIALS OF ANESTHETIC PRACTICE

ESSENTIALS OF ANESTHETIC PRACTICE

STUART C. CULLEN, M.D.
Professor of Anesthesia (Emeritus)
University of California School of Medicine
San Francisco, California
Formerly, Chairman, Department of Anesthesia,
and Dean, School of Medicine

C. PHILIP LARSON, JR., M.D.
Professor and Chairman, Department of Anesthesia
Stanford University School of Medicine
Stanford, California
Formerly, Professor and Vice Chairman,
Department of Anesthesia
University of California School of Medicine
San Francisco, California

YEAR BOOK
MEDICAL PUBLISHERS, INC.
35 EAST WACKER DRIVE/CHICAGO

Library of Congress Catalog Card Number: 73-86838
International Standard Book Number: 0-8151-2052-4

Preface

THE BOOK, *Anesthesia*, edited by one of us (SCC), served a useful function as a manual for the physician obtaining his initial practical instruction in anesthesia, for the non-physician practicing anesthesia, for the physician practicing anesthesia during the course of his general practice and for the student of medicine desiring to learn the fundamentals of anesthesia. This book was first published in 1946, and the sixth (and last) edition was published in 1961. Obviously, this book is 12 years out of date. We believe, however, that there remains a need for a contemporary book similar to *Anesthesia*.

Our efforts, then, in preparing this book were directed toward assimilating and presenting those fundamentals, those items of information and those attitudes and philosophies of anesthesia practice that would be useful to the same group of people for which the original book was designed. This book is not to be construed as a complete text. We have planned, however, for it to be a source of fundamental information sufficient to enable those using it to practice safe, sound anesthesia. We have planned also for it to provide that first overview at clinical anesthesia for those who intend to become specialists in the field. We hope that it will provoke the desire of all who read it to seek more detailed information in those sources that are available. Most of all, we have planned the book to present that sort of philosophy of clinical practice that will foster the approach to the management of anesthesia as an individual problem for each patient. We heartily endorse the policy of trying in every instance to fit the anesthetic management to the special needs of the patient rather than attempting to force the patient to adapt to the anesthetic care that is most familiar, most comfortable or easiest for the anesthetist.

We have consistently approached the presentation of material on a fundamental basis rather than on a "how to do it" basis. This accounts for the fact that the parts and chapters within parts treat fundamentals such as the circulation, respiration and factors common to all anesthetics. We have deliberately avoided attempting to present "anesthesia for the gall bladder patient," "anesthesia for the neurosurgical patient," etc. because we strongly believe that there is no such thing as a "gall bladder patient"—or any other kind of patient linked to a specific surgical procedure. When the surgical procedure requires special anesthetic technics, we have indicated them. We emphasize that patients are individuals with individual mental and physical problems; each is different not only one from another but also different as he or she progresses through various stages of his disease and its management, including anesthesia and surgery. We believe, therefore, it is mandatory to learn fundamentals and relate them to the individual patient in order to safely and satisfactorily manage the anesthesia for the benefit of the individual patient.

If the reader approaches the book in this manner, we think it will provide useful basic information and help to make him or her a better anesthetist.

We are indebted to many of our colleagues for help in preparing the manuscript; especially to Dr. Neri Guadagni, Associate Professor of Anesthesia, for his major assistance in the preparation of Chapter 11, "The Anesthetic Machine," and for his presentation of the appliances used in inhalation anesthesia; to Dr. Ronald Miller for his assistance in the chapter "Muscle Relaxants;" and to Dr. Sol Shnider for his assistance in the chapter "The Obstetric Patient." We recognize also the valuable help of our secretaries, Miss Linda Howard and Miss Gail Teele, and our illustrator, Mrs. Laura Schaubert.

Stuart C. Cullen
C. Philip Larson, Jr.

Contents

PART 1

General Considerations

CHAPTER ONE

Anesthesia— Its Definition and Scope

ANESTHESIA is one of the clinical disciplines in the field of medicine. It has evolved from the courage and ingenuity of men such as Crawford Long and Simpson, the tenacity and adaptability of men such as Morton and Wells, the avariciousness and selfishness of men such as Jackson, the ideas and frustrations of men such as Davy and Hickman and the scientific clinical applications of men such as John Snow. The credit for its conversion in this country from a technical procedure to a broader discipline is due such men as Gwathmey, Guedel, Waters and Lundy.

THE DISCIPLINE OF ANESTHESIA

Anesthesia, as a discipline in medicine, concerns itself with the management of the patient in acute and life-threatening circumstances. The anesthetist is involved in the care of those patients who are unable to establish and/or maintain vital functions such as respiration and circulation. Loss of vital compensatory mechanisms occurs in the state of anesthesia, in disease, in trauma and in surgery. Also, since one of the basic aspects of anesthesia is relief of pain, the control of pain in patients with chronic illness is an element of this specialty. The aspect of critical care in anesthetic practice has evolved from the critical nature of the anesthetic state. In this acute state of dependence, in which the patient's condition is characterized by unconsciousness, insensibility and immobility, the anesthetist becomes responsible for recognizing and promptly treating derangements of respiratory and circulatory functions and of other functions such as acid-base balance, which are induced by iatrogenic or other mechanisms. This familiarity with and knowledge of management of patients in acute and dependent states has led anesthetists to be appropriately involved in the care of patients, for example, in Intensive Care Units (ICU), Respiratory Care Units, Coronary Units, Nursery Intensive Care Units, Emergency Rooms and Drug Poisoning Units. His familiarity with the enigmatic state of anesthesia also makes it appropriate for him to be concerned with pain relief by chemical means or by hypnosis—and, perhaps, by acupuncture.

The involvement of the anesthetist in the acute care of patients is usually on a consultant basis. It is, of course, true that, whether he is administering anesthesia for operative procedures, caring for patients in the ICU, or participating in any other professional activity in which his expertise and interest are useful, he is providing direct care to the patient and exercising his own judgment. The patient is, however, with rare exception, the patient of another physician whom the patient elects to make responsible for his care. The extent and nature of the direct-care responsibility of the anesthetist is dependent upon the delegation of that responsibility by the patient and his primary physician. The delegation of that responsibility is a function of the confidence that the patient and his physician have in the consultant anesthetist. This confidence, especially in the eyes of the patient's primary physician, is developed and attained only by demonstration of competence and interest by the anesthetist. The anesthetist cannot expect to be delegated that responsibility by legislation, by assumption of the specialty of anesthesia or by the granting of the certificate as a diplomate of the American Board of Anesthesiologists. If he is given automatic responsibility through some manipulation in a hospital staff, for example, meaningful responsibility and the confidence of the referring physician can be secured still only by demonstration of competence and interest. We believe, for example, that it will be the infrequent hospital with an ICU that will not delegate major responsibility for that unit to the anesthetist who demonstrates interest, energy, expertise and constant availability. We believe also that the anesthetist who demonstrates his competence and interest will not find it necessary in the interests of good patient care to ask for jurisdictional control of the patients in the ICU. We believe that the patient benefits most from having his care directed by one physician and that that physician in most circumstances welcomes and seeks the assistance of a competent consultant.

The major objective of those in the discipline of anesthesia is to possess knowledge and expertise so that those patients needing assistance in the control of their vital functions on an acute basis, which includes the state of anesthesia itself, can be properly and safely managed through the critical periods of their disability. The knowledge and expertise of the anesthetist is of a special order in that he must be prepared for the unexpected and the unusual. Success is measured by his ability to assess the situation promptly and act on that assessment in seconds or minutes; anesthesia is not a specialty permitting deliberate diagnosis nor therapy taking hours or days. In achieving this objective and to justify assumption of responsibility for patients in critical states, including anesthesia for surgery, anesthetists must be ever alert to the patient as an individual with his own peculiar responses to stress. This means that rigid application of routines for management must be avoided. It means also that management, especially in the anesthetic state, must be related to the individual patient and not to the preferences, convenience or the whims of the anesthetist or surgeon. There can be justification for a specialist in any discipline only if that specialist applies his knowledge and expertise to the successful diagnosis and treatment of the individual as an individual. Surgical anesthetic practice lends itself to the development of rigid routines. The excuse given for this approach is that it is better to know how to apply a few agents and technics well than to diversify in order to meet the challenge of the individual patient's problems. The hazard of the routine approach is that the anesthetist attempts to force the patient to accept the routine rather than attempting to adapt the anesthetic to the patient. Essential to better anesthetic management is the recognition that all patients are not the same. For example, they have different tolerances to drugs and different responses, under stress, of their psychologic and physiologic processes. Furthermore, each patient's condition is not the same at the middle or the end of anesthesia and surgery as it was at the beginning. If one wants to make each anesthetic for each patient as safe and as effective as possible rather than accept success (in terms of morbidity and mortality) on the basis of averages, it is imperative that the anesthetist be prepared to adjust administration of anesthesia to the individual patient.

CLINICAL JUDGMENT IN ANESTHESIA

As in any aspect of medical practice, it is necessary that one have the background, the information and the experience to exercise clinical judgment. Advances in medicine in general and in anesthesia in particular have provided the physician with reliable data that are very helpful in management of clinical problems. However, it is still mandatory that the anesthetist recognize that the "numbers" gained from various measurements of patient response to stress are useful in his managing the patient's problems only if he is able to relate them to what he sees, hears and feels in the patient. Those practicing anesthesia can provide anesthesia that is, in all its aspects, more appropriate and meaningful and more effective and safe anesthesia only if they are prepared with the basic knowledge of the physician as a clinician. Clinical judgment comes, of course, with experience but also only if the anesthetist is able to put together all those aspects of the patient's responses (laboratory data and observation of the patient) in their proper perspective. In these days of reliable instrumentation, the anesthetist is tempted to be inordinately influenced by the "numbers." The successful practitioner of anesthesia, in terms of patient safety, is one who can translate instrumental data and other observations of the patient into appropriate clinical judgment.

Clinical judgment, as defined, must be applied so that the anesthetist is able to induce and maintain a state of anesthesia adapted to the patient, to the surgical procedure, to the attitudes and practices of the surgeon and to the myriad of environmental factors bearing upon the situation on a particular day, in a particular operating room, with a particular set of personnel, etc. This will be discussed later in the section on choice of anesthesia; here, however, it is useful to point out that the state of anesthesia includes three major elements: analgesia, sedation-hypnosis and muscle relaxation. By knowing the particular state of health or mental attitude in the patient and the character of the surgical procedure, one can vary the components to meet the needs of the particular situation. One must learn to recognize the response of the individual patient to the presence (or absence) of pain, sedation-hypnosis and muscle relaxation so that he may administer appropriate drugs in appropriate doses to establish and maintain the desired state.

It is possible, by observing the responses of the patient, to make a distinction between the need of the patient for analgesia, sedation-hypnosis or muscle relaxation.

It is important also in achieving the desired objective in the critical state of anesthesia, as well as in other critical states, to be able to recognize that approaches to therapy that are not based on the use of drugs also may be appropriate. For example, much good can be achieved by establishing mental rapport with the patient for several purposes: to relieve the apprehension, fear and pain that are associated with trauma, surgery and some acute disease states, to improve patient comfort in anesthesia established by conduction methods, to diminish or eliminate the need for preanesthetic drugs in children and to minimize postanesthetic complications. Rapport with the patient can be such that major surgical procedures can be accomplished under hypnosis alone. Other such non-pharmacologic therapeutic methods are, for example, the establishment and maintenance of proper ventilation to compensate for traumatic, surgical or drug depression, or even to provide muscle relaxation without relaxants such as *d*-tubocurarine. Another example is the attention given to establishing and maintaining the correct position not only to facilitate surgery but also to avoid unnecessary impairment of normal respiratory or circulatory function.

With respect to the state of anesthesia itself as a critical and acute problem for the patient, it is important to remember that this iatrogenic disorder includes undesirable influences upon many of the patient's vital functions. There is a price that the patient pays for the benefit derived from the state of anesthesia; for example, the depression of respiration, the depression of heart and peripheral circulation, arrhythmia, the depression of kidney output and the infrequent neurologic sequelae of conduction anesthesia, all of which will be defined more precisely, in the sections on the pharmacology of anesthetic drugs and the influence of various anesthetic systems. The anesthetist must remember that, since he is responsible for inducing and maintaining this state, he is responsible for ensuring that deviation from the normal state is at a minimum. The anesthetist must be acutely aware, for example, that anytime he elects to induce and maintain a state of apnea, either by anesthetic drugs, by relaxants, by conduction anesthesia or by hyperventilation, he then assumes responsibility for a vital function. He then cannot inadvertently, by busying himself with other chores such as blood pumping, changing the light for the surgeon, or even record keeping, ignore the need for ventilation. It is a disconcerting paradox these days that the anesthetist is so used to interfering with adequate ventilation (through the use of drugs, position or paralysis) that he often is callous or indifferent to the constant need for artificial ventilation—with the result that the patient suffers from hypercarbia and hypoxia. To take another example: when the patient is deliberately put in the anesthetic state of dependence upon the anesthetist, the anesthetist must assume responsibility for avoiding such eventualities as burns from cautery or heating and cooling elements, damage to eyes that are left open or from pressure and nerve palsies from undue and prolonged pressure. The anesthetist cannot forget the defenseless state in which he puts the patient and must be ready to be an unrelenting guardian.

Finally, in achieving the objective of caring for the patient in acute states of dependence on expert assistance, one must always keep in mind that, especially in the state of anesthesia, it is the patient who is paying the price of altered and depressed vital functions for the benefit of anesthesia and surgery. As a result, it is mandatory that the decisions regarding management must be made on the basis of the cost to the patient and not on the basis of the convenience, whim, or "standard" practices of the physician.

BENEFIT VERSUS RISK

Throughout this book, an attempt will be made repetitively to measure benefit against risk to the patient. To take three examples: if positive end expiratory pressure (PEEP) is recommended for treatment of respiratory deficiency in the newborn or in the anesthetic state in the adult, one takes into account the disadvantage of reduced venous return to the heart and/or rupture of weakened pulmonary tissue; if vasoactive drugs are used to correct hypotension, the cost of constriction of kidney circulation must be taken into account; and if relaxants are used to still the patient who is moving because of inadequate anesthesia, the cost of not eliminating input of painful stimuli must be recognized.

It is important, then, that the person practicing anesthesia and the care of patients in allied critical states be informed about the basic elements to be described in this book and learn also to apply these basic principles in the safe and successful management of the patient in acute distress. One must be guided by the basic elements, by the basic principles and by the "numbers"; one *also* must be guided by the responses of the patient that can be interpreted only by the application of one's well-developed clinical judgment. We repeat that clinical judgment—that indispensable characteristic of the well-developed physician—can be acquired and maintained only through daily contact with patients and, most importantly, by close observation of the patient as a whole. Both "numbers" and "facts" and that clinical sense derived from observation of the whole patient must enter into the final decision to act appropriately on behalf of that patient.

This, then, is the practice of Anesthesia: the acquisition of knowledge and the application of that knowledge to benefit those patients whose homeostatic mechanisms are critically disordered and who are dependent upon those in the practice of the specialty for diagnosis and treatment. Anesthesia has been described as a practice involving hours of boredom and moments of sheer terror. It is important that those involved in the practice of anesthesia do not submit to boredom because of a failure to be sensitive and responsive to subtle changes of iatrogenic or other origin. In no other discipline in medicine is the patient more dependent upon the knowledge and clinical expertise of those responsible for his care.

PART 2

Factors Common to All Anesthetics

IN THIS PART, we present aspects of the practice of anesthesia that we believe to be common and basic to all anesthetics. We present also our concepts of the manner in which we believe anesthesia should be conducted to ensure safety for the patient and proper working conditions for the surgeon. To accomplish this, we state and reiterate that the approach must involve consideration of each patient, of each anesthetic and of each situation—all as individual problems requiring the expertise of the anesthetist.

Emphasis is placed on the importance of the person in the acute and dynamic process of anesthesia. The patient—as an individual who is faced with a major event in his life and disruption of his normal pattern of living—is the person for whom all efforts must be made. The anesthetist is the scientist-clinician who coordinates the problems of the patient, the surgeon, the procedure and anesthetic management for the best care of the patient. Apparatus is useful in this approach only as it contributes data to be interpreted by the anesthetist and assists him in patient management.

We present the material in this part on a chronologic basis on the assumption that there is a natural sequence to the solution of anesthetic problems which, if recognized and followed, will facilitate the solution and ensure better patient care.

CHAPTER TWO

Preanesthetic Evaluation of the Patient

THE ANESTHETIST AND PATIENT INFORMATION

MOST PATIENTS SURVIVE routine approaches to diagnosis and therapy in medicine. Most patients survive the acute process of anesthetization, even when the anesthetist's management is routine and based on a limited knowledge of the patient and his illness or of the anesthetic agent or technic. If, however, the objective in medical therapy, including anesthesia, is to approach each patient as an individual with problems needing solutions peculiar to his own state of illness and his responses to that illness, it is mandatory that the anesthetist become familiar with the patient as a human being, as a total individual and with his particular disorder (or disorders).

It is essential that the anesthetist know as much as possible about the individual patient not only in order to properly select the anesthetic agent and technic but also to manage anesthesia safely and effectively. Admittedly knowledge of the concomitant presence of such disorders as a hernia, hemorrhoids or a lipoma in many circumstances will influence little the selection and management of an anesthetic for a patient who, for example, is to undergo gastric resection. All of us, however, have known of situations in which patients came to major surgery (such as laminectomy) with undiagnosed cancer of the large bowel or significant but unrecognized deficiencies in cardiac or pulmonary function. These deficiencies may have been "overlooked" because, for example, a low hemoglobin value was ignored, no effort was made in the history to elicit complaints other than those related to back pain, and complete physical examinations were not done. We hold no brief, for example, for the policy of withholding anesthesia or surgery, or both, simply because the hemoglobin value is below some arbitrary level. We do hold, though, that it is essential to make every effort to find out why the hemoglobin value is low. As another example, we do not propose to interdict anesthesia if the patient has a cough. We do, however, believe that with such a patient every effort should be made to determine the significance of the symptom rather than offhandedly assign it to cigarette smoking. Similarly, as a final example, we see no reason for arbitrarily cancelling a tonsillectomy and adenoidectomy in a child on account of a slight elevation of temperature on the morning of the operation. It is mandatory, however, that meaningful inquiry be made into possible causes for the elevation in temperature and that appropriate action be taken on the basis of the cause rather than on the temperature elevation itself.

The anesthetist must be a part of this total information-gathering process. If the anesthetist assumes any responsibility for the care of the patient, as he should, he is then obligated to help ensure that the history, physical examination and laboratory testing are all appropriately complete. In the best interests of the patient, the anesthetist is obligated, of course, not only to ensure that as much as possible becomes known about the patient's state of health but also to learn these things in order to manage the anesthetic properly. In assisting in this information-gathering process, the anesthetist is obligated to review the information available in the chart and to interview and examine the patient. Usually, the examination of the patient by the anesthetist is limited to those critical areas such as respiration and circulation but, if review of the chart or the interview with the patient alerts the anesthetist to other investigative possibilities, he is obligated to pursue them or to see to it that they are pursued. Because the anesthetist functions ordinarily as a consultant, obtaining additional information about the patient is necessarily referred to the patient's primary physician; but with mutual understanding between the patient's primary physician and the anesthetist, some anesthetists assume the responsibility for the preoperative preparation of the patient. The anesthetist must be discreet about revealing information to the patient prior to consulting with the patient's physician. It is unwise also to order directly any additional investigations without consulting the patient's physician or adhering to some previous arrangement with him. Such factors as cost to patient and the possible presence of such information in office records must be taken into account.

It is important that the anesthetist visit with the patient before the day of operation so the patient can identify the anesthetist as a real person who is interested in the patient's welfare rather than a "ghost" of some sort seen in a hazy and confused state immediately prior to anesthesia. Such a "ghost" is often brought to reality only when the patient receives the statement for professional services.

REASSURANCE OF THE PATIENT

Most patients are concerned about the anesthetic process and many have well-established ideas about what they want and do not want. They may be thoroughly misinformed by friends, relatives and others who are full of "old wives' tales" about anesthesia. Many patients are not at all well informed about the total anesthetic and surgical experience, including the periods of preparation, surgery and recovery. Many are uninformed about the nature and extent of any discomfort they may have. Many are also uninformed about the need for simple exercises such as moving, leg bicycling, coughing, and deep breathing. All these things, together with others, can be explained in a relatively short interview, with the result that, because the patient is now informed, he often is substantially relieved of many unnecessary worries and better prepared for anesthesia and surgery.

This sort of rapport with the patient is especially beneficial in the preparation of youngsters. Youngsters as well as adults are more afraid of the unknown than the known, and it has been clearly established that any child with whom one can communicate, however young, is much less apprehensive at the time of induction if he is made aware of what goes on. It is often useful, for example, to have the child visit the operating room area or, at least, to bring to him some of the paraphernalia of anesthesia such as a mask. The need for heavy premedication is substantially diminished by acquainting the child with as much of the procedure as possible. Even so, it is important not to attempt to hoodwink the youngster. For example, if he will smell something strange as he goes to sleep, if he will be stuck with a needle or if he will be a little sick to his stomach after the operation, he should be told about these things. If a child has been told that he can have ice cream after his tonsillectomy, when he finds out both that he cannot have ice cream after the operation and that it is not palatable, he is going to be very disturbed. Even more important, in the future he is going to be distrustful of anything that has to do with doctors and nurses and the practice of medicine in general. This may be manifested by sequelae such as bed-wetting, nightmares and withdrawal.

In addition to obtaining information about the physical state of the patient from the record and any additional personal examinations desired, it is critically important to assess the patient's attitude about the whole surgical situation. This information will not only assist the anesthetist to select the appropriate anesthetic agent and technic but also will make it possible for him to attempt to relieve distress by answering questions, providing information and, in general, assuring the patient that things are expected to go well. Such assessment of the patient's reactions and responses to this stressful situation will also help to determine the nature and extent of premedication. Finally, the patient's knowledge that his anesthetic will not be managed by a total stranger but rather by someone with whom he has had contact and conversation is in itself one of the most significant and important features of the evaluation and preparation process.

EVALUATION OF THE PATIENT

During the visit to the patient, the anesthetist can also evaluate other physical aspects that are often critical in determining management of anesthesia. For example, it is useful to know if the patient is obese and how the fat is distributed. If the neck is excessively fat, one might anticipate some difficulty in managing the airway and take appropriate steps to minimize the difficulty. If the arms and legs are excessively fat, one can anticipate difficulty in establishing an intravenous line and take necessary steps to ensure a stable line by prior cut-down if indicated. One can also expect that exercise and ventilation of the lungs will be compromised and steps can be taken to ensure extra attention to obese patients in order to diminish the likelihood of a complication such as atelectasis.

The anesthetist can also observe the shape of the mandible, the oral opening, the presence or absence of protruding upper teeth and the presence or absence of dentures or capped or loose teeth. If there are, for example, carious and loose teeth or teeth with caps, it is wise to alert the patient to the possibility that these may be damaged during intubation. A narrow and receding mandible suggests there may be difficulty with intubation of the trachea; one might be well advised to prepare for nasotracheal instead of orotracheal intubation and to provide optimum position, relaxation and depth of anesthesia for intubation. Likewise, one can inspect the abdomen to advantage. If the abdomen is protuberant, one can be prepared to provide appropriate relaxation and working conditions for the surgeon by selecting spinal or epidural anesthesia or by being prepared to use generous amounts of relaxant. If the abdomen is scaphoid, one can anticipate that providing good working conditions within the abdomen will be not difficult and that any appropriate agent and technic will usually suffice.

If one plans on using conduction anesthesia (i.e., spinal, epidural or regional block), it is wise to examine the site of needle placement to determine, for example, the presence (or absence) of bony landmarks or infection.

It is wise, of course, to make special inquiries into items pertinent to anesthesia selection and management that often are overlooked in the standard history and physical examination. For example, it is useful to know what drugs patients have been or are taking. Of particular interest are antihypertensive drugs, various drugs used in the treatment of diabetes mellitus, tranquilizers, narcotics (for pain or due to addiction), barbiturates, and mind-affecting drugs such as LSD and amphetamine. It is useful also to know if the patient has any general allergic tendencies or any known specific allergy, especially to drugs. Inquiry into the family history is useful. For example, a family sensitivity to succinylcholine or a family trait of unusual response to drugs such as morphine or anesthetics may be elicited. It is also useful to inquire into previous experiences with anesthesia. By so doing, one may learn about difficulties that arose, special reactions that developed and, of course, personal dislikes or preferences of the patient. Fortunately, modern anesthetic records detail patient responses that provide useful clues for subsequent management. Although the phenomenon of sensitivity to halothane (or similar fluorinated agents) is not unequivocally established, one should inquire as to its previous use in the patient so that whatever steps each individual anesthetist elects to take can be planned.

It is useful also for the anesthetist during the preanesthetic visit to assess the overall impression that the patient gives. For example, does the patient look older (or younger) than the age given? Does the patient seem to be putting on an air of bravado and be inwardly tense with fear? Is the patient stoical and so more suitable for conduction anesthesia or is he so apprehensive that, even if he were to accept conduction anesthesia, the reactions would make such anesthesia unsatisfactory? Making these overall assessments enables the anesthetist to anticipate responses, to make appropriate adjustments and to be prepared for reactions. This overall assessment is often given a number and is designated usually as the risk or physical status. The anesthetist can assign a number to the physical status if he wishes; what is important, however, is that he arrive at an assessment that gives him a working basis for managing the anesthetic. Risk is another thing;

risk takes into account not only the physical state of the patient but a host of other factors such as competence of surgeon and anesthetist and all others involved in the care of the patient, the quality and quantity of equipment and the familiarity of personnel with that equipment, the frequency with which the particular operative and anesthetic procedure has been done by those involved, the mental attitudes and physical conditions of the persons involved (one of whom may, for example, have a cold or have kept late hours on the day before operation), the experience of the surgical team in working together and the environment in the operating room (e.g., whether the air conditioner is working). Risk also involves the patient's mental state: whether he is cooperative and ready to do all he can to survive with minimal morbidity, whether he can be expected to be unwilling or afraid to take deep breaths, cough and move and, finally, whether he is in such a state that he is ready to die and will make little or no effort to avert a fatal outcome.

After having made the preoperative evaluation, it is vital that the essence of the evaluation, including especially such details as notable features of the patient's illness, physical build (e.g., obesity or muscularity), dental condition (poor or false teeth) and previous anesthetic history, be noted in the chart. This notation can be combined with a note concerning the selection of anesthetic and patient's agreement to it.

THE NEED TO INFORM THE PATIENT

In view of patients' awareness of the medicolegal aspects of the practice of medicine, it is important also to inform the patient as completely as is feasible and prudent about the possible complications of anesthesia. In doing so, of course, the anesthetist must be aware of the nature and extent of information about the operation that the surgeon intends to impart to the patient so that there is no inadvertent conflict in the information provided by anesthetist and surgeon. Attorneys, of course, insist that the patient must be "completely" informed in order to give "informed consent" to anesthesia and operation. It is not possible within the scope of this book—nor for that matter in any treatise—to define "informed consent." The anesthetist must use his own judgment, after assessing the patient's reaction to the anticipated stress of anesthesia and operation, as to the nature and extent of information about anesthesia he will impart to the patient. Thus, it may be appropriate, based on the anesthetist's own philosophy and his assessment of the patient's reactions, to inform the patient as to the relative chances of cardiac arrest. Certainly, it is usually wise to tell the patient that he may have respiratory complications such as atelectasis (or pneumonia) if he does not cough and move about in the postoperative period. The patient should be informed also about the likelihood of phlebitis and the necessity for leg movements after operation. Probably the type of anesthesia that is more critical in requiring the anesthetist to impart information is conduction anesthesia; spinal and epidural anesthesia seem to be more susceptible to litigation. As a result it is important to inform the patient about the incidence (which is very low) of neurologic complications such as paresthesias and localized paralysis. Headache, of course, should be mentioned even though its mention may increase the chances of its occurring. What is most important is to emphasize to the patient that these things may occur in the presence of excellent management and that their appearance does not automatically indicate poor management. What is exceedingly important in all of this is that the instructions and the information given to the patient and the patient's responses be written in the record at the time the information and response take place. Information given and responses obtained after the patient has received premedication are less valid.

It can be seen, then, that in practicing the individual approach to the care of patients in acute states including anesthesia, the preanesthetic evaluation of the patient through the mechanism of direct personal contact is essential. No patient can be managed successfully, especially in cases of acute disease or traumatic process, without direct personal contact; anesthesia care is no exception to this rule.

CHAPTER THREE

Preparation of the Patient for Anesthesia

PREPARATION AND SUBSEQUENT MANAGEMENT of the patient are influenced significantly by results of the evaluation. In this chapter, we will elaborate on various aspects of the preparation of patients for anesthesia and operation. Many of the factors included in the preparation of the patient for anesthesia are also vital to preparation of the patient for surgery. The fundamental objective is to prepare the patient so that he has the best chance for complete recovery from both anesthesia and surgery.

THE MILIEU OF THE OPERATING ROOM

In order to prepare the individual patient, the anesthetist must not only know about problems peculiar to that patient but also be familiar with the many characteristics of the surgeon: his personality, competence, dexterity, speed (or slowness) of work, attitude under stress of work, peculiarities of technic and personal preferences and dislikes. It is often said that a poor surgeon needs a competent anesthetist and the good surgeon deserves one. Obviously, it is the patient who needs all the competence of those responsible for his acute care. In a situation such as anesthesia and surgery, it is vital to the patient's welfare that anesthetist and surgeon recognize and adjust to each other's personalities and ways of working.

In addition to the surgeon and anesthetist knowing each other, it is important that the anesthetist know the operation. He then will be prepared to provide suitable working conditions at minimal physical and mental cost to the patient. The anesthetist also will be prepared to anticipate and plan for changes in the physical state of the patient caused by the operative procedure. For example, blood or other appropriate fluids can be made ready, appropriate vasoactive agents such as phentolamine (Regitine) can be made available in cases of pheochromocytoma and arrangements can be made for appropriate monitoring with technics such as blood-gas analysis, electrocardiography and central venous pressure.

In preparing the anesthetist so that he can prepare the patient properly, some other items are important. For example, the anesthetist needs to know whether, at the time of operation, he should consider electrical hazards such as cautery, special lights, saws and static electricity. If an explosive agent is deemed the best solution to the particular anesthetic problem, it is necessary for the anesthetist to plan for appropriate adjustments in the operating room milieu pertinent to electrical hazards.

SPECIFIC PREPARATION OF THE PATIENT

Now that we have outlined the elements that enter into the preparation of the anesthetist, the surgeon and others and that bear on the preparation of the patient, we can consider some of the more specific items pertaining directly to the patient and his mental and physical state.

Laboratory Examination

A necessary part of a complete preoperative examination is the basic laboratory panel of hemoglobin, hematocrit, red and white cell counts and urinalysis. By determining these values, one establishes a base line for further reference and one can recognize and correct deficiencies. Some of the deficiencies, such as a low hematocrit, can be corrected more efficiently and more safely a day or more prior to operation than on the eve or the day of operation. The hazards of ignoring the basic blood and urine examination are the likelihood of subjecting patients to surgery and anesthesia that may adversely affect an unrecognized disorder and overlooking a disorder that may unfavorably influence anesthesia or surgery. For example, early or occult forms of sickle cell anemia or porphyria may be detected.

Temperature Elevation

A common problem is the slight elevation of temperature that appears the evening before or on the morning of operation. We hold that a slight elevation of temperature by itself has little influence on the choice of anesthesia or its management (in the absence of malignant hyperthermia) but that its origin must be investigated. The classic example is the slight elevation of temperature appearing in the youngster scheduled for tonsillectomy. The elevation may be due simply to mild dehydration or the effect of premedication with belladonna preparations or it may be the prodrome of an upper respiratory infection or an acute exanthema. One must, of course, be influenced by the economics of the situation; hospital costs are such that a waste of a day's hospital costs through cancellation and deferment is important. However, such costs must be weighed against the cost to the patient of exacerbation of an unrecognized or incipient disorder by proceeding with elective surgery—the end costs may be substantially greater by taking the latter course. The special problem of malignant hyperthermia is discussed in Chapter 28.

Nutrition

The general state of nutrition of the patient must be assessed and steps taken to improve any deficiency. Unfortunately, even with the use of hyperalimentation solutions, the process of restoration of nutrition is slow. One can hope only to correct the existing deficiencies as effectively as possible by appropriate alimentation in the optimum time that is available.

A significant problem related to nutrition is obesity. Ample evidence indicates that obesity materially increases the incidence and severity of complications associated with anesthesia and surgery. The obese patient often has significant cardiac and respiratory deficiencies and these may be exaggerated during operation and in the postoperative period. Obviously, whenever possible, the patient should be strongly urged to reduce prior to surgery and anesthesia.

Assessment and Management of the Diabetic Patient

A specific nutritional problem is that of the diabetic patient. After the diagnosis of diabetes has been made and its nature and extent established, it is necessary, of course, to prepare the patient for surgery and anesthesia and to manage the diabetic condition during the operative and postoperative period. One must first stabilize the diabetic state as well as possible during whatever time period is available before operation. This may mean, in emergency circumstances, the appropriate balancing of glucose intake and insulin needs parenterally. Each physician seems to have his own routine for management of diabetes in the surgical patient, and the anesthetist is well advised to consult with the physician managing the diabetes. There is, however, reasonable consensus that there should be minimal deviation from the established pattern of diet and insulin. In most patients this means continuing administration of the same type of insulin, the dose usually being decreased just before anesthesia and surgery. It means also that the diabetic patient is scheduled for surgery preferably in the early part of the schedule so that there is time during the remainder of the day to make necessary adjustments in insulin and glucose intake, either by the intravenous route or by restoration of oral intake. Probably an insulin reaction, rather than inadequate control of glucose metabolism, is the greater problem that may be encountered.

Assessment and Management of Circulation

In patients with known cardiac and peripheral vascular disease, it is necessary to assess the nature and degree of circulatory deficiency by means of history, physical examination, ECG, transaminase studies, serial weighing and electrolyte studies. It is necessary also to obtain a history of responses to whatever drugs have been used, such as digitalis, diuretics and potassium. In brief, an objective is to establish some reasonable steady state; the problems of assessment and management of circulation are discussed more completely in Chapter 20.

Position is an important factor in cases of circulatory impairment. It is useful to determine from the patient what position he finds most comfortable and what positions he cannot tolerate, and to avoid using the latter positions in the anesthetized patient. Although it is rarely done, useful information about the patient's tolerance can be obtained by placing him in the anticipated operative position prior to anesthetization. By so doing, one can establish the response of the patient (e.g., arrhythmias, dyspnea and hypotension) in the absence of complicating factors such as depression from the anesthetic, blood loss and surgical manipulation. Patients for whom assessment of responses to various positions is useful are as follows: 1) those with occlusive disease of the head and neck vessels, who have learned by experience in what positions they cannot place the head or neck without loss of consciousness; 2) patients with large bullae of the lung who may have learned that they cannot lie in certain positions without severe impairment of ventilation; 3) patients with orthopnea from severe heart or lung disease, who obviously cannot tolerate lying flat; 4) some patients who react to the traditional position for renal surgery with pronounced hypotension; and 5) the pregnant patient, at or near term, who often may have hypotension when lying supine because the vena cava becomes compressed by the uterus.

Assessment and Management of Respiration

For patients with known or suspected pulmonary deficiencies, special investigations are needed in the preparation period. The methods for making the special assessments and the evaluation of those measurements are described in Chapter 19; here it is sufficient to state that precise knowledge of the state of lung function is necessary for preparation of the patient, proper selection of agent and technic and proper management during and after operation. Many steps can be taken to improve lung function materially and to set the stage for improved postoperative care. Thus, for a patient with bronchiectasis a program of lung drainage can be used to remove secretions. The condition of a patient with obstructive lung disease can be improved sometimes by the application of intermittent positive pressure or end-expiratory positive pressure. The patient is thus also instructed on such technics for use after operation. There is good evidence, especially from the Scandinavian countries, that training in breathing exercises (i.e., deep breathing, holding an inspiration, breathing with the chest versus the diaphragm and even lateralizing the breathing) not only improves lung function preoperatively but also, more importantly, prepares the patient for useful lung exercises after operation. Patients should be informed in the preanesthetic period of the need for procedures such as proper and adequate breathing, coughing and changes in position so that they can prepare themselves, not only as indicated above but also mentally for such maneuvers in the presence of pain.

Medications

Many patients before entering the hospital are receiving some form of drug therapy, and many of these drugs affect total body function and, indirectly or directly, the management of anesthesia. Two of the more important of these drugs used by many patients are corticosteroids and antihypertensives. Currently, younger patients are often taking such drugs as LSD, amphetamine and various barbiturates. Marijuana, however, we discount as having little or no impact on the patient's reactions to surgery or anesthesia, unless it has been used excessively and for an extended period of time (i.e., for years).

CORTICOSTEROIDS.—Our practice with respect to corticosteroids is to determine what drug is being used, for what purpose, for how long and with what effect. Such knowledge alerts us to the nature and extent of the disease for which the drug is being used and the progress of that disease. Generally, we make no effort to discontinue the drug but rather to continue the same drug at the usual dose throughout the surgical and anesthetic experience. Of course, if the drug has influenced the fluid and electrolyte balance significantly, it is necessary in the preparation of the patient to assess such changes and to attempt to restore a normal balance prior to anesthesia and surgery.

ANTIHYPERTENSIVE DRUGS.—Our practice is similar with respect to antihypertensive drugs. Most patients receive the same drug in the same dose before, during and after anesthesia and surgery. Hypotension of varying degrees, augmented perhaps by the drug, may be anticipated; therefore preparation should include establishment of reliable intravenous routes and the availability of appropriate drugs to counteract hypotension. Fortunately, in most patients taking antihypertensive drugs, a complete loss of epinephrine stores does not occur, and drugs working through catecholamine mechanisms remain effective. In the presence of a significant loss of epinephrine, any vasoactive drug working as an alpha-adrenergic stimulant will be effective.

It is important to remember that a patient with long-standing hypertension (from any cause) has diminished plasma volume; as a result, shock may develop more readily with relatively minimal losses of blood and fluid. Moreover, certain anesthetic drugs and technics (e.g., halothane and spinal anesthesia) induce pronounced hypotension by relaxing the vascular system and thereby create a discrepancy between plasma volume and vascular capacity. A patient whose vascular tension is suddenly lessened, as in surgical sympathectomy or the removal of pheochromocytoma, needs to have the plasma volume restored to compensate for the increased vascular capacity.

BARBITURATES AND OTHER DRUGS AFFECTING THE CENTRAL NERVOUS SYSTEM.—If the patient has been taking barbiturates, one can be prepared for residual depression from the drugs. If the barbiturates have been taken intermittently or in relatively heavy doses for some time, one may anticipate withdrawal symptoms from the lack of drug during hospitalization. A patient taking various hallucinatory drugs may be expected to show an affect that is different from normal and his emotional reactions to planned anesthesia and surgery may be unpredictable. Flashbacks from previous use of these drugs may be expected and may influence the anesthetist's selection of a technic such as regional anesthesia. If a patient has been on recent protracted or repeated "trips," one may also expect some deficiency in nutrition and fluid intake.

For the patient addicted to narcotics or barbiturates there is no virtue in attempting therapy at the time of surgery. It is better to continue the usual intake of the particular drug. For such patients narcotics and/or barbiturates may be given if these are indicated as part of premedication or the anesthesia itself. If the patient has been permitted to continue taking his usual dose, the dose for premedication or during surgery or for pain relief is the same as for the non-addict. Likewise, patients (especially those on psychiatric therapy) who have been taking large doses of mood-changing drugs, such as chlorpromazine (Thorazine), should preferably continue taking the same drug in the same dose.

ALCOHOL INTAKE.—If the patient is in the acute phase of alcohol ingestion, one must try to discover whether the patient is a chronic alcoholic. For an acute phase in a nonalcoholic patient, an important consideration is whether the stomach is full. The management of this problem is discussed in Chapter 26. There is no need to attempt to sober the patient; indeed, the acute state serves as reasonable premedication. If the patient is belligerent, sedation with a drug like thiopental may be needed. Chloral hydrate can be used, but it functions essentially no better than a barbiturate; paraldehyde is unpleasant, no more effective than thiopental and it may produce pulmonary microemboli.

If it is determined that the acute phase is only another episode in the life of a chronic alcoholic, additional inquiry and correction is needed in relation to a likely deficiency in the nutritional and fluid state. One can, of course, suspect severe impairment of liver function. To some extent, augmented glucose and protein intake can compensate, but the anesthetist should be alerted to avoid anesthetic agents and technics that may worsen liver damage. All involved should be alerted to the possible development of hepatic coma after operation and to the possibility of the need for treatment of delirium tremens before, during and after surgery and anesthesia. Susceptibility to delirium tremens appears to be greatest in the chronic alcoholic. This is especially so in those patients who participate in intermittent bouts of drinking and who have had no alcohol intake for a period of 24-72 hours. The chronic alcoholic who continues to drink alcohol up to the time of anesthesia and surgery seems less susceptible to delirium tremens, provided that his intake is not interrupted during the hospital stay. As with the narcotic or barbiturate addict, treatment at the time of surgery is not worth attempting.

PREMEDICATION

Pre-"medication" is the traditional label for the drugs used in the final step of preparation of the patient to make him tranquil and relatively indifferent to the stress of confrontation with a new and often frightening situation. Drugs are used also to decrease the level of general metabolic activity and thereby to decrease concentration and total amount of anesthetic drug needed.[1,2,3] If the patient is in pain, analgesic drugs are a proper part of premedication. Drugs are used also to suppress reflex responses or to eliminate or minimize the effects of anesthetic agents. For example, atropine can be used to block bradycardia and/or hypotension due to carotid sinus or celiac plexus manipulation or bradycardia due to halothane or cyclopropane.

TABLE 3-1.—CHEMICAL DIVERSITY OF COMMONLY USED SEDATIVE-HYPNOTICS(a)

CHEMICAL CLASS	REPRESENTATIVE EXAMPLES
Barbiturates	Hexobarbital (Evipal) Pentobarbital (Nembutal) Phenobarbital (Luminal)
Thiobarbiturates	Thiopental (Pentothal) Methohexital (Brevital)
Piperidinediones	Glutethimide (Doriden) Methyprylon (Noludar)
Carbamates	Ethinamate (Valmid) Meprobamate (Miltown)
Benzodiazepines	Chlordiazepoxide (Librium) Diazepam (Valium)
Quinazolones	Methaqualone (Quaalude)
Alcohols	Chloralhydrate (Ethanol) Chlorobutanol (Chloretone)
Cyclic ethers	Paraldehyde

(a) Reproduced, with permission, from Way and Trevor.[4]

The first objective (i.e., tranquility and sedation) can be achieved in large part without drugs by establishing rapport with the patient.

Pharmacokinetics

For the anesthetist to use drugs properly and effectively, it is important that he understand the pharmacokinetic aspects of drug action. Pharmacokinetics is the measurement of concentrations of a primary drug and its metabolites in body fluids and tissues with respect to time. The overall pattern of distribution of a drug (absorption, distribution, metabolism and excretion) is influenced by its physicochemical properties. To act within the central nervous system, a drug requires a suitable combination of properties, including a relatively high lipid:water partition coefficient and a low degree of ionization at body pH. Most sedative-hypnotics are either weak acids (e.g., barbiturates) or weak bases (e.g., diazepam [Valium]) or neutral compounds (e.g., carbamates such as meprobamate [Miltown] or paraldehyde). Lipid solubility plays a major role in determining the rate at which drugs penetrate and leave the brain. For example, pentobarbital (Nembutal) has a much lower partition coefficient than thiopental (Pentothal) and penetrates the blood-brain barrier much more slowly.

Since sedative-hypnotics are often given orally, it is useful to know that in the stomach (pH near 1), weakly acidic drugs (e.g., barbiturates and glutethimide [Doriden]) are almost completely nonionized and hence are absorbed at rates dependent upon lipid solubility through the "lipid sieve" of the epithelial lining of the gut. For example, barbital (Veronal) is 40 times less soluble in lipid than is amobarbital (Amytal) and, although both drugs have essentially the same degree of ionization, amobarbital is absorbed more rapidly. Some degree of water solubility is also critical in the absorption of drugs from the gastrointestinal tract. Sodium salts of most barbiturates, including thiopental, are more water-soluble and are therefore readily absorbed from the stomach. Weakly basic drugs, such as chlordiazepoxide (Librium) and diazepam (Valium), are most effectively absorbed at or near

TABLE 3-2.—PHARMACOLOGIC PROPERTIES OF SEDATIVE-HYPNOTICS AND TRANQUILIZERS(a)

PHARMACOLOGIC PROPERTY	SEDATIVE-HYPNOTICS	TRANQUILIZERS
Sedation (low dose)	Yes	Yes
Easy arousal (higher dose)	No	Yes
Antipsychotic effect	No	Yes
Anticonvulsant effect	Yes	No
Extrapyramidal effects (Parkinsonism-like symptoms)	No	Yes
Anesthesia	Yes	No
Autonomic effects		
Anticholinergic	No	Yes
α-Adrenergic blockade	No	Yes
Respiratory depression	Yes	No
Physical dependence	Yes	No

(a) Reproduced, with permission, from Way and Trevor.[4]

neutral pH in the small intestine or colon. This must be taken into account if one anticipates that stomach mobility is diminished or absent when oral medication is given.

During transport of a drug in blood, a dynamic situation develops in which drug molecules enter and leave tissues at rates primarily dependent upon blood flow, concentration gradients and permeabilities; this is a process that is discussed more fully in the case of anesthetic agents (Chapter 15). The intensity of drug action is a function of dose but duration of action largely depends on the pattern of redistribution. For example, rapid redistribution of drugs to lean body tissues (tissues with relatively high blood flow) is primarily responsible for short duration of hypnotic action. Metabolic inactivation and excretion are of marginal significance in influencing the degree of sedation but do influence to some extent the degree of post sedation hangover.

Types of Drugs Available

Tranquility and sedation can also be achieved by several types of drugs: (1) sedative hypnotics, (2) tranquilizers and (3) narcotics. It is pertinent to establish what we consider to be the difference between sedative-hypnotic drugs and tranquilizers. We consider that a sedative drug is expected to calm the patient and allay anxiety yet not to abolish easy arousability, coordinative and motor ability and mentation. It is critical, however, to realize that actions of drugs are dose-dependent and that sedative-hypnotic drugs can, in larger doses and with respect to age, physical state and interaction with other drugs, for example, go beyond the optimum point just outlined. Table 3-1 lists commonly used sedative-hypnotics[4]; Table 3-2 lists basic differences between the sedative-hypnotics and tranquilizers. We hold that sedative-hypnotic drugs are more appropriate for premedication than tranquilizers. As Table 3-2 indicates, sedative-hypnotic drugs and tranquilizers share only sedation. Tranquilizers have the apparent advantage of easy arousability and absence of respiratory depression or physical dependence. The arousability, though easy, is often associated with a "startled" reaction.

The sedative-hypnotics (in doses used for premedication) cause minimal respiratory depression and physical dependence is not a factor. Furthermore, the sedative-hypnotics do not cause extrapyramidal effects nor do they introduce the elements of anticholinergic action or alpha-adrenergic blockade.

SEDATIVE-HYPNOTICS AND TRANQUILIZERS.—In the past, it has been customary to classify barbiturates (as one class of sedative-hypnotics) according to their length of action. Now it is apparent that length of action is a function largely of distribution and absorption. As a result, it is more meaningful to *classify* the barbiturates in terms of absorption and distribution; furthermore, it is more meaningful to *apply* the drugs on the basis of absorption and distribution as influenced by the properties of the respective drugs and factors in the patient such as intestinal activity and the state of competence of circulation. If, however, one desires prompt action of short duration, one can select a drug such as thiopental that is rapidly absorbed in the stomach and rapidly redistributed. For more prolonged action, one can use a drug that passes more slowly through the lipid barrier in the stomach and has different concentration gradients and permeability.

In preparing a patient for the experience of anesthesia and surgery, the anesthetist should take into account the problem of sleep and rest during the night prior to the procedure. In arriving at a reasonable solution to this problem, it is useful to determine if the patient's normal sleep pattern involves difficulty in getting to sleep but no problem in staying asleep or whether the pattern is the reverse. For the former, a short-acting agent like thiopental might be indicated; for the latter, a longer-acting drug like secobarbital (Seconal) or diazepam (Valium) might be indicated.

Determination of dose.—Dose, of course, is a critical factor in producing the desired effect, and in determining dose one must take into account the apparent degree of apprehension and anxiety of the patient and any history one may obtain about any previous response to similar drugs. Naturally, one considers the age of the patient, the general state of well-being and special circumstances, such as porphyria, that preclude the use of barbiturates.

One common practice is to select the dose of a drug based on body weight. This practice is useful for sedating or anesthetizing animals but it is not applicable to the premedication of human beings prior to anesthesia or for the production of sleep. Factors such as we have mentioned—age, state of well-being, degree of anxiety, previous experience with drugs, influence of drug on anesthetic management, interaction with longstanding drug use or interaction with drugs such as amphetamine—are the important factors in determining dose. Of these factors, age is probably the major determinant of dose.[5,6] The use of weight as the determinant leads to gross errors in dosage. For example, the obese patient may have a sluggish circulation with consequent slower distribution. Metabolic activity also may be low and the need for drug diminished on this account. On the other hand, a larger dose may be needed for a patient of the same age who is thin, wiry and very active with high blood flow and rapid distribution of drug.

Choice of sedative-hypnotic.—Choice of a sedative-hypnotic, then, depends on one's ability to assess the factors mentioned. Although the various drugs have different times of onset and lengths of action, probably the most significant feature is dosage, and one needs to be aware of all the factors that influence the amount of drug to be given. One can be somewhat precise in prescribing a sedative-hypnotic. For example, if in the premedication period one needs to produce only a short period of sleep with a minimal effect thereafter, including an impact upon anesthetic agent and technic, one can use thiopental by mouth. If, however, one wants a somewhat longer action with minimal impact on the anesthetic and is somewhat concerned over one's ability to decide on an optimal dose, one can use diazepam (Valium), which has a longer action and a rather flat dose-response curve and which permits wide variations in dose.

Finally, the interaction of sedative-hypnotics with other drugs should be considered. Although there are a number of questionable interactions of varying degree with other drugs, from a practical standpoint, one probably needs only to be interested in a negative interaction that may occur between sedative drugs and amphetamines. The former drugs may "turn off" or slow down the reaction to amphetamines. However, it has been noted that, in the patient constantly taking high doses of amphetamine intravenously, the barbiturates may augment violent aggressive behavior.

NARCOTICS.—In achieving the objectives that have been outlined, narcotics are useful not only in producing or adding to the sedative-hypnotic effects but also in diminishing the level of metabolic activity and in eliminating or minimizing pain. This latter ability of the narcotics is useful in premedication to relieve distress of the patient in pain from his disorder and to minimize the discomfort associated with the induction of conduction anesthesia. Pain relief is useful also in minimizing distress associated with procedures that may be part of the induction of inhalation anesthesia; for example, the insertion of needles for intravenous fluids or medications, the introduction of catheters for arterial or central venous pressure and the placement of the patient in position on a hard or cold operating table.

Narcotics also contribute to the state of tranquility in patients who do not have existing pain. Although dysphoria develops in some patients after the administration of a narcotic—as evidenced by nausea, emesis and an ill-defined state of mental uneasiness—most patients find that their stressful situation becomes ameliorated by a sense of warmth, relaxation and indifference to surroundings. This, we believe, contributes to the desirable pre-anesthetic state. As with other classes of drugs, the desirable effect is highly dose-dependent and, in general, one needs only to give relatively small doses. For example, in the absence of pain the average adult will need doses such as 5–10 mg of morphine, 50 mg of meperidine (Demerol) and equivalent doses of any other narcotic one may elect to use. As in the case of the sedative-hypnotics, it is necessary to assess the patient's tolerance to the drug that is to be used, adjust the dose accordingly and avoid the use of weight as a criterion only insofar as it reflects the general well-being of the patient and the uptake and distribution of the drug.

The narcotics also contribute to the anesthetic state itself by decreasing the level of metabolic activity. This means, for example, that induction and maintenance concentrations of anesthetic agents may be less than those needed if a narcotic has not been used. This was established for ether in

1957 by Taylor, *et al.*,[1] for halothane in 1964 by Saidman and Eger[2] and for fluroxene in 1965 by Munson, Saidman and Eger.[3] With doses of approximately 10 mg in adults, there was a 15% decrease in the concentration of ether required to produce the same EEG level, a reduction from a MAC value of 0.74 to 0.69 of halothane and a reduction from a MAC value of 3.4% to 2.9% of fluroxene. Thus, if one intends to maintain anesthesia with a combination of a narcotic and nitrous oxide, the first stage in the process can be begun with the premedication.

There are disadvantages, of course, to the use of narcotics in premedication. They contribute to respiratory and circulatory depression in varying degrees according to the dose used, the physical state of the patient and his individual degree of susceptibility to the narcotic. They (especially morphine) may also cause contraction of the sphincter of Oddi (a condition that simulates gallbladder colic), nausea, emesis and relaxation of the bowel. In practice, most anesthetists who plan to use anesthetic agents such as halothane and cyclopropane do not use narcotics as premedication because those agents have little or no stimulating effect on respiration. The use of a narcotic then would often cause slowing of induction. Likewise, maintenance of a satisfactory anesthetic state is impeded.

Choice of narcotic.—Many narcotics may be used for premedication. These include morphine, alphaprodine (Nisentil), meperidine (Demerol), fentanyl (Sublimaze) and pentazocine (Talwin). There are relatively few differences between them and the choice of one or the other depends largely on the personal preference of anesthetist or patient. Differences in duration of action are of some significance; fentanyl and alphaprodine have a very short duration of action. Pentazocine is not subject to the control of addictive drugs and is effective orally. In some patients alphaprodine, fentanyl and meperidine have the unusual property of producing severe stiffness of the chest, which sometimes prevents ventilation even with extreme inspiratory pressure. This can be overcome by administering nalorphine (Nalline), levallorphan (Lorfan) or naloxone (Narcan). Patients may have individual differences with respect to the incidence and degree of nausea, respiratory depression and circulatory depression. If the likely occurrence of such side effects from a narcotic can be determined by a history of personal previous experience of the patient with a narcotic, it may be useful to use a different narcotic. Formerly, it was believed that morphine had a more significant impact upon the patient's reaction to pain—that the drug had more of a "central" action than, for example, meperidine. Investigations have shown, however, that such a difference, if it does exist, is minimal.

Although we are opposed, in principle, to premixed combinations of drugs, there are advantages in premedication and during conduction anesthesia to using the combination of fentanyl and droperidol (Innovar). Droperidol tends to diminish nausea and emesis and makes the patient less aware of the environment. The anesthetist must be cautious in repeating the combination because droperidol produces an appreciable residual mood change (e.g., confusion). With the combination of a narcotic (unless this is considered a disadvantage as, for example, prior to the use of halothane) and a barbiturate or diazepam one can produce most of the elements of satisfactory premedication. It seems to bring the patient to the operating room in the desirable state of comfort, lack of pain, sedation-hypnosis and indifference to the proceedings without any unnecessary difficulty in arousal and with minimal respiratory and circulatory depression.

NARCOTIC ANTAGONISTS.—Highly efficient antagonists to narcotics are sometimes useful in premedication as well as in the inclusion of narcotics as part of the total anesthetic. These agents are capable of reversing all aspects of narcotic action, especially respiratory depression and analgesia. There is, however, clinical evidence that reversal is dose-dependent; in other words, it seems possible to reverse respiratory depression satisfactorily without eliminating analgesia. This property of the antagonists is useful in those circumstances in which respiratory depression occurs out of proportion to depression of pain stimuli.

The narcotic antagonists include nalorphine (Nalline), levallorphan (Lorfan) and naloxone hydrochloride (Narcan). The usual dose for complete reversal is 5 to 10 mg of nalorphine, 0.5 to 1.0 mg of levallorphan and 0.3 to 0.4 mg of naloxone hydrochloride. Effective reversal of respiratory depression can be achieved often by doses of 1.0 mg of nalorphine, 0.1 mg of levallorphan and 0.02 to 0.05 mg of naloxone hydrochloride. Nalorphine and levallorphan seem to act as narcotics when used in larger doses than those recommended for complete reversal, and one may then anticipate added depression rather than reversal. Naloxone hydrochloride, on the other hand, is not only exceedingly potent but does not contribute to depression in larger doses.

Attempts have been made ever since the introduction of antagonists to narcotics to develop an optimal mixture of narcotic and antagonist that will provide pain relief without respiratory depression. Generally, such mixtures have been unsatisfactory because all patients do not react to narcotics (or antagonist) in the same manner.

BELLADONNA DRUGS.—The remaining objective of premedication—minimizing or eliminating reflexes—is usually accomplished by the use of either scopolamine or atropine. Formerly, when anesthesia was produced most often by ether, induction was slow owing to the inefficiency of the technic (i.e., open drop) and the high solubility of ether. The slow induction permitted the patient to remain in a level of depression in which mucus production was not only not inhibited but probably enhanced. Under such circumstances scopolamine or atropine was useful in diminishing the output of secretions. Nowadays, because of more effective technics and faster-acting agents, induction is rapid, and inhibition or reduction of secretions is no longer the primary function of the belladonna drugs in premedication.

Atropine and scopolamine still are useful in blocking vagal transmission. Hence, bradycardia due to agents such as cyclopropane and halothane can be alleviated, and bradycardia and hypotension due to physiologic responses such as carotid sinus or celiac plexus stimulation can be controlled. We believe that, for premedication, scopolamine is superior to atropine because scopolamine contributes to the patient's state of indifference to surroundings and amnesia whereas atropine contributes only to the patient's discomfort by

Table 3-3.—Dose Ranges of Drugs Used in Premedication

AGE OF PATIENT (YR)	DRUGS AND DOSE RANGES: MORPHINE(a) (MG)	SECOBARBITAL PENTOBARBITAL (MG)	DIAZEPAM (MG)	ATROPINE (MG)	SCOPOLAMINE (MG)	FENTANYL & DROPERIDOL [INNOVAR] (ML)
0-1	0	0	0	0.05-0.1	0	0
1-2	0.5	0-5	1-2	0.05-0.1	0	0
2-5	1-2	10-25	2-3	0.1-0.2	0.05-0.1	0
5-10	2-5	25-50	3-5	0.2-0.3	0.1-0.2	0.5
10-15	5-8	50-100	5-10	0.3-0.4	0.2-0.3	0.5-1.0
15-60	5-15	100-150	5-10	0.3-0.6	0.3-0.4	1-2
60-75	5-10	50-100	5-10	0.3-0.4	0.2-0.3	0.5-1
75+	2-5	25-50	3-5	0.1-0.3	0.1-0.2	0-0.5

(a) Dose-equivalents of narcotics (mg) to 10 mg morphine: fentanyl, 0.05; pentazocine, 30; alphaprodine, 40; meperidine, 100.

dryness of the throat. Among some anesthetists scopolamine is in disfavor as a premedicant because it is claimed that the drug contributes to aberrations in behavior prior to and after anesthesia. We submit this is a function almost exclusively of the use of too large doses. As a blocking agent, scopolamine is as effective or more effective than atropine, and smaller doses can be given. In addition, if the vagal block is inadequate, atropine always can be added to achieve the desired objective. The postanesthetic delirium that is often attributed to scopolamine is due to the patient's reaction to pain in the presence of incomplete recovery from the mental inhibiting effect of the anesthetic agent. As a guide to dosage, we suggest that for the average adult in good condition 0.4 mg of scopolamine is the maximum dose—0.3 mg would be satisfactory; for the elderly or very young 0.1 mg often suffices.

Summary of Doses of Drugs Used in Premedication

We have repeatedly referred to the importance of the dose of a drug and to the many factors that influence dosage. We have emphasized age as being probably the most critical factor. Dose ranges of the various drugs are presented in Table 3-3 with the proviso that the dose ranges of premedicant drugs must be adjusted to the individual patient, the type of anesthetic agent and technic and the situation in accord with the factors we have already outlined. We do not believe that we can formulate a foolproof pattern when so many variables are involved. As a result, we urge the reader to use Table 3-3 in relative rather than absolute terms.

Timing of Premedication

Almost as critical in achieving the desired effect as dose is timing. All too often in the busy and unpredictable operating room schedule, premedication is ordered "on call." Unless the anesthetist is alert to progress of the schedule, premedication is often forgotten and given to the patient subcutaneously on the cart on his way to the operating room. Obviously, this is often not only ineffective as a means of bringing the patient to this important experience in his life in a tranquil state, but also it may add to the difficulties and hazards in managing the anesthetic in that depression from the premedication occurs later in the early or middle stages of the anesthetic. If the premedication is poorly timed, all the efforts to achieve the objectives of premedication are wasted and the patient is subjected to discomforts and apprehensions that the anesthetist seeks to avoid or diminish. The anesthetist, with his awareness of the progress of the operating room schedule, should ensure that the drugs are given at a time that permits maximum effect prior to induction of the anesthetic state.

Route of Administration of Premedicant Drugs

In view of the factors of absorption and distribution, the intravenous route obviously ensures better absorption and the impact of distribution is more immediately evident and assessable. If other routes are used (i.e., oral, subcutaneous or intramuscular), one must be aware of the differences in absorption and subsequent distribution as well as the ability of the drug itself to be absorbed. One must be aware of these differences not only to get the most efficient absorption and distribution for each drug but also to ensure the development of a maximal effect prior to anesthesia; that is, to have the drugs provide the premedication. In general, the oral route is the least predictable with respect to absorption, especially when the normal process of absorption from the stomach or small bowel is impaired because of disease or apprehension. The subcutaneous route is more predictable and constant but somewhat slower than the intramuscular route. The latter route, depending upon the proximity to and availability of blood vessels at the site of injection, approximates the intravenous route in speed and predictability of absorption.

In concluding our consideration of the problems of preparation of the patient, we reiterate that the period of preparation of the patient gives the anesthetist the opportunity to acquaint the patient with his identity, to further acquaint himself with the patient's mental and physical state, to inform the patient about the upcoming experience in anesthesia and surgery and to prepare the patient for the events of the immediate postanesthetic and postoperative period. As in other aspects of the practice of anesthesia and the practice of medicine in general, one can resort to routines and get by with it with most patients; but there is no substitute for individualizing each patient's problem and attempting to solve the problem according to each individual patient's needs. Only by so doing can one expect to achieve the best results for each patient—and what other excuse is there for developing a well-informed, competent and conscientious physician?

REFERENCES

1. Taylor, H. E., Doerr, J. C., Gharib, A., *et al.*: Effect of preanesthetic medication on ether content of arterial blood required for surgical anesthesia, Anesthesiology 18:849, 1957.
2. Saidman, L. J., and Eger, E. I., II: Effect of nitrous oxide and of narcotic premedication on the alveolar concentration of halothane required for anesthesia, Anesthesiology 25:302, 1964.
3. Munson, E. S., Saidman, L. J., and Eger, E. I., II: Effect of nitrous oxide and morphine on the minimum anesthetic concentration of fluroxene, Anesthesiology 26:134, 1965.
4. Way, W. L., and Trevor, A. J.: Sedative-hypnotics: a review, Anesthesiology 34:170, 1971.
5. Bellville, J. W., Forrest, W. H., Jr., Miller, E., *et al.*: Influence and age on pain relief from analgesics, J.A.M.A. 217: 1835, 1971.
6. Sherman, E. D., and Robillard, E.: Sensitivity to pain in the aged, Can. Med. Assoc. J. 83:944, 1960.

CHAPTER FOUR

Choice of Anesthesia

ALTHOUGH THERE MAY BE few positive indications, if any, for any particular anesthetic agent and technic, there are some absolute or relative contraindications. As a result, it is necessary that the anesthetist persist in the individualistic approach to solving the anesthetic problems he encounters; he must take into account not only the factors pertaining to the evaluation and preparation of the patient already outlined but also those pertaining to the patient's physical state and the properties of the various agents. It is necessary also that the anesthetist be familiar with administration of a wide variety of agents and technics so that he can meet the challenges of the requirements and contraindications safely and satisfactorily. The challenges are oriented toward the patient, the operation, the disease, the anesthetist, the surgeon and the environment.

We are aware of the cliché that agent and technic are secondary in importance to the talent of the anesthetist. We have no quarrel with this premise, but we hold that the talented and informed anesthetist becomes so because he is aware of and takes into account in his expert management the differences that exist in the patient, in himself, in the surgeon, in the operation and in the environment. We urge that both the experienced anesthetist and the beginner or part-time anesthetist avoid the pitfall of using a single agent or technic simply because it solves most (not all) of his anesthetic problems and because he thinks his special proficiency (by reason of exclusive use) compensates for his lack of diversity and adjustment to the particular requirements or contraindications that do exist. Establishment of such a comfortable rut seems to have been enhanced by the introduction of halothane. This agent's favorable properties have led many anesthetists to abandon attempts to develop experience and proficiency with other agents and technics. By so doing, they have permitted themselves to become unable to cope with situations in which other agents and technics might be more suitable and safer for the patient. As with all agents, it is now apparent that halothane is not without hazard in some circumstances and those anesthetists who have limited themselves now find that they are ill-equipped to resolve safely some of the anesthetic problems with which they are confronted.

Factors bearing on the choice of agent and technic, then, include the patient's desires and his disease, the anesthetist's preferences, dislikes and competence, the surgeon's requirements and preferences and the environmental situation. Probably the most significant indications are strong personal preferences by patient or surgeon, or both, provided, of course, there are no contraindications to these preferences. Often the patient's preference is associated only with the induction period and is expressed as a desire for "pentothal." This does not, of course, limit the choice of agent and technic for other than the induction period. The patient's preference may be expressed also as a desire not to know anything about what is going on and to be assured that he will feel no pain. Such a preference does not necessarily preclude conduction anesthesia because appropriate medication can satisfy the desire; usually it means that inhalation anesthesia is indicated. On the other hand some patients wish to be aware of what is going on and have a fear of "going to sleep"; such preferences can be met with conduction anesthesia. Generally, it is unwise to "talk a patient into" a form of anesthesia that he does not prefer; this is especially true of spinal or epidural anesthesia.

The surgeon's preferences should be expressed in terms of the need for proper operating conditions rather than in terms of specific agents or technics. The surgeon should indicate such requirements as the degree and length of relaxation, a quiet lung, a certain position, high urinary output, cautery, deliberate hypotension and hypothermia. Likewise, he should indicate the possibility of complications such as air embolism, fat embolism, excessive hemorrhage and brain stem damage.

The major factor influencing choice of agent and technic comprises contraindications. As we have emphasized consistently, it is critical that the anesthetist be familiar with the patient and his disease, the surgeon and his operative requirements, the environmental elements (e.g., time of day, state of well-being of personnel and availability of equipment) and all the agents and technics in modern anesthesia. It is not enough, in the interests of patient safety, to have the anesthetist attempt to adjust his "usual" agent and technic to the particular problem when the problem can be better and more safely resolved by an agent and technic that is not absolutely or relatively contraindicated.

In this chapter, rather than discuss all the numerous potential contraindications, we will present only a few examples to illustrate the point. There are few absolute contraindications to the use of particular agents or technics. Examples are the following: (1) barbiturates in the presence of porphyria; (2) halothane after a history of unexplained fever, eosinophilia or jaundice following a previous exposure to halothane; (3) high concentrations of anesthetics (e.g., nitrous oxide) in circumstances in which high oxygen concentrations are needed, as with patients who have cyanotic heart disease or severe lung disease, and with moribund patients; and (4) explosive agents in the presence of ignition sources. Relative contraindications are legion and reflect in part an anesthetist's personal knowledge and experiences; they include the following examples: (1) highly fat-soluble agents for prolonged anesthesia in obese patients; (2) conduction anesthesia (i.e., spinal) for patients with disease of the central nervous system; (3) conduction anesthesia for patients to be placed in an uncomfortable position such as the lateral position for a nephrectomy; (4) spinal or epidural anesthesia for patients in shock; (5) halothane for therapeutic abortion; (6) ketamine in adults; and (7) dislike on the part of patient or surgeon for particular agents or technics.

At the risk of overemphasis, let us repeat that we believe the patient benefits by having the anesthetist fit the anesthesia to the patient and his disease, to the surgeon and his requirements, and to the environment rather than trying to fit all these factors to one agent or technic and the anesthetist's lack of diversity. The talented and well-informed anesthetist always can improve his standard of safe and satisfactory anesthesia by applying his judgment and knowledge to the conditions he deals with in his anesthetic practice.

CHAPTER FIVE

Monitoring

MONITORING IS A VITAL FUNCTION of the anesthetist through which he pursues and extends the policy of individualizing the management of each patient. It is critical to the success of monitoring, however, to adopt and apply the concept that the monitor is the anesthetist. By functioning as a monitor, the anesthetist can determine the responses of each patient so that he can (1) become aware of early signs of change, (2) make second-to-second adjustments in anesthetic management, and (3) predict subsequent changes and anticipate appropriate therapy. The various methods and devices that are improperly labeled as monitors are simply means of providing information about the patient to the monitor (the anesthetist). These methods and devices cannot substitute for the indolent, indifferent and inept anesthetist. The methods and devices cannot interpret; they can only provide data which the anesthetist must then interpret and so institute appropriate adjustments. These methods and devices, furthermore, should function to enhance the scientific knowledge and clinical judgment of the anesthetist; in presenting data, they should enable the anesthetist to sharpen his clinical abilities so that in time he can detect changes almost as readily as the devices. One of the major hazards of widespread application of devices is a tendency on the part of the anesthetist to become dependent upon the gadgetry and to "untrain," or cause to lie dormant, his senses used to evaluate patients. In functioning as a monitor, the anesthetist pays special attention to various aspects of the cardiovascular, respiratory and central nervous systems.

There are a number of simple and reliable methods for obtaining information about changes in the major organ systems. We shall detail these for each system not only to emphasize their usefulness, reliability and ease of application but also to establish the basic concept that the monitoring function is not limited to or primarily a matter of gadgetry.

THE CARDIOVASCULAR SYSTEM

Simple Methods

AUSCULTATION OF THE HEART.—*The stethoscope and heart sounds.*—A stethoscope applied to the chest can provide useful and constant information about the rate, the quality of heart sounds and any irregularity of heart action. In the case of air embolism, it can provide also the characteristic sound of air in the heart chambers. The anesthetist should train himself to detect changes in heart sounds. It has been established that not only the intensity but also the nature of heart sounds change with alterations in the concentration of anesthetic drug to which the heart is exposed.[1] With higher concentrations, the heart sounds become muffled ("mushier") and, even more significantly, the relative emphasis of the first and second sounds changes.

In addition to the traditional stethoscope, useful modifications are available. First, there are simple heavy metal open-sided pieces that function as stethoscopes when placed either on the chest over the heart or on the trachea suprasternally. Placed in this latter spot they also provide information about respiration. The advantage of the latter simple devices over the traditional stethoscope piece is the weight, which permits placement without taping. Second, one of the most useful simple devices for obtaining information about heart (and respiration) is the esophageal stethoscope. This consists of a catheter fitted with openings in the terminal 2 to 3 cm over which is fitted a loose balloon. If the stethoscope is properly positioned in the esophagus, the anesthetist can listen through an ear piece to the sounds of the heart and breathing. The esophageal scope is especially beneficial in those circumstances in which placement of the stethoscope on the chest or trachea is precluded by position or the operative site. Third, an ear piece can be fitted for the individual anesthetist. Such ear pieces can be fashioned by technicians familiar with the making of ear pieces for patients with hearing aids. They remain in position, they permit mobility of the anesthetist by attachment of long leads of tubing, they ensure constant attention to cardiac and respiratory sounds, and they allow the anesthetist to have one ear available for attention to other necessary sounds and conversation in the operating room. Many anesthetists find it convenient also to arrange with appropriate bidirectional valves from intravenous sets to connect both blood-pressure apparatus and the chest or esophageal stethoscope to the ear piece (Fig. 5-1).

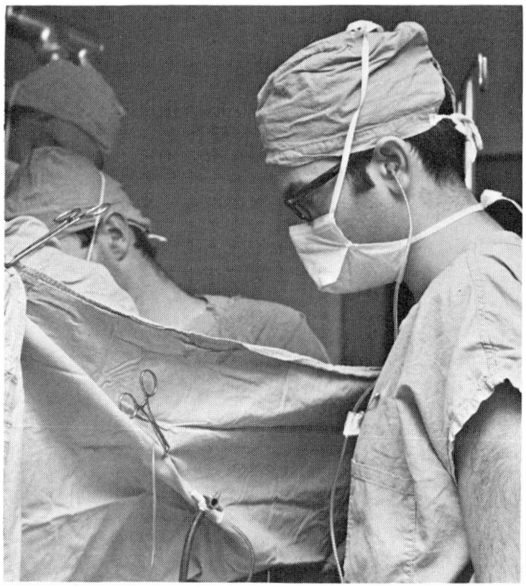

Fig. 5-1.—Ear piece in place connected to a three-way valve connected to esophageal stethoscope (or chest piece) and the stethoscope for blood-pressure measurement.

PALPATION OF THE PULSE.—An "educated" finger on the pulse can detect changes in rate, quality and regularity. The finger may not be able to calibrate the quality or determine the nature of the irregularity but it certainly can alert the anesthetist to a change that can be verified by the ECG and measurement of blood pressure. A disadvantage is that palpation is often discontinuous and some adaptation occurs.

MEASUREMENT OF BLOOD PRESSURE.—The traditional method of measuring the blood pressure is by means of stethoscope and cuff. Usually, it is convenient and more stable to place the stethoscope underneath and at the distal edge of the cuff, the tubing generally being directed toward the head of the patient. It is important that the cuff be the width of two thirds of the diameter of the arm; an excessively wide cuff will result in an abnormally low absolute reading and a cuff that is too narrow in either adult or child will result in an abnormally high absolute reading. Many anesthetists find it just as informative and simpler to use only the cuff and make readings from the "bounce" of the needle in an aneroid manometer. This is probably satisfactory if one is interested in approximate rather than absolute values for arterial pressure. Most anesthetists prefer the aneroid to the mercury manometer because of its smaller size, greater mobility and greater oscillation. The aneroid manometer, however, is more prone to loss of calibration and more subject to damage (e.g., by being dropped onto hard floors).

Instruments are now available that use the Doppler effect. Changes in blood flow introduced by compression of the artery by a blood pressure cuff can be transmitted to the instrument from a sensor located over an artery and translated into sound signals. The instrument is remarkably insensitive to movement and extraneous currents. It is especially beneficial in measuring blood pressure in infants and small children and in situations like hypothermia in which the usual cuff method is unreliable.

EVALUATION OF COLOR AND THERMAL CHANGES.—It is important for the anesthetist to train himself to recognize subtle as well as gross changes in color. These changes give useful clues to the state of the heart and peripheral circulation. One needs to be able to distinguish between the pale color of shock and the ashen color of near total or total circulatory collapse. A simple test for the adequacy of peripheral circulation and return of blood is the application of digital pressure to the skin and determining the speed of return of color to the blanched area. Quick return of a pink color in an area blanched by digital pressure suggests that the peripheral circulation is adequate, provided that the skin temperature is reasonably normal (i. e., not cool and sweaty). If, on the other hand, the patient looks pale, the return of blood to a blanched area is slow and the skin is cool and sweaty, one should be alerted that the peripheral circulation may be inadequate. One should not take any one aspect of a change in any body system as the sole determinant for diagnosis and action. Evaluations of this sort, as with most assessments of body functions, are more informative when performed serially.

DETERMINATION OF URINARY OUTPUT.—Assuming that renal function is normal, urinary output can be a useful measure of the competency of the circulation. Obviously, urinary output reflects many other factors that bear on it such as input of fluid, nature of fluid input and increased excretion of antidiuretic hormone caused, for example, by narcotics. All these must be taken into account in assessing the meaning of changes in urinary output.

Assessment of mentation.—If the patient is awake, as with conduction anesthesia, the celerity of response and the orientation of the patient's verbal responses are useful in assessing the nature and degree of deterioration of the heart and peripheral circulation. Also to be taken into serious consideration is the patient's preference as to position. A desire, for instance, to have the head elevated gives clues not only to the state of heart and circulation but also to the optimum position to be maintained, if possible, during the anesthesia and surgical procedure.

Complex Methods

In this chapter, only an outline of complex methods of monitoring is presented. Each is discussed in more detail in Chapter 20.

Electrocardiography.—The ECG is, of course, the most commonly used device to provide data on the heart during anesthesia. This apparatus, however, reflects only the electrical events occurring in the heart and it is not a measure of heart function. Furthermore, it has been demonstrated repeatedly that a normal ECG complex can be seen on the oscilloscope or tracing of a heart that, for practical purposes, is totally nonfunctional and even in apparent asystole.

The instrument that is adaptable to use in the operating room is capable of displaying a tracing that is useful in practice only for detecting changes in rhythm. Because it is built to withstand the rigors of functioning in an operating room, the instrument lacks some sensitivity to the heart's electrical changes (other than those of rhythm) and is not too reliable in representing changes in the complex due to such factors as hypoxia, alterations in potassium concentrations and infarction. To permit continuous observation, the instrument represents the electrical output of the heart by an oscilloscope tracing. Some instruments have a built-in direct writing device but, because of the built-in diminished sensitivity, these instruments are still unable, especially if multiple leads are not used, to depict changes that can be seen on the standard ECG apparatus.

Instruments suitable for use in the operating room should incorporate circuitry that allows the sweep to center itself if it becomes displaced from the screen because of loose leads or use of the electrosurgical unit, for example. These instruments also should permit adjustment in the intensity and height of the tracing to facilitate identification in the brightness of the operating room and to compensate for low-voltage input, for example, from poor leads; they also should permit the speed of the oscilloscope sweep to be adjusted to facilitate counting of the rate and to permit better analysis of the complex and rhythm changes. Inclusion of an integrating device to display a read-out of the heart rate is useful but not mandatory.

Instruments used in the operating room are often designed to allow one to use leads that can be fitted to needles placed subcutaneously. However, because current becomes concentrated in the needles if ground connections of other electrical apparatus are faulty and because needles are more painful to insert, it is preferable to use contacts made of small conductive discs, which are applied to the skin of the patient by means of larger foam rubber discs with built-in adhesive. The conductive discs have leads attached to a junction box. The junction box is then connected to the oscilloscope unit through an appropriate lead to a jack.

The ECG can also be monitored by means of telemetry. The leads are placed in the usual manner but are connected to a small transmitter. The transmitter sends a signal to an FM tuner, the output of which is picked up by an oscillosope. A significant advantage of telemetry is the elimination of the likelihood of grounding of other electrical energy such as from an electrosurgical unit. Moreover, the oscilloscope does not respond to the currents generated by other electrical sources. Telemetry is, however, responsive to transmitters within the range of abutting operating rooms and the oscilloscope may display the ECG transmitted from another room. Also, the FM tuner may be out of tune; the oscilloscope then displays a spurious tracing.

Because interest in the operating room is confined almost exclusively to changes in rhythm, the leads need be placed only in such a manner as to give an identifiable complex which, for convenience, has the R wave upright. As a result, the leads are often placed with the two active contacts on either side of the upper chest and the third (ground lead) on the anterior axillary line caudal to the upper chest lead. In modern instruments the leads and junction box are color-coded to facilitate placement.

Whenever an instrument such as the ECG is used at the same time as another electrical unit, especially the electrosurgical unit, one must guarantee a ground connection for the unit.[2,3] Deliberate decrease of the input resistance of the ECG facilitates the passage of current through the leads if the ground connection of the electrosurgical unit is faulty or inoperative. Current then is concentrated at the needles or disc contacts, and severe burns may result.

MEASUREMENT OF CENTRAL VENOUS PRESSURE.—Determination of the central venous pressure (CVP) is a well-established method of assessing one of the critical elements of the circulation. Essentially, CVP measures the ability of the heart to take care of the venous load to which it is exposed. A rising venous pressure is a sign that the heart is incapable of managing the load. CVP is an index of the pressure in the venous system at its central point; ideally, this point is the right atrium. In practical use, however, the superior vena cava at its entrance into the atrium is equally satisfactory, and this position may be better for removal of air. Measurement of venous pressure at any other site introduces the possibilities of complications such as venospasm, changes in position with distortion of veins and interruption of venous connection to the central pool; as a result, the measure is unreliable and not useful in assessing the state of heart function.

The preferred technic of determining CVP is as follows: A long plastic catheter (an infant feeding catheter is useful) is introduced through the left antecubital vein and threaded centrally. With the catheter connected to a

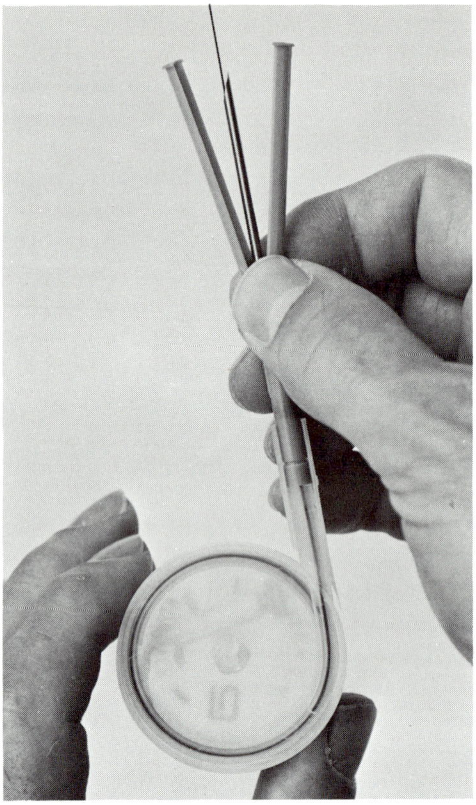

Fig. 5-2.—Example of package of needle, catheter and guards for central venous pressure line.

strain gauge and the output of the gauge depicted on an oscilloscope tracing, the catheter can be advanced until the tip is in the right ventricle as shown on the oscilloscope by the pressure swings generated in the ventricle. The catheter is then withdrawn until the pressure swings disappear and only the smaller swings of pressure produced by the changes in intrathoracic pressure from respiration are evident. In the absence of an oscilloscope, one looks for the unimpeded pressure swings due to respiration. Available for CVP measurement now is a device incorporating a large-bore needle and a length of catheter that can be advanced up the vein by means of a reel which can be unwound. The assembly then comes apart and the needle removed so that all but the catheter is left in place (Fig. 5-2). A reasonable approximation of central venous pressure can be secured by inserting the standard intravenous plastic cannula into the superior vena cava through the external jugular vein. The technic of venous catheter or needle placement is described in Chapter 12.

Measurement of CVP can be made in several ways. The simplest is to arrange, by means of bidirectional valves and ordinary intravenous tubing, a column of fluid (whatever fluid one elects to use intravenously) which, when connected to the tubing in the vein, reflects venous pressure. This simple and homemade arrangement can be substituted by a ready-made assembly of tubing and stopcocks and an attached scale reading in centimeters of water. The zero point is established by lowering or raising the column and attached scale so that the zero point is at heart level. If this is not done or if the position of the patient is changed, the readings obtained are, of course, not absolute but only relative. Venous pressure measurement can be accomplished also by connecting the venous catheter to a strain gauge, the output of which is represented on an oscilloscope tracing. As for the simpler method, the strain gauge must be open to atmosphere and adjusted to heart level in order to obtain absolute values for venous pressure. Occasional flushing of the venous line with fluid or with fluid containing a small amount of heparin may be necessary to keep the line open.

Some assessment of venous pressure can be made in the absence of an intravenous line by observation of the peripheral veins, especially the jugular veins. Skin color is another useful sign. If the skin is suffused or cyanotic and this clears with rubbing, one can suspect an increased venous pressure. Obviously, these changes may be due to interference with venous return from factors such as pressure and position, but if the signs described do appear and there is no obvious interference with venous return, one is well advised to use a direct technic of measurement.

The CVP line is useful for the removal of air in cases of air embolus. Prompt diagnosis through the esophageal, tracheal or chest stethoscope of the presence of an air embolus and the immediate removal of the air through the CVP line has undoubtedly saved the lives of many patients. It is, therefore, considered a mandatory item in cases in which air embolism is a potential complication, as with posterior craniotomy in the sitting position.

DIRECT MEASUREMENT OF ARTERIAL PRESSURE.—It is standard and useful practice to establish an intra-arterial line to obtain information on the second-to-second changes in systolic, diastolic and mean pressure. This method of measurement of arterial pressure is particularly useful in certain circumstances: (1) when measurement by cuff is not possible (e.g., hypothermia, burns and intensely constricted peripheral vessels); (2) when the anesthetist is performing other tasks such as pumping blood; (3) when data on reactions to surgical manipulations are needed on a second-to-second basis; (4) when deliberate hypotension is desired; (5) when measurement of pressure in another vessel, such as the carotid or renal artery, is needed in relation to systemic arterial tension; and (6) when systemic pressure changes occur rapidly as in cardiac and vascular surgery.

The practicing anesthetist can be expected to be proficient in making an arterial puncture and in establishing and interpreting the measurement made via transducer and oscillographic representation. Instruments useful for direct measurement of arterial (or venous pressure) under the conditions of the operating room are now reliable and relatively simple to operate. As described for the ECG apparatus, the instrument should have an oscilloscope display that is self-centering and has variable intensity and speed of sweep; also, calibration and zero-setting should be simple. Useful also is the incorporation of a scale capable of depicting mean pressure, as well as systolic and diastolic, and the pulse rate.

The arterial line is connected to a strain gauge. The strain gauge is left open to the atmosphere for establishment of the zero level. Strain gauges used either for CVP or arterial pressure must be filled carefully to avoid air in the chamber over the sensing element. The strain gauge is connected to the oscilloscope through an appropriate lead and connection. An appropriate system of intravenous tubing, pressure tubing (from arterial catheter to strain gauge), stopcocks, and a pressure bulb (such as used for blood pumping) is arranged so that a weak solution of heparin can be easily flushed through the arterial line.

After the needle or catheter, or both, has been placed successfully in the artery, the catheter is connected to a strain gauge through more rigid pressure tubing and the tracing is observed. If the tracing is free and undamped, the catheter and tubing can be secured. If the tracing is damped, sometimes changing the position of the hand and wrist or the catheter results in a free tracing. Flushing of the line with the heparin solution often clears the line and allows an undamped tracing. If the tracing repeatedly becomes damped or is especially sensitive to position, it is wise to start the whole procedure over again and to obtain a free tracing. On occasions, the upswing of the oscilloscope tracing is so pronounced that there is a spurious high reading. If so, it is useful to introduce a small bubble of air in the line to damp the oscillations slightly.

Whenever the needle or catheter is removed, pressure should be applied to avoid a hematoma. Nothing is more exasperating in a situation in which one depends upon direct arterial measurement than to have an erratic and undependable tracing due to impeded blood flow. If the blood flow is unimpeded at the start and the tracing later becomes damped, there is either clotting in the line, which requires flushing, or a pronounced change in position has partially occluded the catheter or the line. Adjustments have to be made, of course, if changes in the position of the patient alter the zero level. If one carefully ensures proper placement of the catheter, secures it well, balances the instrument and flushes the line occasionally, direct arterial measurement by this method is remarkably effective.

Use of pulse rate integrators.—At one time, pulse rate integrators were more popular than they are today. They were capable of translating changes in density of tissue or changes in volume of tissue into a pulse rate that could be displayed as a number. Now, these instruments limited to measurement of pulse rate have been displaced by integrating units on the ECG that display the heart rate. More importantly, by means of the ear piece and the chest piece or esophageal scope, the anesthetist can monitor the heart rate constantly and has little need for the integrator. Furthermore, the heart rate is of substantially less significance than the quality of heart tone, and aberrations in the ECG complex and the integrator do not provide that information.

THE RESPIRATORY SYSTEM

Simple Methods

The character of the respiratory pattern.—The pattern of respiration in anesthesia represents the classic situation in which the anesthetist must train himself by constant observation of the patient to detect subtle but meaningful changes in the respiratory pattern. The nature of respiratory movements is useful in assessing not only depth of anesthesia (see Chap. 7), but also the nature and extent of air movement. The anesthetist must constantly relate chest movements to movements of the breathing bag, respirometer or ventimeter. By so doing, a reasonably accurate judgment can be made of the nature and degree of respiratory obstruction. We emphasize the necessity for correlating chest and bag movements. All too often the anesthetist limits his observations to the breathing bag or respirometer, and by so doing he fails to obtain information vital to a correct assessment of the situation and, more importantly, fails to train himself to detect most useful information from observation of the patient rather than the apparatus. In addition, the anesthetist can sharpen his clinical judgment of the degree of ventilation by checking his observation and assessment of ventilation with blood-gas analysis.

The observations to be made (which will be elaborated in discussions of measurement of depth of anesthesia and management of airway) include rate, depth, regularity, relation of inspiration to expiration, pauses at end of inspiration and expiration, presence or absence of intercostal activity, lower chest flaring, nasal flaring, force of expiration and sounds associated with inspiration and expiration.

USE OF THE VENTIMETER.—The ventimeter is a bellows device that gives a visual clue to the nature and extent of respiratory movements and measurement from direct calibration. The device may be separate but usually is incorporated into the gas machine itself or into a mechanical respirator.

USE OF RESPIROMETER.—Another relatively simple and useful device is the respirometer, a small unit that can be inserted into the inspiratory or expiratory line to measure tidal volume and accumulate minute volume. These devices include the Wright, Drager and Monaghan respirometers (anemometers, ventilation meters). They measure breath-by-breath tidal volume. The breath-by-breath volume accumulates to provide measurements of the minute volume. These measurements accurately represent tidal and minute volumes only if the system is leakproof except through the normal vent valve in the high-flow system. If there is a leak about the mask or endotracheal catheter, the flow through the meter is diminished and does not measure the tidal volume. Since respirometers measure, in the usual high-flow system, the movement of air in the circuit, it is necessary in order to get an absolute measure of tidal volume to interrupt temporarily the input of gases from the machine. The devices are usually subject to deterioration in function from moisture accumulation in the gears.

USE OF OXYGEN ANALYZERS.—Oxygen analyzers may utilize the unique ability of oxygen to deflect a galvanometer; the galvanometer responds only to oxygen in mixtures of other gases. The classic example is the Pauling meter. Other instruments using special sensors permit continuous analysis when inserted into the external circuit of a gas machine. The instruments are sensitive to moisture and repeated calibration with air is necessary to ensure reliable measurement.

Complex Methods

More complicated means of obtaining information about respiratory function are as follows:

ANALYSIS OF INSPIRED AND ALVEOLAR CARBON DIOXIDE.—The CO_2 analyzer is designed to provide dynamic analysis of CO_2 in the air passing through it. Analysis is possible because of the ability of carbon dioxide in respired air to impede the transmission of infrared light compared to transmission through glass cells containing carbon dioxide and air. The device has a frequency of response that permits breath-to-breath analysis. A reasonable approximation of alveolar carbon dioxide is obtained by analysis of end-expiratory gas. The device is placed in the expiratory side of the breathing circuit in an anesthetic apparatus to permit analysis of expired air. Readings are taken at the point at which a plateau appears in the curve of changing concentrations. Alveolar sampling is more accurate either if the patient forces air out as in a vital capacity measurement or if, in the anesthetized patient, pressure is applied to the chest to remove air so that the FRC is approached. The apparatus necessary for dynamic analysis, however, is cumbersome. Furthermore, the circuitry is such that stability is possible only if the apparatus is allowed to "warm up" to a stable operation.

The usefulness of and the problems associated with analysis of carbon dioxide in the respired atmosphere are outlined in Chapter 19.

BLOOD-GAS ANALYSIS.—Measurement, in either arterial or venous blood (preferably arterialized), of Po_2, Pco_2, and pH with calculation of base excess is a well-established and essentially mandatory practice in the measurement of respiratory efficiency. No anesthetist can unequivocally assess with accuracy the state of respiratory function without blood-gas analysis to back up his other observations. As in other measurements mentioned here, blood-gas analysis is discussed in detail in Chapter 19. Arterial blood is preferred for blood-gas analysis because arterial blood more accurately reflects the blood-gas values, the pH, and the base excess (or deficit) to which the tissues of the body are responding. Venous blood, particularly if arterialized, can be used but the values obtained need to be translated into arterial values. The values so obtained are often inaccurate because venous blood reflects the area from which it comes and also, in essence, the impact of tissues on the venous blood rather than the potential impact of the arterial blood on tissues.

Arterial sampling is easily done. With the apparatus currently available, reliable analysis can be done on small samples (2 to 5 ml). It is advisable to heparinize the syringe by rinsing the syringe and needle with heparin. A 25-gauge needle is then introduced into an artery, usually the radial at the wrist. Blood from the artery is identified by the red color and the force with which the blood fills the syringe. Identification and fixing of the artery for sampling is done in the same manner as for placement of arterial catheters. Pressure is applied to the artery after sampling to diminish leakage.

The apparatus for blood-gas analysis uses the electrodes developed by Clark and Severinghaus. The apparatus has been developed so that, with minimal "cookbook" type instruction and experience, reliable analysis can be obtained. Base excess (or deficit) is calculated from nomograms prepared by Siggaard-Andersen and Rattenborg.[4-7]

THE CENTRAL NERVOUS SYSTEM

We shall now consider what the anesthetist has available to him for monitoring of the central nervous system. Some of the changes or reflex actions in the central nervous system, of course, are reflected in the heart and peripheral circulation and in the respiration. These changes, such as bradycardia, arrhythmia, elevation or depression of arterial pressure, changes in peripheral tone of vessels, apnea, and irregular respirations can be identified by the means already discussed.

ELECTROENCEPHALOGRAPHY (EEG).—Some direct measurement of central nervous system function can be accomplished with the EEG. The changes in amplitude and character of the brain waves in various areas of the brain associated with the changes taking place during anesthesia and surgery are generally useful only to those anesthetists who have undertaken a special effort to recognize and interpret these waves. Changes in the brain waves relating to the level of depression by agents such as ether and thiopental have been reasonably well established; the patterns for other agents, however, are not as clearly defined. In general, increasing depth of depression of the brain is reflected in an increasing frequency of brain waves and the appearance of delta waves. Transplantation of organs has led to the acceptance of the lack of brain waves (flat line) in the EEG as the determinant of death. Electroencephalography is, of course, an expensive and cumbersome means of acquiring information about the patient and in general is not satisfactory in the complicated milieu of the operating room. Also, the many factors associated with anesthesia and surgery, such as changes in the cerebral circulation induced by shock, alterations in P_{CO_2} and P_{O_2}, anesthetics (such as halothane), and anatomic defects (congenital or acquired) in the vascular supply to the brain make interpretation of EEG patterns most difficult.

PUPILLARY REACTION.—To some extent, the pupillary reaction to light is a measure of brain function. If the brain is not functioning because of hypoxia, for example, the pupils often become dilated and unresponsive to light. If they contract and become responsive to light, this reaction is probably as reliable an indication of returning brain function as the EEG.

OBSERVATION OF MUSCLE RESPONSE.—Muscle twitching and convulsions are an infrequent response to anesthesia. Divinyl ether has the peculiar property of inducing "running movements," and this is a unique response to this agent. Twitching and convulsions are, of course, a sign of toxicity reaction to local anesthetics; this is amplified in Chapter 8. The occasional wrinkling of the brow and the occasional random and non-purposeful movement of the hand or arm, in the absence of light anesthesia, reflect some sort of central nervous system response. What it is, no one seems to know. What is important is that the movements not be interpreted always as light anesthesia and anesthetic agent unnecessarily added in response to these movements.

DETERMINATION OF TEMPERATURE CHANGES.—Hypothermia and hyperthermia can be considered to be functions of central nervous system activity. These aberrations are discussed more fully in Chapter 28; here, it is important to emphasize that the anesthetist is well advised to monitor the temperature during anesthesia and surgery. This is especially true in patients in whom malignant hyperthermia may be anticipated and in infants and small children. Ambient temperature, use of drapes, exposure of bowel, exposure during grafting or burn debridement can effect pronounced changes in temperature in children, and routine measurement is mandatory.

Esophageal temperature recording is a reliable means of measuring the core temperature; thermistor probes likewise can be placed with ease, comfort and stability on the tympanic membrane. Evidence indicates that recording of temperature at this site reflects blood (core) temperature and is as reliable, if not more reliable, than recording of esophageal temperature. Rectal temperature gives a somewhat lower value and is slower in responding to core-temperature changes. Since the critical changes take place in heart and brain, the core temperature is more meaningful.

Simple, relatively inexpensive and small units are available for constant temperature measurement. These can be readily calibrated to room temperature and are stable in operation. Thermocouples or thermistor probes, which can be inserted in the esophagus, the rectum, or on the tympanic membrane (or at any point where a temperature reading of meaning can be secured), are connected to the instrument through a jack plug. The instruments are usually self-contained, having batteries as the source of energy. If such devices are not available, the temperature can be monitored by use of the rectal, axillary, or oral clinical thermometer.

If heating (or cooling) pads or blankets are used, it is advisable to monitor the temperature of the pad or blanket with a mercury thermometer placed next to the pad or blanket. The regulatory thermostats of these heating or cooling units often are unreliable and direct monitoring of the temperature is necessary to avoid burns.

Other central nervous system responses are usually those associated with changes in the depth of anesthesia; these are considered in Chapter 7.

BLOOD LOSS

Monitoring of blood loss is essential to continuous estimation of blood loss. Blood loss is estimated as follows: (1) observation of the amount of loss on drapes at the site of the operation; (2) weighing of sponges and "lap" pads (a quick estimate of loss through sponges and pads can be made by assigning, on the average, 10 ml to each sponge and 50 ml to each lap pad); and (3) measurement of blood in the suction bottle. In making this last measurement, it is convenient to insert a calibrated trap-bottle in the suction line. Correction can be made for use of irrigating solutions by means of a hygrometer on the blood-fluid mixture in the bottle and by keeping a record of the volume of the irrigating solution used. The anesthetist can usefully keep his own record of blood loss, but a more graphic and visible record displayed on the wall of the operating room is a convincing reminder of blood loss. This record can be revised every 15 to 30 minutes, depending upon the rate of loss. Monitoring of blood loss is critical not only to ensure more accurate replacement but to permit more precise control of fluid and blood replacement in infants and small children and in patients with incompetent hearts.

Monitoring pertinent to use of muscle relaxants is detailed in Chapter 18.

In conclusion, we emphasize again that the important monitor is the anesthetist. He is the one who watches and he is the one who is capable of interpreting the signs and symptoms and of providing warning and appropriate action. Whatever devices he may elect to use to enhance his clinical ability should be recognized as being capable only of adding to his knowledge. The information provided by the devices should be considered to be only a portion, and most likely a small portion, of the data necessary to critical evaluation of the patient's condition. Unwarranted reliance on monitoring devices can result only in restricted information, misleading information (at times), and deterioration of clinical acuity.

REFERENCES

1. Rence, W. G., Cullen, S. C., and Hamilton, W. K.: Observations on the heart sounds during anesthesia with cyclopropane or ether, Anesthesiology 17:26, 1956.
2. Bruner, J. M. R.: Hazards of electrical apparatus, Anesthesiology 28:396, 1967.
3. Walter, C. W.: Electrical Hazards in Hospitals, Proceedings of a Workshop. National Academy of Sciences, 1970.
4. Siggaard-Andersen, O., and Engel, K.: A new acid-base nomogram, Scand. J. Clin. Lab. Invest. 12:177, 1960.
5. Severinghaus, J. W., Stupfel, M., and Bradley, A. F.: Variations of carbonic acid pK with pH and temperature, J. Appl. Physiol. 9:197, 1966.
6. Current concepts of acid-base measurement, Ann. N. Y. Acad. Sci. 133:3, 1966.
7. Rattenborg, C. C., El Etr, M., Salem, R., *et al.*: A New Acid-Base Slide Rule, Research in Surgery, University of Chicago (January 13) 1968.

CHAPTER SIX

Management of the Airway

IN ANESTHETIZING A PATIENT, the anesthetist assumes a major responsibility for the establishment and maintenance of adequate respiration. The surgeon similarly must take into account the impact on respiration of, for example, whatever position or surgical procedure he proposes. Indeed, all those concerned with the correction of respiratory deficiencies—on a short-term acute resuscitation basis, on a somewhat more extended basis as in intensive care units or in the treatment of long-term deficiencies—must be aware of all factors bearing on the establishment and maintenance of adequate respiration. Most critical to adequate and properly functioning respiration is the airway. The anesthetist is most often especially concerned with the airway because of the impact of anesthesia and associated relaxation, but airway management is a vital element in many other problems of respiratory deficiency. For example, many patients suffering from drug depression, diabetic coma, alcoholic stupor, head injuries and stroke die not directly from the disorder but indirectly from the consequences of an inadequate airway. We emphasize, therefore, that all persons responsible for the care of patients be aware of the possibilities for airway obstruction, alert to the sites at which it may take place and experienced in correcting the impairment. We believe that the principles of airway management as set forth here for anesthetic practice are applicable to all situations in which the airway may be involved in an overall respiratory deficiency.

No anesthesia is safe or satisfactory unless diligent efforts are made toward maintenance of a functioning airway. There is no anesthetic agent or technic that guarantees a good airway. There are no shortcuts to avoid constant attention to the patency of the airway. Any attempts to supplant close supervision of the airway by mechanical contrivances and any neglect of the airway soon will be reflected in increased anesthetic morbidity and mortality. Deaths from inadequate control of the airway are usually inexcusable and avoidable.

TOTAL AIRWAY OBSTRUCTION

Total airway obstruction is characterized by complete obstruction of air movement between the external or ambient atmosphere and the lungs. The obstruction may prevent air moving in either direction, but usually the obstruction is such that it prevents inspiration. Total obstruction may occur at any of the sites where partial obstruction may occur, but most often obstruction occurs in the upper airway and is due to occlusion of the pharyngeal air space by relaxation of the mandible and consequently the tongue. Total obstruction occurs also as a result of complete laryngospasm and the presence of foreign material (either causing laryngospasm or mechanically blocking entrance of air into the larynx).

A characteristic of total airway obstruction is the lack of any breath sounds coupled, usually, with continuing but ineffectual efforts at breathing. Inexperienced persons, unfortunately, interpret the chest and abdominal movements as "respiration" or the movement of air. Respiratory movements associated with complete obstruction are characterized by obvious strenuous effort, flaring of nostrils and a pronounced retraction of the thoracic cage and excessive diaphragmatic movement. Checking for actual air movement is mandatory and can be done by using the stethoscope (on the chest or on the trachea in the neck), by placing the ear at the chest or the mouth, by feeling with the hand for air movement or the warmth of air from the lung and by observing movements of breathing bag if the patient is connected to an anesthetic or resuscitative apparatus. Obviously, a state of asphyxia develops promptly with total airway obstruction and immediate measures must be taken to relieve the obstruction. Those measures are the same as outlined for partial airway obstruction.

PARTIAL AIRWAY OBSTRUCTION

A free airway can be defined as one through which inspired air passes, without obstruction, from outside the body into arterial blood and through which waste gases can pass, without obstruction, from venous blood to the external atmosphere. The airway includes the nasopharynx and oropharynx, the larynx, the trachea, the bronchi and all the subdivisions and alveoli. It is evident that opportunities for interference with patency of the airway are numerous and that awareness of the possibilities for obstruction is essential to a complete appreciation of problems involved in control of the airway. Partial airway obstruction is a common problem in patients under anesthesia, including conduction anesthesia. It is also an important problem in patients with other disorders causing depression of the central nervous system.

We now outline the effects, signs and treatment of airway obstruction. What we outline is applicable to any form of airway obstruction; it is included here because partial obstruction is the more frequent problem.

Effects of Partial Obstruction

A partially obstructed airway causes several undesirable effects: (1) an increased respiratory effort is required by the patient; (2) induction and maintenance of sufficient and even anesthesia is difficult; and (3) oxygen supply and carbon dioxide elimination are seriously impeded.

INCREASED EFFORT BY THE PATIENT.—Physiologic economy is centered around a constant intake of oxygen and elimination of carbon dioxide. Any interference with this process results in an attempt by the body to reestablish normal supply and removal of these gases. Obstruction of the airway makes increased demands on muscles of respiration because moving a mass of air becomes more difficult. The additional effort required to move air past an obstruction tires the patient, makes him less capable of tolerating the surgical procedure and adds to the demand for oxygen.

There is reason to believe that strenuous respiratory (inspiratory) efforts may provoke or, at least, enhance the development of pulmonary edema. Certainly, the profound extra work of breathing against an obstruction—especially an inspiratory obstruction—accentuates the deficiency in oxygen supply and augments the amount of carbon dioxide that has to be eliminated. Partial inspiratory obstruction of the upper airway, especially in infants and small children, often augments the aspiration of air into the esophagus and stomach, which enhances thereby the development of gastric dilation and the possibility of regurgitation and emesis.

DIFFICULTY IN INDUCING AND MAINTAINING ADEQUATE AND EVEN ANESTHESIA.—It is particularly true of inhalation anesthesia that the anesthetic state cannot be achieved unless the agent reaches the blood stream in sufficient quantity and concentration to effect the desired depression. The anesthetic state cannot be maintained if it is impossible to maintain a certain concentration of the agent in the blood, and an excessive blood concentration of the agent is difficult to avoid if elimination is blocked. Prolonged induction of inhalation anesthesia is often the result of airway obstruction, which slows down the attainment of an adequate blood concentration. In cases of uninhibited use of thiopental (or other similar short-acting intravenous agents) and relaxants to cover deficiencies in the management of induction by inhalation, the hazards of giving an overdose in order to avoid excitement produced by airway obstruction (or leaks in the system) are augmented. If induction is delayed because of airway obstruction and the inability therefore to achieve a satisfactory blood concentration of an agent by inhalation, one should certainly not compound the problem by further diminishing the patient's ability to breathe by introducing a depressant or relaxant drug intravenously. Similarly, the abrupt production of high blood concentrations from a sudden correction of an airway obstruction (e.g., the free flow of potent anesthetic gases and accentuated ventilation) may cause severe respiratory and circulatory impairment, including cardiac arrest. Many patients who are alternately coughing in light anesthesia and then not breathing in excessively deep anesthesia are often alternately deprived of and provided with a good airway. The classic example of uneven anesthesia is inhalation anesthesia by insufflation with a poor airway in the patient undergoing tonsillectomy.

Muscular relaxation is not easily accomplished in the patient with an obstructed airway. Operating conditions in the abdomen are particularly unsatisfactory because the muscles are tense and abdominal contents heave because of excessive diaphragmatic action. These working conditions are often misinterpreted as being the result of insufficient depth of anesthesia. Frantic attempts to improve the state by increasing the concentration of the agent serve only to aggravate matters and too frequently are a cause of death. Countless patients have lost their lives because of the unfortunate response of inept anesthetists to the imperious demands, "Get him deeper, get him deeper" or "relax him," when the real trouble was an obstructed airway. Inadequate operating conditions associated with obstruction of the airway are often covered, inappropriately, by the administration of a relaxant. If a relaxant is used in such a circumstance, it should be used only to facilitate the improvement of the airway (e.g., by the insertion of an endotracheal catheter) and not to diminish the muscular effort and poor conditions for operating within the abdomen associated with airway obstruction.

IMPAIRMENT OF OXYGEN SUPPLY AND CARBON DIOXIDE ELIMINATION.—Body physiology depends on an uninterrupted supply of oxygen and elimination of carbon dioxide. No provision is made for storage of oxygen. This lack of oxygen reserve makes it imperative that the airway be preserved at all times. The patient may tolerate the increased effort occasioned by an imperfect airway and he may not suffer too greatly from an uneven and inadequate anesthesia, but he will die if the airway obstruction is great enough or prolonged enough to impede his oxygen supply and carbon dioxide removal. One can, of course, correct the oxygen deficiency by increasing the concentration of oxygen in the inspired atmosphere. One does this *only* as a temporary measure until the airway obstruction can be relieved or in circumstances in which the airway obstruction cannot be corrected. An unobstructed airway is an integral part of satisfactory ventilation. The significance of adequate ventilation is discussed in Chapter 19.

Sites, Signs and Treatment of Upper Airway Obstruction

The patient with partial upper airway obstruction shows the following signs: (1) diminished tidal exchange; (2) retraction of the upper chest; (3) restriction of air movement with inspiration; (4) excessive diaphragmatic activity; (5) prolonged inspiration; (6) various characteristic sounds (to be described); (7) diminished breath sounds heard either in chest or over trachea; (8) discrepancy between the movements of the breathing bag and the chest; and (9) ultimately the signs of asphyxia (tachycardia, hypertension, cyanosis, etc.).

We emphasize particularly the need for recognizing these signs, with special emphasis on the correlation of respiratory effort with air movement. One must be concerned not only with deciding whether or not air is being moved but how much is being moved. In making this latter assessment, useful technics are noting the movement of the breathing bag and listening by an ear at the mouth for the volume of air moved. One must be aware that a stethoscope on the chest or over the trachea in the suprasternal space will indicate whether air is being moved but auscultation is unreliable in making an assessment of the volume of air being moved.

OROPHARYNX.—Obstruction of air flow occurs most frequently in the oropharynx. The interruption is usually due to relaxation of the jaw and tongue, which fall back to occlude the space between the posterior pharyngeal wall and the base of the tongue. This process is popularly termed "swallowing the tongue." There is either no sound at all, which indicates complete obstruction, or a rough, irregular and stuttery noise, which indicates incomplete obstruction. "Stertorous" respiration is often obstructed respiration of this type. This type of obstruction is serious because of the degree and frequency of respiratory impairment so caused.

Oropharyngeal obstruction occasionally may be caused by foreign bodies, such as dentures, gum or a cud of tobacco. The signs and symptoms are similar to those appearing with obstruction by the tongue. Tumors also may cause oropharyngeal obstruction.

Interruption of air flow in the oropharynx can be corrected without mechanical aids by preventing the mandible from falling back and by not allowing the tongue to sag. The fingers must be placed behind the angle of the mandible so that forward motion can be applied (Fig. 6-1). It is useful also to open the mouth slightly with the thumbs. The common mistake is to apply pressure along the ramus of the mandible—this maneuver not only does not facilitate forward displacement of the mandible but it often accentuates the obstruction by pushing tongue and other soft tissue into the oropharynx. This is particularly true in infants and small children. As a matter of fact, infants and small children often maintain their own oropharyngeal airway very well even under anesthesia and oropharyngeal obstruction is often due to interference by the anesthetist. The tongue can also be displaced forward by grasping the mandible at its midpoint between thumb and forefinger and pulling forward. Traction on the tongue with fingers, suture, or forceps relieves the obstruction but is more traumatic and no more effective than the other two methods.

Fig. 6-1.—Correct method of manual control of airway. Note placement of forefinger and second finger behind angle of jaw; thumb is placed so that slight forward motion opens the mouth.

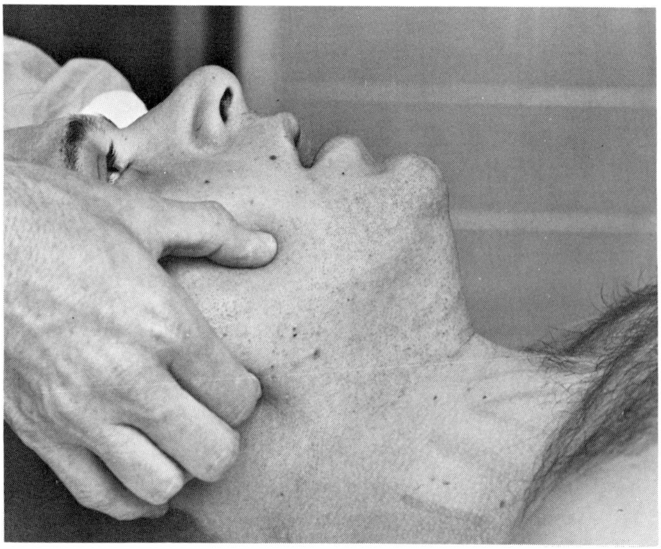

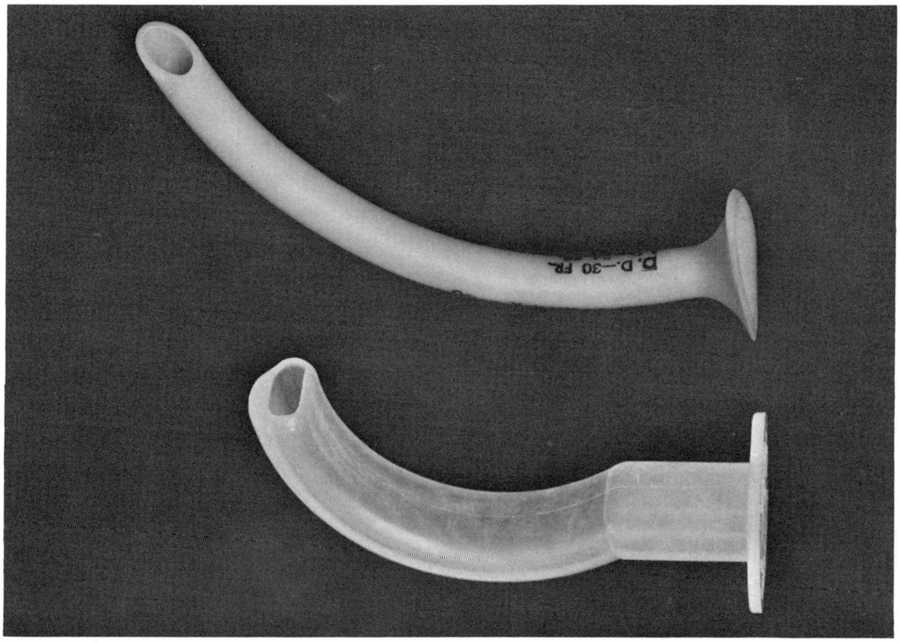

Fig. 6-2.—Oropharyngeal (*lower*) and nasopharyngeal or Robertazzi (*upper*) airways. These come in different sizes appropriate to the patient.

Position of head.—The head of the relaxed patient is in the optimal airway position when it is slightly extended. It must not be forgotten that, in many patients with impeded air flow in the oropharynx, just turning the patient's head to the side will often lead to improvement of the airway. It is wise to remember also that turning the patient into a lateral position often leads to improvement of the airway; the lateral position also facilitates drainage of mucus and blood, for example, from the pharynx.

Evidence accumulated during the course of investigations into the optimal position of the head and neck for expired-air resuscitation (e.g., mouth-to-mouth breathing) indicates that the tendency of the tongue and jaw to occlude the airway can be effectively prevented in most patients by hyperextending the head and forcing the mandible forward. This is a useful maneuver as an emergency or temporary measure during anesthesia, but the airway can be established and maintained with other methods more efficiently; in this way one can avoid producing the neck ache that patients may complain of after anesthesia and that may occur with severe hyperextension over a protracted period.

Oropharyngeal pressure.—Another method that is at times effective in correcting or compensating for obstruction in the oropharynx is the establishment and maintenance of increased oropharyngeal airway pressure. This can be effected simply by distending the breathing bag with the anesthetic mixture or oxygen and maintaining an increased end-expiratory pressure; pressure with the hand on the bag is also effective but it is less constant and often less effective than overdistention of the breathing bag. A slight head-down position is also helpful in establishing and maintaining a patent airway. Unless under direct control, the patient's head should not be placed in a position with the face up. A pillow may be used if it is placed well under the shoulders and the head is not flexed.

Oropharyngeal and nasopharyngeal airways.—Two mechanical contrivances are often used to correct obstruction of air flow in the oropharynx (Fig. 6-2). One is the oropharyngeal airway, of which there are several types; the other is the nasopharyngeal airway. Of these, the more satisfactory from the standpoint of restoring a patent airway with the least trauma is the nasopharyngeal (Robertazzi) airway. It is easily introduced, it seems to be better tolerated (there is less gagging) in light anesthesia or light coma and it introduces fewer of the problems associated with the introduction and retention of the oropharyngeal airway. Such airways are commercially available in different sizes and lengths and are made of rubber with a flange to prevent their sliding down the nose and to facilitate securing them. They are introduced with the aid of a lubricant through the most patent naris and extend into the pharynx sufficiently to provide an air passage past the tongue.

On occasion, the nasopharyngeal airway either does not relieve the obstruction or constriction at the nares does not permit introduction. In these circumstances an oropharyngeal airway may be useful.

The oropharyngeal airway is constructed of metal, rubber or plastic. It is shaped to be placed between the teeth and the lips, to fit over the curve of the tongue and to rest on the posterior wall of the oropharynx between it and the base of the tongue. It is usually hollow and a certain amount of air goes through it when in place, but its primary function is not to provide an artificial air passage but to keep the tongue off the posterior pharyngeal wall and to permit free flow of air around as well as through the device.

Fig. 6-3.—Method of inserting an oropharyngeal airway. The forefinger of the left hand is placed between the buccal surface and the alveolar ridge behind the last tooth and gently rotated. The airway is inserted with a rotating motion over the tongue.

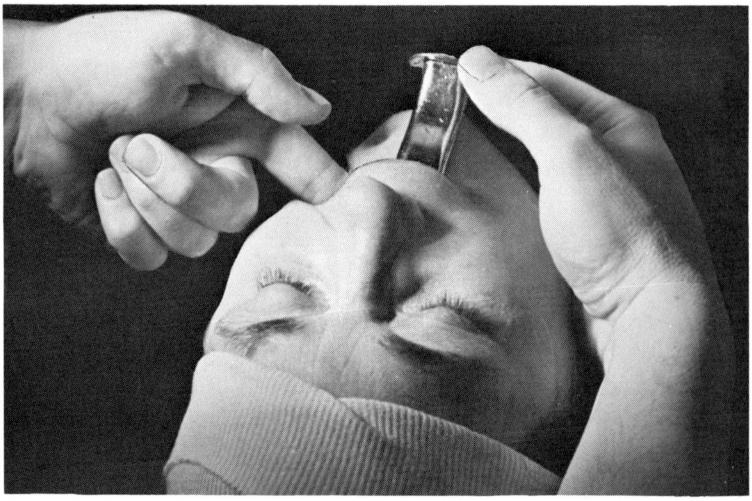

An oropharyngeal airway can be introduced easily and without trauma. With one hand the instrument should be grasped at the lip end (which usually has a flange on it), while the forefinger of the other hand slips down outside the teeth and inside the cheek of the patient until it slips into the space behind the last molar. With a gentle rotating motion of the forefinger and slight pressure on the midpoint of the mandible, the mouth can be opened, even in patients with spastic masseter muscles; pressure on the midpoint of the mandible alone is usually an ineffective means of opening the mouth. After the mouth has been opened, the airway is passed over the tongue by a rotating motion until the tip of the appliance comes to rest on the posterior wall of the pharynx behind the base of the tongue (Fig. 6-3). Efforts to push the airway straight in are traumatic and increase the obstruction. An oropharyngeal airway may be introduced also by placing a tongue blade over the tongue and passing the airway over the tongue blade. Still another method that precludes placing either finger or tongue blade in mouth is introduction of the airway by inserting it past the teeth and over the anterior tongue 180 degrees out of its ultimate position and then rotating it as it reaches the midpoint of the tongue and advancing it to its optimum position in the oropharynx. If both the airway and the tongue are dry, wetting the airway with water facilitates its introduction; it need not be lubricated with petrolatum or similar material. If the airway is metal, it is advisable to cover the portion of it that lies between the teeth with rubber to minimize damage to the teeth, should the patient bite down on the airway.

One must be aware that during the stage of awakening and before the patient is sufficiently awake to maintain a patent airway, the jaw may tighten down on an oropharyngeal airway sufficiently to loosen teeth or dislodge dentures. If possible and within the limits of safety for the patient, it is advisable to remove the oropharyngeal airway before the jaw tightens. If air flow is still unsatisfactory, a nasopharyngeal airway may be used.

The placing of an oropharyngeal or nasopharyngeal airway does not guarantee an unobstructed air flow. It may still be necessary to support the mandible at its midpoint by forward traction or at angles by forward pressure. Every physician in general practice will find it advisable to carry several sizes of an oropharyngeal or nasopharyngeal airway in his bag. In anesthetic practice the airway is used optimally after pharyngeal and laryngeal reflexes are obtunded by the anesthetic agent. Introduction of an oropharyngeal airway before these reflexes have been depressed may precipitate gagging, emesis and laryngospasm. Induction of anesthesia often has been spoiled by introduction of an oropharyngeal airway too early. If obstruction of air flow in the oropharynx occurs before the reflexes have been eliminated, maintenance of a patent airway is best achieved by use of external mandibular support or a nasopharyngeal airway, or both.

THE LARYNX.—An important function of the vocal cords is protection of the lower respiratory tract from foreign material. The vocal cords are capable of forceful partial or complete adduction, a state known as laryngospasm. Since the cords are adapted to prevent contamination of the lower respiratory tract, any obstruction is usually to inspiration. Varying degrees of laryngospasm cause varying degrees of sound, but the usual sound associated with laryngospasm is a high-pitched whistle or squeak. Total absence of sound may indicate complete adduction of the cords. The signs are those of upper respiratory obstruction. Laryngospasm may be precipitated by high concentrations of inhalation agents, foreign material or bodies or stimulation of the recurrent laryngeal nerve directly or reflexly—for example, by stripping off the costal periosteum, dilating the rectum or manipulating around the celiac plexus. Barbiturates such as thiopental sodium (in light doses) do not obtund the laryngeal reflex, and laryngospasm frequently accompanies use of these drugs, if precipitating factors such as mucus or foreign bodies are present.

Clearing of airway at the larynx.—The best treatment for laryngospasm is prophylactic. Laryngospasm usually can be traced to errors of omission or commission in administration of anesthesia. Sudden high concentrations of anesthetic agents should be avoided, and foreign material should be kept out of the oropharynx. If there is to be contamination of the oropharynx (as in surgery about the head and neck), if there is to be reflex initiation of laryngospasm, or if there is to be vocal cord adduction by recurrent laryngeal nerve stimulation (as in some neck dissections and occasionally in thyroidectomy), it is better to prevent adduction of the cords by introducing a tracheal tube. At times—as in anesthesia induction, insufflation anesthesia for tonsillectomy, laryngoscopy and circumstances that do not permit oral or nasotracheal intubation—inhalation anesthesia can be established and maintained provided the level of anesthesia is deep and the oropharynx is kept clear of foreign material (mucus, blood, etc.).

Laryngospasm.—Laryngospasm not infrequently occurs also during inhalation induction if induction is too slow. The slow development of an adequate blood concentration of an anesthetic agent, which results from leaks in the anesthetic system, vaporizers not functioning properly, or the anesthetist being deliberately slow in increasing the inhaled concentration, permits the patient to stay in a light level of anesthesia and in a state in which mucus is produced and the larynx is susceptible to stimulation. If anesthesia is administered carefully and causes for laryngospasm are anticipated, the anesthetist will have little difficulty from obstruction of the airway at this point. If, however, the anesthetist is inept, careless and unaware of the possibilities for laryngospasm, spastic adduction of the vocal cords can occur frequently and be most distressing and extremely hazardous.

Laryngospasm must be treated promptly and effectively. The cause or causes of the spasm must be determined and treated immediately. The concentration of the inhalation anesthetic agent must be decreased by diluting the inhaled atmosphere with oxygen; manipulations that may be inciting the spasm reflexly or directly must be discontinued; and foreign material in the oropharynx must be removed. It is important, however, to be exceedingly brief in the use of aspiration during laryngospasm; this maneuver removes vitally needed oxygen and diminishes the time during which high concentrations of oxygen can be applied to the oropharynx.

A mask can be fitted snugly to the face and strong intermittent pressure applied, by hand, to a bag full of oxygen connected to the mask directly or

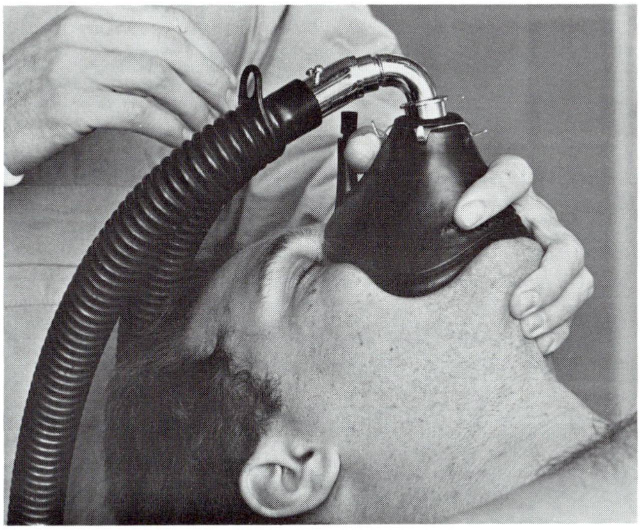

Fig. 6-4.—Optimal all-purpose placement of mask, for induction of inhalation anesthesia, application of positive pressure, resuscitation, etc. Note that fingers are positioned to maintain tight mask fit and forward position of mandible.

through a circle system (Fig. 6-4). In these circumstances, "strong" pressure means as much pressure as can be applied by one or two hands and arms and within the limits of tolerance of the breathing bag. No regard should be paid to traditional limits of pressure applied to airway and lung. If the oropharyngeal airway is patent, it is often possible to force oxygen through the spastic cords by using this simple but effective resuscitative maneuver. The contour of stomach must be watched closely during this procedure because oxygen may be forced down the esophagus. This complication is, however, no contraindication to use of oxygen under pressure through a bag and mask if the anesthetist is succeeding in getting even a small amount of oxygen into the lungs. After a little oxygen is forced past the adducted cords, the spasm often relaxes and efficient gas exchange is resumed. The bag and mask should be left in place and oxygen in excess supplied until one is certain that anoxia has been completely relieved. Many anesthetists find that firm forward displacement of the mandible often relieves laryngospasm. We recommend forward displacement together with the administration of oxygen by mask under pressure.

This method of control of laryngospasm is usually sufficient. There is always a strong temptation in these circumstances to attempt tracheal intubation. This temptation should be rigorously avoided because the time taken to make the attempt prolongs the duration of hypoxia and may be the critical factor in a serious outcome. In cases of severe spasm of the cords, glottic structures are often also in spasm and definition of the glottic opening is difficult. When glottic structures become identifiable, usually from asphyxial relaxation, ventilation can be accomplished easily by bag and mask and intubation is not necessary. Unless there is mechanical obstruction, tracheotomy is likewise usually unnecessary. Tracheotomy, as a means of relieving laryngospasm, is reserved exclusively for those situations in which a foreign object located between the cords cannot be removed. If direct access to the trachea is needed as an absolute emergency (i.e., acute complete obstruction of the upper airway), we strongly recommend making the opening in the cricothyroid membrane. This area is easily accessible and, in the life-threatening situation to which we refer, there is not time enough to expose and search for trachea below the larynx.

Manual methods of artificial respiration are ineffective in the presence of a severe laryngospasm and should not be used. Deflation of the lungs by pressure on the chest during the spasm will evacuate what little oxygen is present and air will not enter the lung on release of the chest wall pressure.

Atropine in large doses (0.0012 gm to adults, given intravenously) is sometimes effective in counteracting reflex laryngospasm. The foregoing means of combating the spasm should be used in addition to administration of atropine.

Muscle relaxants, especially succinylcholine, are used for prevention and relief of laryngospasm. These agents are effective; but there is, however, good reason to doubt that use of muscle relaxants for the deliberate purpose of reducing laryngospasm associated with improper use of agents is good practice. There is no doubt about the effectiveness of a drug such as succinylcholine in relieving severe laryngospasm. However, the measures outlined should be instituted first. Laryngospasm is often severe but brief, and relief is effective by the measures outlined. The induction of paralysis often only adds an unnecessary complication. We also believe that there is sufficient evidence that succinylcholine, especially in the state of asphyxia associated with laryngospasm, may provoke severe cardiac arrhythmias. If succinylcholine is used, it should be injected by someone other than the anesthetist; his attention should be paid to establishing and maintaining a good oropharyngeal airway and pressure with 100% oxygen. Since succinylcholine is so effective in relieving laryngospasm there is an unfortunate strong tendency for anesthetists to use the drug as a "crutch" and, as a result, they make little effort to learn why the laryngospasm developed and to take appropriate preventive measures.

Sometimes a slight degree of laryngospasm persists in spite of efforts to remove inciting causes. In such circumstances, positive pressure in the anesthetic system often alleviates the difficulty. Certainly, one should attempt this simple maneuver before resorting to tracheal intubation.

THE GLOTTIS.—Glottic restriction of air flow most often is due to foreign bodies that are small enough to pass the base of the tongue but too large to enter the larynx. These foreign bodies may include large food particles, bridgework, gum, and chewing tobacco. A large floppy epiglottis may cause obstruction of the glottic opening under the circumstances of anesthesia and relaxation. Obstruction may be due to edema or infection in glottic structures and the epiglottis. Partial obstruction may precipitate edema of these structures. The obstruction is usually complete, and therefore there is no sound. The signs are those of upper respiratory obstruction.

Clearing of airway at the glottis.—The airway at this point is usually cleared by removing foreign bodies with fingers, forceps or suction. It is often advisable, and sometimes necessary, to expose the glottis to direct vision by means of a laryngoscope.

Infrequently, glottic obstruction may be due to impaction of a long flabby epiglottis in the glottis. This impaction must be dislodged by forceps used under direct vision. On other occasions the glottic obstruction may be due to edema of structures surrounding the laryngeal opening. Edema may follow partial obstruction, instrumentation or infection in that area (particularly in young children), or it may be due to anaphylaxis. Epiglottitis is not an infrequent cause of obstruction at this site. One must be prepared for tracheotomy if more conservative measures fail, keeping in mind always that the margin between adequate airway and an inadequate one may disappear precipitously. Interference of this type is best treated by either tracheal intubation or tracheotomy, or in acute states, cricothyrotomy.

THE LIPS.—Hindrance to flow of air past the lips occurs in persons with full lips. The interference is most noticeable in the expiratory phase of respiration and is accompanied by a low-pitched, rough, fluttery sound. The tidal exchange is not appreciably reduced, and this type of obstruction is of little consequence except for the annoying sound. Restriction of air flow past the lips may occur in individuals whose dentures have been removed. The lips fall in and sometimes coapt. This is particularly true in elderly people whose mandibles have shrunk. Interference with the passage of air in this circumstance takes place during inspiration, and there is little or no hindrance to air flow during expiration. The patient manifests the typical signs of obstruction of the upper respiratory tract. Obstruction occurs early in the development of narcosis with minimal loss of muscular tone and may appear following the administration of therapeutic doses of depressant drugs.

In infants and small children, obstruction at the lips is common. If nasal or nasopharyngeal obstruction is present (as from adenoids), it is often advisable to keep the mouth open. Contrary to the practice in adults, in children it is often better to relax pressure on the jaw, which permits the lips to part and secures a better airway. Obstruction in infants and small children often is due to unnecessary and misplaced pressure on the soft tissue under the jaw. Pressure applied here compresses the tongue against the palate and obstructs the oral airway. Support when necessary must be applied to the mandible at midpoint or behind the angle of the jaw. Choanal atresia is a possible contributor to mouth-breathing and consequently the necessity for attention to the details of management we have outlined must be borne in mind.

A not uncommon form of airway obstruction at the lips is that due to the drapes, the surgeon's and assistant surgeon's hands and arms and large surgical instruments. This type of obstruction happens many times during anesthesia by topical, infiltration, or regional methods for operations about the head and neck. The sound usually associated with this type of interference with the airway is the voice of the patient complaining. If the patient is heavily premedicated, he may be asleep and severe asphyxia may develop before obstruction is observed. Both inspiration and expiration are impeded, and the signs are predominantly those of upper respiratory obstruction. Surgeons working about the head and neck of the patient under topical, infiltration or regional anesthesia should be alert to this cause of obstruction.

Clearing of airway at the lips.—Obstruction to airflow by thick lips can be relieved by the introduction of either an oropharyngeal or a nasopharyngeal airway. In infants, as has already been emphasized, it is possible to improve the airway by relaxing mandibular support.

Hindrance to air flow in the edentulous patient whose lips fall together can be corrected by leaving the dentures in place and taking care to see that they remain in place. It can be corrected also by wetting two gauze squares or sponges, wadding them and placing them in the space between the inside of the cheek and the alveolar ridge. This procedure is also helpful in filling out the cheek and in assisting in the air-tight application of a face mask. Strings should be tied to the gauze and taped to the outside of the cheek to prevent aspiration of the gauze and to serve as a reminder to remove the gauze at conclusion of the anesthesia.

Obstruction of the airway at the lips by drapes, assistants' arms and hands and surgical instruments can be corrected only by constant attention to this possibility by the surgeon, his assistants and the surgical nurse. If the site of surgery permits, it is advisable to place an instrument table or similar device over the patient's nose and mouth. Assistants can lean on this, drapes can be placed over it and instruments can be placed on it without discomfort or danger to the patient.

Sites, Signs and Treatment of Lower Airway Obstruction

The signs of lower respiratory restriction of air flow are present during both inspiration and expiration. They are (1) diminished tidal exchange; (2) excessive costal and diaphragmatic activity; (3) active inspiration and expiration; (4) increased pulse and respiratory rates; (5) cyanosis; (6) thrill to chest-wall palpation; and (7) coarse bubbling rales, rhonchi or wheezing on auscultation. Here again the movements of the rebreathing bag and chest and diaphragm must be correlated. Classically, with lower respiratory obstruction, the bag empties slowly and refills slowly; if one feels the bag, one senses the slowness with which the gas is being moved in both directions. Listening devices also assist materially in defining the site, obstruction degree, and nature of the obstruction.

The trachea and large bronchi.—Obstruction at this point is usually due to foreign material or bodies. The sound associated with it is rattly or sloshy, owing to the passage of air over or through moist material.

Relief of blockade of the airway at this point usually entails the removal of foreign material such as blood, pus, mucus, vomitus and foreign bodies. This may be accomplished by bronchoscopy, but in emergencies the insertion of a tracheal tube, through which a suction catheter can be directed, is quite effective and often lifesaving. As a matter of fact, a rather thorough job of tracheal and bronchial aspiration can be done with the adept use of a tube and the use of a suction catheter, and bronchoscopy can be reserved for those cases in which more definitive aspiration is indicated.

It is, of course, advisable to put the patient in a head-down position with the head turned to the side. However, there is ample evidence to indicate that the head-down position does not prevent aspiration and perhaps does little in minimizing aspiration. Until tracheal intubation or bronchoscopy can be done, tracheal drainage is best accomplished with the patient in the lateral or prone position with the head low. Pounding the patient on the back will sometimes assist him in expelling foreign bodies. Infants and small children can be held by the feet in a completely inverted position for short periods to facilitate drainage of the tracheobronchial tree.

THE BRONCHIOLES.—Bronchiolar constriction is detected chiefly by active expiration, wheezing rales and diminished tidal exchange. This type of obstruction is usually found in asthmatics. However, except in the relatively clear cut circumstances of asthma or an unequivocal allergic response, much of what has been interpreted as bronchospasm under anesthesia is more likely a function of a diminished lung volume with consequent decrease in size of bronchial and bronchiolar passages and increase in resistance to air flow. We believe that true bronchospasm is a rare circumstance under anesthesia. If the signs and sounds of restriction of air movement in bronchial or bronchiolar passages are elicited, one should think rather of other possibilities for the impairment of air flow than bronchospasm. The etiology, signs, and symptoms of reduced lung volume are discussed more fully in Chapter 19.

Clearing of airway at the bronchioles.—If constriction of air flow at the bronchioles develops, as in rare circumstances and except for the asthmatic patient, therapy is directed at relieving the constriction specifically with drugs. Isoproterenol (Isuprel) given intravenously in doses of 0.002 gm, diluted to 10 ml, may help. Aminophylline, in doses of 0.5 to 1.0 gm given slowly intravenously, may help also. Hypotension may follow the administration of either drug. However, if the diminution in small air passage air flow is due to other factors such as small lung volume (atelectasis, stiffness of the chest wall, etc.), therapy is directed at relief other than by direct use of drugs for an effect on the bronchioles. This problem is more fully discussed in Chapter 19.

THE ALVEOLI.—Alveolar obstruction causes the classic signs of lower respiratory obstruction. It may be due to pneumonic consolidation or similar pathologic processes or to emphysematous changes. Atelectasis is a type of alveolar obstruction. Alveolar obstruction can be detected during anesthesia by an increased pulse rate, decreased tidal exchange, lag of the chest wall on the affected side, shift of the mediastinal structures to the affected side and cyanosis. Carbon dioxide retention, as in obstruction from emphysema, can be manifested by dulled responses (or even unresponsiveness), maintenance of anesthesia with unusually low concentrations of agent, elevation of blood pressure, perspiration and, in the absence of depression from drugs or relaxants, early increased ventilation due to increased tidal exchange.

In states of atelectasis or similar conditions in which there is perfused but non-aerated lung, the abnormal condition is usually more effectively detected by blood-gas analysis, which reveals the shunt. This problem is discussed more fully in Chapter 19.

Obstruction of air flow in alveoli is significant in anesthesia because of the delay in gaseous exchange between alveoli and arterial blood. This delay not only interferes with oxygen and carbon dioxide transport but also impedes the flow of anesthetic gases or vapors and retards induction of and recovery from inhalation anesthesia.

In regard to airway obstruction at the alveolar level, the anesthetist must be especially alert to the problems imposed by increases in dead space such as in emphysema and lung cysts. In such circumstances the transfer of gases is seriously impeded between alveoli and blood. One must adjust for this defect by allowing time for transfer. This means that it is unsafe to yield to the temptation to increase the concentration of agent when confronted with an abnormally slow induction. One can increase the concentration *but only* if one recognizes the delay in gas transfer and reduces the concentration several minutes before the desired level of anesthesia is reached. One must, of course, be aware that the recovery process is similarly delayed so that the removal of the agent can be started sooner than usual and appropriate adjustments made for the care of the patient postanesthetically.

Similar problems in gas transfer may occur as a result of reduced pulmonary blood flow. This problem will be discussed in Chapter 20.

Assisted or controlled ventilation, or both, may in a sense induce airway obstruction. Two changes may take place: (1) artificial ventilation may be inadequate in tidal and minute volume, which induces deficiency in oxygen supply and carbon dioxide removal and also may tend to induce development of atelectasis, and (2) atelectasis may develop also in the presence of adequate tidal and minute volume if the ventilation pattern is unaltered. Although there is some debate about the need for "deep breaths," there is reasonable evidence to indicate that "deep breaths," "sighs" or, at least, a change in the pattern of respiration is useful. Assisted or controlled ventilation may also produce an abnormal distribution of air (or anesthetic gas mixture) with preferential channeling, so that substantial segments of the lung are not aerated. It may be that the ventilation required for assisted or controlled ventilation is greater than it is in normal undepressed voluntary respiration. This topic also is discussed more completely in Chapter 19.

Use of Suction in Preventing and Relieving Airway Obstruction

One of the most effective, simple and important aids to establishment and maintenance of an airway is suction. No anesthesia, whatever the technic, should be induced, maintained or terminated in the absence of an immediately available source of suction. The need for removal of foreign material from the pharynx, larynx or tracheobronchial tree always must be anticipated; and ready, dependable suction is the most effective method of handling this need. Frequent and effective aspiration in patients in coma or with neurologic defects involving the upper air passages is undoubtedly a lifesaving procedure.

A number of different types of catheters for aspirating purposes are available. Most of these are made of plastic and have several holes near the distal end and a hole near the proximal end to be closed by a finger when suction is needed. In emergency circumstances, of course, an ordinary urethral catheter can be used. The evidence is incontrovertible that infection can be introduced or transferred from patient to patient or from personnel to patient by poor attention to aseptic handling of catheters for aspiration, especially of the lung. The catheters should be prepared and packaged in a sterile manner and handled as aseptically as possible. Preferably a catheter should be used only once. Metal suction tips (e.g., a tonsillectomy suction instrument) may be used but may be more traumatic and use should be restricted to circumstances in which direct observation of the oropharynx is possible and large volumes of material are being aspirated.

The catheter, when used, may be introduced either through the nose or mouth. To avoid nasal trauma (e.g., a nose bleed) and because the nares are often too constricted to permit passage of a catheter of a satisfactory size, oral entry is preferred. Often it is easy to continue passage of the catheter into the trachea and this maneuver often obviates the need for bronchoscopy. The catheter should be well moistened with some of the patient's mucus, water or a water-soluble jelly in order to minimize trauma to mucous surfaces and facilitate its passage. Liquid petrolatum accelerates deterioration of rubber catheters. It is wise to interrupt suction while the catheter is being inserted and to aspirate only on withdrawal. In patients who require repeated aspiration of upper and lower air passages, such as those in coma and with upper airway paralysis, it is essential that trauma be minimized by attending to the detail of introducing the catheter with the suction interrupted and aspirating only when the catheter is being moved, usually on withdrawal. Even with several holes in the catheter tip, strong suction can result in aspiration of mucosal surfaces into the openings, with subsequent hemorrhage or edema.

The metal aspirator and the catheter should be cleared frequently by dipping in water because they are easily occluded by mucus, blood, vomitus and other foreign material that may be aspirated. A glass or clear plastic connecting tip between the catheter or metal appliance and the remaining suction line permits observation of material being removed and aids in determining whether or not the suction line is functioning.

Prolonging the time during which suction is applied in any aspirating procedure may produce two undesirable effects. One is the collapse of alveoli and small bronchioles, with consequent atelectasis. This complication is especially hazardous in patients unable by reason of their disease (for example, paralyzed or comatose patients) to reexpand these areas. The second undesirable effect is hypoxia. In patients breathing room air, oxygen is removed from the lung by suction applied particularly in the trachea and bronchi. If extensive and protracted aspiration is needed, prior oxygenation with a high concentration of oxygen is advisable. Reinflation of the lungs after aspiration is indicated to diminish the tendency for atelectasis.

ENDOTRACHEAL INTUBATION

There is a widespread tendency to consider the introduction of a large-bore tube through the larynx into the trachea as something other than simply another means of establishing and maintaining an airway. Except for the fact that considerably more training and experience are required to introduce an endotracheal tube adeptly and atraumatically, there is no reason for separating this means of securing an airway from the other effective methods. The use of an endotracheal tube is often erroneously referred to as "endotracheal anesthesia." An endotracheal tube has but one function, and that is to provide a patent airway. It is not a method of anesthesia.

A tube passed by the translaryngeal route into the trachea and kept free from kinks and having a clear lumen is a guarantee against obstruction of air flow at the lips, the nasopharynx, the oropharynx, the glottis and the vocal cords. The endotracheal tube is therefore useful whenever interference with air flow at any of those points may be anticipated or be present. Although most of the trauma associated with introduction of an endotracheal tube is due to inept instrumentation by the endoscopist, there is no evading the fact that passage of an endotracheal tube presents more opportunities for trauma than simpler methods of securing an airway. Therefore, anesthetists should resist the temptation to introduce an endotracheal tube simply because it makes things more convenient for them or because they are too inept or too lazy to maintain an airway by simpler means.

Indications for Use of Endotracheal Intubation

The use of an intratracheal tube is usually reserved for situations in which simpler methods of airway control are inadequate. These situations are as follows:

1. The position of the patient's upper respiratory tract which may make the tract inaccessible to the anesthetist.
2. Contamination of the upper or lower respiratory tract, current or in the future.
3. Normal or pathologic anatomy of the upper respiratory tract that precludes satisfactory control of the airway by simpler methods.
4. Greater convenience to the surgeon because the anesthetist and his major equipment are no longer near the head and neck of the patient.
5. Surgeon and anesthetist working in the same area.
6. A prolonged surgical procedure (long mask pressure may induce ischemia or reaction to contact).
7. The need for controlled and/or artificial respiration (with or without muscle relaxants).

POSITION OF THE UPPER RESPIRATORY TRACT.—The upper respiratory tract usually is inaccessible when the patient is in the prone position, and particularly when the head is in a cerebellar head rest. The upper respiratory tract may be inaccessible also during surgical manipulations about the head and neck.

CONTAMINATION OF THE UPPER AND LOWER RESPIRATORY TRACT.—Contamination of oropharynx, larynx, trachea, and bronchi may be the result of operations in these areas. Blood can be prevented from entering the trachea and bronchi and can be removed from the trachea and bronchi if an endotracheal tube is in place. The oropharynx of a patient whose stomach is not empty may be contaminated with material that is vomited, regurgitated, or otherwise introduced into the pharynx by relaxation of the cardiac sphincter. In such a patient, intubation should be used to prevent contamination of the lower respiratory tract. Some anesthetists prefer to intubate the trachea of the awake patient (with or without topical analgesia) and inflate the balloon (cuff) to prevent aspiration. Topical analgesia of the larynx may be accomplished by the transoral introduction of the analgesic agent by sprays or nebulizers. It may be introduced also by transtracheal instillation; this method is effective and efficient, but needles introduced through the cricoid membrane have been broken and serious infection at the injection site has been reported. Topical anesthetization of the larynx prior to intubation seems to be useful in diminishing reaction to the catheter during anesthesia. Lighter levels of anesthesia may be possible in the presence of an endotracheal tube and undesirable "bucking" and straining can be diminished.

In patients with bronchiectasis, lung abscess, or pulmonary edema and patients undergoing pulmonary resection an endotracheal tube should be passed in order to facilitate aspiration and ventilation. The tracheal tube can be fitted with an inflatable balloon, which takes up the space between the tube and the tracheal wall and impedes entrance of material from the upper into the lower respiratory tract. A small suction catheter can be introduced through the endotracheal tube and foreign material aspirated from the lower respiratory tract. There are special double-lumen tubes (e.g., the Carlens tube) that can be used in circumstances in which it is useful to block off one lung and achieve ventilation with the remaining lung. Selective aspiration of either lung can also be accomplished. The use of such tubes is limited, however, primarily because of difficulty in placement and also because the respective lumens are relatively small.

INADEQUATE CONTROL DUE TO ANATOMIC ABNORMALITIES.—Endotracheal intubation is usually required in patients with a receding mandible, a narrow mandibular arch, a large tongue, a bull neck, an ankylosed mandible or neck, a tumor encroaching on the oropharynx, trachea or larynx, a long epiglottis or a paralyzed vocal cord in order to prevent obstruction of the airway. Anesthetists should learn to recognize those anatomic features that make intubation difficult. By so doing, one can prepare for a difficult intubation and arrange for alternatives such as an awake nasotracheal intubation or tracheotomy. Rapid induction with paralysis should be effected with caution if difficulty in tracheal intubation is suspected.

CONVENIENCE TO THE SURGEON.—It is possible for the anesthetist to remove himself and the major portion of his equipment from the operative site when an endotracheal tube is in place to ensure an adequate airway. Geographic removal of the anesthetist does not eliminate the necessity for maintaining contact with the patient.

THE NEED FOR CONTROLLED RESPIRATION AND ARTIFICIAL RESPIRATION.—Controlled or assisted respiration and artificial respiration (with or without relaxants) are performed most efficiently with an endotracheal tube

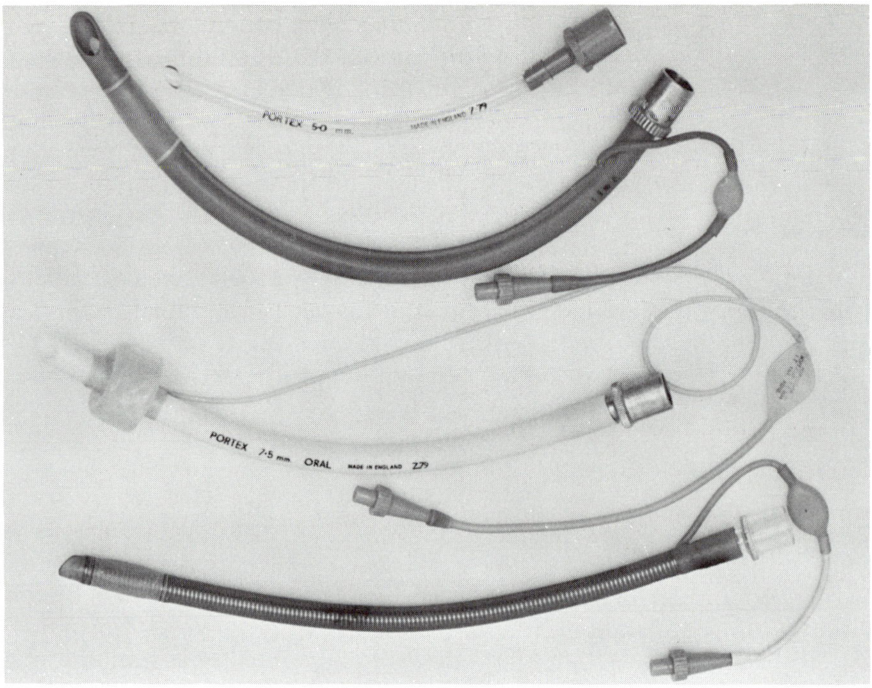

Fig. 6-5.—Various types of endotracheal tubes. The *uppermost* tube is plastic and not equipped with a balloon; it is often used in children. The other three tubes are fitted with balloons (cuffs). Of these, *center tube* is fitted with low-pressure cuff, and *lower tube* is "LA" or "anode" tube incorporating spiral of wire which diminishes opportunity for kinking. Note pilot balloons on tubing from cuff; these pilot balloons give indication of competency of cuff and degree of inflation.

in place, because patency of the airway is ensured, distention of the stomach is prevented, and the lungs can be inflated easily.

Elements for Successful Intubation

The introduction of an endotracheal tube can be accomplished with dexterity and without trauma only after considerable training and experience and with meticulous attention to details. The inexperienced individual will cause much trauma to lips, teeth, oropharynx, nasopharynx, glottic structures, larynx and trachea by rough and inept handling of laryngoscope and tube.

NATURE OF TUBE.—An endotracheal tube is a large bore catheter made of rubber, rubber-covered metal, or plastic. It is flexible and has a relatively thin but sturdy wall. Sizes vary from F 14 (Magill 00), suitable for small children, to F 40 (Magill 12), for large adults (Fig. 6-5). To avoid unnecessary resistance to air flow, a tube approximating the size of the laryngeal opening should be used. It is unwise and unnecessary, especially in children, to use an endotracheal tube that is too large and has to be forced through the laryngeal opening. The decrease in resistance afforded by the large tube is

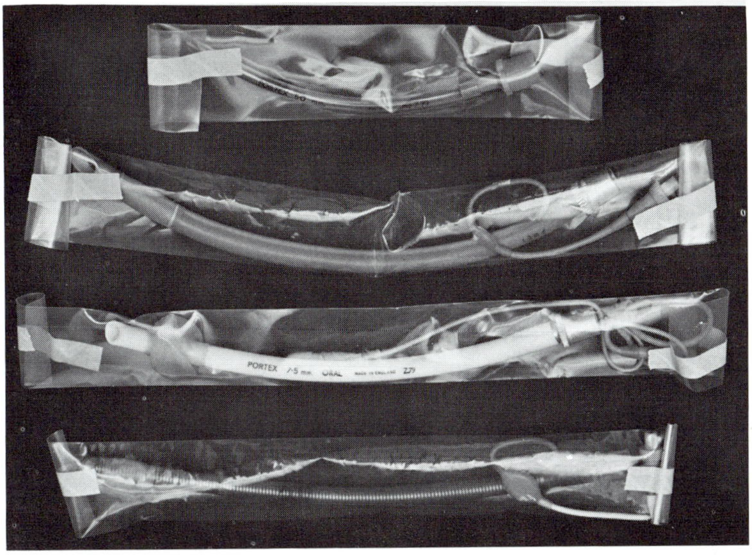

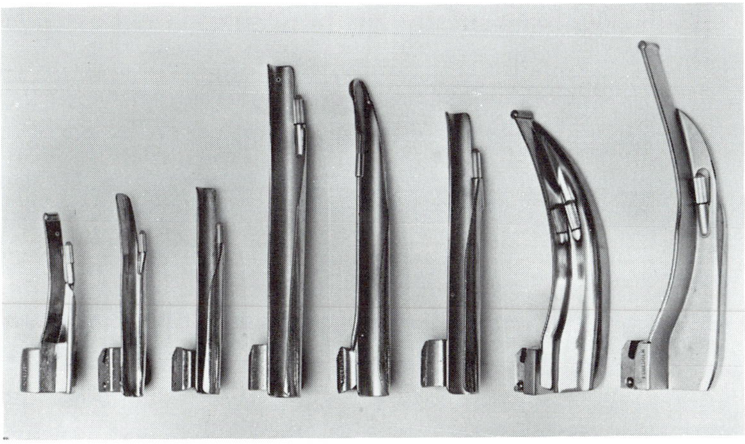

Fig. 6-6 (top).—Endotracheal tubes packaged in plastic containers, in which they can be sterilized and maintained aseptically prior to use.

Fig. 6-7 (bottom).—Various types of blades available for laryngoscopy. Each blade can be attached to universal handle, usually powered by batteries.

not of sufficient magnitude to compensate for the damage to laryngeal and tracheal structures. It should be remembered that in children the narrowest portion of the larynx is at the cricoid cartilage; a catheter that enters the upper portion of the larynx thus may be too large for the portion surrounded by the cricoid cartilage. In small children (to the age of 5 years) it is advisable to avoid using a tube with a cuff and to insert a tube of a caliber that permits a small leak around the tube. By so doing one can appreciably diminish the glottic and laryngeal edema frequently encountered in children of this age. By eliminating the cuff one can use a tube that is one size larger.

Although rubber tubes are still widely used and are satisfactory, tubes made of various types of plastic have apparent advantages in that they (1) seem to be better tolerated (less local tissue reaction), (2) mold better to the trachea and oral airway and (3) permit observation of any material that may come from the lungs. The endotracheal tube may be introduced either through the oropharynx into the trachea or through the nares, nasopharynx and oropharynx into the trachea. Introduction through the oropharynx is more common than the nasal route and this approach will be discussed first.

Orotracheal Intubation

The endotracheal tube is introduced through the oropharynx with the aid of a laryngoscope, which permits one to visualize the glottic opening and the structures proximal to it. Except in small children, the tube passed through the oropharynx usually carries a cuff.

As has been mentioned, endotracheal intubation has inherent opportunities for trauma and infection. As a result, it is important that care be taken in the technic and we will attempt to outline here some of the general principles and basic technic of intubation. Obviously, one can learn how to intubate successfully and atraumatically only by instruction and actual practice.

CONTROL OF INFECTION.—As in the circumstance of aspiration by catheter, it is clearly established that the endotracheal apparatus, especially the tube itself, constitutes a source of transmission or introduction of infection, or both. As a result, it is mandatory that the apparatus be clean, the tubes aseptic and the technic as aseptic as possible. This means, for example, that the apparatus used (e.g., laryngoscope and fittings) be laid out not on the dirty top of a gas machine but on a clean towel. The tubes themselves should be thoroughly cleaned prior to packaging in individual paper or plastic containers. The package with enclosed tube is then sterilized most effectively by gas sterilization (Fig. 6-6).

LARYNGOSCOPE AND TUBE SIZE.—Figure 6-7 shows the common types of blades available for laryngoscopy. It is important to assess the situation requiring intubation and select appropriate equipment. For example, if the patient's head is in severe flexion, it may be wise to use an "armored tube" (L.A. tube), a tube containing a built-in coil of wire that discourages kinking or occlusion from bending of the tube; such a tube also may be useful in anesthesia for esophagoscopy so that the esophagoscope does not compress the endotracheal tube. If the patient is a small child, it is wise to have at least three tubes available for use; one that the anesthetist estimates is the proper size and one larger and one smaller. Upon visualization of the glottis, the apparent proper size can be selected and then checked for leaks. If the tube is too large or too small, the change can be made immediately. A convenient rule of thumb for estimating tube size (French) in children is to add age in years to a no. 18 French catheter.

ELEMENTS PERTINENT TO SUCCESSFUL ORAL INTUBATION.—The importance of learning to assess the anatomic make-up of the patient's neck, oral opening, jaw, and teeth has been emphasized. Difficult intubation by the oral route can be anticipated if (1) the patient's neck is thick and short, (2) the tissue from mandible to sternum is in a straight line (fullness), (3) the jaw recedes ("Andy Gump" type), (4) the upper teeth override, (5) the oral opening laterally is narrow (small mouth), (6) the patient can open his mouth only slightly, (7) the teeth are "buck" type or some are loose and (8) the mobility of the neck is limited (arthritis, cervical tumor, etc.).

Certain basic elements are essential to successful and atraumatic intubation by the oral route. A tube can be of any type and size that is appropriate for the individual patient. Connecting fittings may be curved or straight as needed for the particular situation. The tube cuff should be checked to determine if it leaks or bulges unequally. Although most cuffs are built into oral tubes and most of these are small requiring high pressures to inflate, we prefer the larger low-pressure balloons. Evidence is more than adequate to indicate that small high-pressure cuffs produce ischemia at the site of contact, often inflate unevenly, sometimes protrude over the end of the tube and may rupture producing a high-pressure jet effect on adjacent tracheal tissue. Lubrication of the tube is best limited to the terminal 3 cm. We believe that petrolatum jelly is a better lubricant but it does cause rubber to deteriorate; water-soluble lubricants or ointments containing a local anesthetic also may be used. With a local anesthetic, one should be careful to determine if the patient is sensitive to that local anesthetic and one should be aware also that most of the local anesthetics incorporated into the lubricants are relatively poor topical agents with a relatively short action.

Selection of the type of laryngoscope blade largely depends on the personal preference of the anesthetist. We prefer the straight blade for routine use and reserve the curved blade for use in patients whose glottis we assess by observation to be likely difficult to expose. We prefer a straight blade for three reasons: (1) it gives a less limited view of the glottic opening, (2) there is more room within the oral cavity to introduce the tube and, as a result, to observe and direct its actual entrance into the glottis, and (3) there is less need to have the tube curved so that it can be introduced into the anteriorly situated glottic opening.

We use a stilette in a tube at all times when a curved laryngoscope blade is used because the glottic opening is often anterior and one must pass the tube along the curved route made by the blade. A stilette may be made of any malleable metal. It should be well lubricated; nothing is more exasperating than to be unable to remove a stilette from an endotracheal tube after a difficult intubation. Curved tubes can be used and intubation often done without a stilette, but too often intubation has to be interrupted and the patient reanesthetized or relaxed, just so the stilette can be put in the tube. We submit this is an unnecessary maneuver that does the patient no good. We use a stilette also in introducing the armored tube because its flaccidity makes it difficult to direct. Especially with the armored tubes, one should always be careful to see that there is no weak area that will permit kinking and obstruction between fitting in the tube and the rest of the tube.

Except in circumstances that have been described (e.g., in the presence of a full stomach) we believe that intubation is more easily accomplished with the patient well anesthetized. Actually, we believe that intubation should be accomplished with the patient in the deepest plane of anesthesia

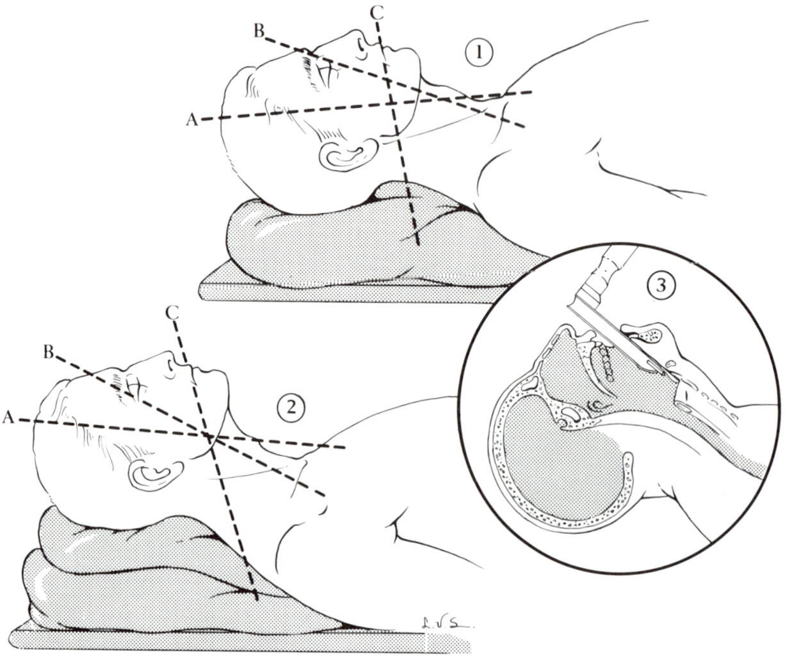

Fig. 6-8.—Positions of head for laryngoscopy and intubation. **1**, Usual position with slight or no elevation of occiput. *A*, axis of pharynx; *B*, axis of trachea and *C*, axis of oral cavity. **2**, Increasing elevation of occiput, as on pillow or several towels, increases visualization of glottic opening and alignment of axis of trachea more nearly to that of position of laryngoscope. **3**, Extension of head tends to move laryngeal opening forward and more difficult to enter.

that may be necessary at any time during the operation and that the concentration of the anesthetic must be maintained at its highest until just prior to intubation. This makes bucking, which does not benefit the patient, less likely and probably diminishes the incidence and severity of cardiac irregularities associated with intubation. If intubation is to be done by the inexperienced anesthetist or if intubation is expected to be difficult, it is wise to administer oxygen in a high concentration for a few breaths prior to intubation. Relaxants are useful in facilitating intubation. Ordinarily, succinylcholine is used because short intense relaxation is often all that is needed.

We abhor the practice of "crash" induction and intubation with combinations of thiopental and succinylcholine followed by the introduction by artificial respiration of potent inhalation agents. With this technic, the patient is often inadequately anesthetized and not only tries to move during the procedure of intubation but may be more susceptible to cardiac irregularities. Even more significantly, as has been demonstrated too often, cardiac arrest follows this technic because the use of artificial ventilation exposes the patient to too much potent agent in too short a time with no sign of loss of tolerance until arrest occurs.

TECHNICAL PROCEDURE OF INTUBATION.—As in blind nasotracheal intubation, the head should be in the sniffing position (Fig. 6-8). This is particularly true if the curved blade is to be used; extending the head will only accentuate the anterior position of the glottic opening and enhance the difficulty of exposure. The sniffing position will also diminish the need for a stilette when the curved blade is used. Extending the head, too common a practice, also makes alignment of the trachea less satisfactory.

The laryngoscope blade is held in the left hand (blades for left-handed anesthetists are available). Ideally the blade is held with the hand at the junction of the blade and handle; in this position the hand can rest on the patient's upper jaw and thus stabilize the laryngoscope when it is properly placed for exposure of the glottic opening; there is also less tendency for the anesthetist to pry with the handle. The mouth is opened by pulling with the forefinger of the right hand on the upper teeth to the right of the midline. Some anesthetists also use the thumb to push on the lower jaw, but we believe this maneuver adds little to the mouth opening process and often the thumb is in the way of proper introduction of the laryngoscope. The blade is introduced in the right side of the oral cavity so that the tongue can be kept entirely to the left. Many unsuccessful or difficult intubations are due to the fact that the tongue flops over the blade on the right side, thus establishing a "tunnel" through which attempts are made to introduce the tube blindly. All of the tongue must be to the left of the blade. The blade is further introduced until the epiglottis is visualized. As the blade is introduced, the jaw is also lifted forward. This can be done with the blade (lifting, not prying on the upper teeth) and the forward motion of the mandible can be facilitated by grasping the lower teeth and jaw with the right thumb and forefinger and pulling it forward.

At this point, the technic depends upon the type of blade that is used. If the straight blade is used, the blade is advanced so as to put the tip of the blade under the epiglottis. It is then lifted forward to expose the glottic opening. With the curved blade, one advances the blade so that its tip engages in the vallecula (anterior to the base of the epiglottis); further advance of the blade lifts the epiglottis and exposes the glottic opening. With either blade one remembers that it is useful to keep the handle and the blade in a vertical position, not tipped to either side; also, the blade must be in the midline. The tendency is to have the blade directed to the right and advanced too far, which exposes not the glottis, but the opening of the esophagus. The two openings are differentiated as follows: (1) the esophagus is located to the right and posteriorly; (2) the esophagus opening is round and puckered with no structures around it; (3) the glottis is triangular; (4) the glottis is located in the midline; (5) the glottis contains arytenoids posteriorly (these appear as prominent knobs in difficult intubation and may be the only clue to glottic opening); and (6) the cords and dark cavern of the trachea can be seen beyond the glottis.

Once the glottis is exposed (and the tongue is out of the way), the endotracheal tube is introduced by picking it up as if it were a pencil, with the built-in curve so directed that the tip of the tube tends to move forward into the glottic opening. Preferably one brings the tube in from the right side and not down the blade, so that one can observe the tube entering the glottic opening. Sometimes it is useful to slide the tip of the tube down the underside of the blade (coming from the right side) so that it enters the glottic opening directly off the end of the blade. If one holds the tube so that the natural curve is to the right the tendency is for the tip to enter the esophagus rather than the glottis. Once the tube has entered the glottis, especially if one is using a stilette, the tube should be rotated 90° to the right; this brings the plane of the tube into alignment with the plane of the trachea. The tube is advanced until the cuff just disappears in the glottic opening. Sometimes it is not possible to expose the glottis entirely. In such circumstances, one can sometimes see the arytenoids or the epiglottis, or both. With an appropriately curved tube or a stilette in the tube curved at the end, one can introduce the tube under the epiglottis, lift the epiglottis, and pass the tube past the arytenoids into the glottis.

The laryngoscope is then removed unless one wants to use it to facilitate introduction of an esophageal monitor. The tube is secured by one hand, which rests on the patient's jaw. Unless the tube is thus secured prior to taping in place, there is a strong tendency for the tube to be unwittingly advanced several centimeters into a bronchus. The patient also may cough at this point and, unless the tube is secured, one may find it has been coughed out of the trachea and intubation has to be repeated. Some anesthetists inflate the cuff at this stage but unless there is a large leak preventing inflation of the lungs there is no immediate need for so doing except to prevent aspiration. It is, however, wise to insert a bite block at this stage to prevent the patient from clamping down on the tube as he awakens or as the relaxant wears off. The tube also should be secured well with tape. Four-point placement of the tape (using benzoin to insure sticking of the tape) makes it less likely that the tube will come out during the surgical procedure. A final check on tube placement should be made by listening to the chest to determine if endobronchial intubation occurred. A simpler and yet more positive means of determining the location of the tube in the trachea and of preventing endobronchial intubation is to inflate and deflate the cuff while palpating in the neck at the level just below the larynx. If the cuff is properly placed on the tube and inflation of it can be felt just below the larynx, one can be reasonably certain (more certain than by listening to the chest) that the tip of the tube has not been placed endobronchially inadvertently.* Hearing uniform breath sounds throughout all lung fields is not a guarantee that the tube does not lie in a bronchus, and if there is any question one should retract the tube about 1 cm. The breath sounds can then be rechecked. This is especially true in infants and small children, in whom breath sounds are easily transmitted. In critical situations, it may be advisable to check position of the tube by x-ray. Finally, one must remember that the tip of the tube placed in the trachea of infants and small children may be advanced if the head is flexed and retracted or if the head is extended or turned sharply to the side, and that turning the head to the side also may cause the opening of the tube to impinge on the side of the trachea.

*The authors are indebted to Dr. Wendell Stevens for this simple yet effective test.

Nasotracheal Intubation

If orotracheal intubation is not feasible, introduction of an endotracheal tube via the nose, nasopharynx oropharynx is possible and useful. Nasotracheal intubation is particularly useful if the operative procedure is to be in the oral cavity or if long-term access to the tracheobronchial tree and lung is needed (long-term artificial ventilation, removal of secretions, etc.), for the tube introduced nasotracheally is more stable.

SELECTION OF TUBE.—Introduction of a tube via the nose, however, often means that the lumen becomes compromised by the narrowness of the nasal passage or by a kink at the junction of the posterior nares and nasopharynx. Nasotracheal tubes also may occlude the eustachian tubes and middle ear infection may develop. It is necessary to have tubes that are curved so that the tip tends to enter the glottic opening. The curve must not be too acute, or the tip of the tube tends to be too far anterior and does not engage in the glottic opening; a suitable curve is that obtained by storing tubes in a can previously used for 5 lb. of bonbons. Furthermore, the tube preferably should have a reasonably long bevel; a stubby bevel does not engage in the glottic opening as well as a longer bevel. The tube caliber should be somewhat smaller than that of a tube selected for oral intubation, so that the nasal opening is not dilated too much and movement in and out and laterally is facilitated. Usually, red rubber or neoprene tubes are more satisfactory than plastic tubes for nasotracheal intubation because they are firmer. The tubes may carry cuffs, but the cuffs often bulge somewhat and necessitate a reduction in tube size to permit passage through the nose.

Selection of the tube size, curve, and consistency is critical to success in nasotracheal intubation. One need not feel constrained to use the largest tube that will pass through the nose; smaller tubes may be quite satisfactory from an airway standpoint and be infinitely easier to introduce. Tubes of different sizes and curves should be available.

TECHNICAL PROCEDURE OF INTUBATION.—The patient can be anesthetized topically or by inhalation. In any event, it is preferable to cocainize the nose to shrink the mucosa and diminish the opportunity for bleeding. Cocainization is accomplished most satisfactorily by insertion of pledgets attached to applicators. Spraying by atomizer usually anesthetizes and shrinks only the anterior portion of the nasal cavity and fails thereby to provide optimum effect. Time is important also; adequate time should be allowed to permit complete anesthetization. The larynx may be anesthetized topically by oral introduction of local anesthetic or by transtracheal instillation. If general anesthesia is used, it is important that respiration not be depressed, because deep breathing is essential to successful blind nasotracheal intubation. It is even sometimes beneficial to add carbon dioxide to the inhaled atmosphere to stimulate breathing; the deeper breathing assists in helping to identify the location of the glottic opening as will be mentioned later.

The patient's head is then placed in the "sniffing" position: the occiput raised approximately 10 cm from the table and the eyes looking to the ceiling. The terminal 3 cm of the tube is then well lubricated, preferably by a thick coating of petrolatum jelly. Lubrication of more than the terminal 3 cm of the tube is unnecessary and disadvantageous; as the tube enters the nose, the lubricant on the tip will lubricate the remainder of the tube. Water-soluble lubricants are definitely less satisfactory; they tend to disappear and leave a sticky tube that does not move easily in and out. The side of the nose with the largest aperture is then selected and the tube introduced past the nasopharyngeal junction into the oropharynx. If resistance is encountered in getting the tube past the nasopharyngeal junction, it can be rotated 90° in either direction. If the tube cannot be passed, one should try the other nostril or then use another tube. It is most important that one be aware that it is entirely possible, with not too much force, to have the tip of the tube break the nasopharyngeal mucosa and burrow under it.

Once the tube is in the oropharynx, one attempts to align the tip of the tube with the glottic opening. This is best done by listening to the volume and quality of sound of air moving through the tube. This is why it is necessary to have the patient breathing deeply. When the tip of the tube is directly in front of the glottic opening, one hears (and feels) a large volume of air with little noise coming through the tube. One then times the advance of the tube into the glottic opening to coincide with or just precede inspiration. The tube is advanced quickly and with a "full" motion, not gently and slowly. Timing is critical because the cords are open at inspiration and perhaps the position of the glottic opening is more favorable for entrance of the tube. Some anesthetists prefer to advance the tube slowly until it enters the glottic opening. The incidence of success with this technic will be less than with that just described primarily because advantage is not taken of the change in position of the glottic opening and its patency at time of inspiration. Entrance of the tube is determined by a continuation of the air movement through the tube, by a cough, or by vigorous bucking. On occasion, the tip of the tube just enters the glottic opening and stops anteriorly. This can be determined by noting the movement of the larynx externally in the neck and sometimes by a peculiar brassy sound coming through the tube. If this occurs, it is sometimes useful to flex the head and so bring the plane of the trachea into more direct line with the plane of the tube. Sometimes one can dislodge the tip and have it continue into the trachea by gently moving the larynx externally. Failing this, one retracts the tube and reintroduces it usually with the head flexed. If the tube fails to enter the glottic opening, the position of the tip of the tube is shifted laterally in either or both directions by rotating the tube; hopefully this lines up the tip with the glottic opening. One of the major reasons for failure of blind nasotracheal intubation is the introduction of the tip of the tube too far; it is necessary to hear the rush of air through the tube and the tube should be retracted until this is heard. Movement of the head, usually flexion, can be accomplished while attempting to advance the tube by placing the left hand under the occiput. One can also observe the neck to determine whether the tip of the tube passes to the right or left of the larynx.

Unless exposure of the larynx is difficult or impossible because of the various factors outlined, one can use relaxants and introduce the nasotracheal tube under direct vision if it is not possible to introduce it blindly. By so doing, in the learning process one can sometimes find out what errors are being made in placing the tip of the tube blindly. If nasal bleeding occurs, it is probably wise to leave the tube in place to act as a tamponade; perhaps if the bleeding is severe, the tube can be retracted and the cuff inflated to act as a tamponade. Especially with small children and if short tubes are used, it is wise to remember that flexion of the head tends to push the tube further into the trachea whereas extension of the head tends to pull the tube out of the trachea.

Extubation

Except in those circumstances in which the anesthetist desires to leave the tube in place during the postanesthetic or postsurgical period, extubation may take place at any appropriate time in the surgical and anesthetic procedure; usually this is at or near termination of the anesthetic. We believe that when it is possible to maintain an airway and anesthetic by mask, it is preferable to remove the tube with the patient in moderately deep anesthesia. This diminishes the likelihood of coughing and laryngospasm as the tube is removed as well as of bucking; abdominal wall sutures have been known to break under the stress of bucking. The pharynx is suctioned prior to extubation to remove accumulated secretions that might enter the trachea or provoke coughing or laryngospasm. Unless there is evidence of material in the trachea or lungs, it is doubtful whether it is necessary or advisable to risk introducing infection by aspirating the trachea through the tube. If one anticipates temporary interference with ventilation because of obstruction or laryngospasm or breath holding as the tube is removed, it is probably advisable to give the patient several breaths of 100% oxygen prior to extubation. There is no special trick to extubation. One must remember, of course, to deflate the cuff. Some anesthetists prefer to remove the tube while pressure on the breathing bag is being applied. If the tube is removed in light anesthesia, severe laryngospasm may follow extubation; this is especially true of children. Prior oxygenation then is useful and the anesthetist must be prepared to cope with laryngospasm.

Complications of Intubation

We have mentioned several complications of endotracheal catheterization such as coughing, bucking, laceration of pharyngeal mucosa, kinking of the tube, endobronchial placement, displacement of the tube, and increased resistance to breathing. The laryngoscope itself may loosen or dislodge teeth, and cut or bruise lips. Edema of the larynx also may occur. If this does occur or if it is expected, one should put the patient in a high-humidity atmosphere and administer steroids. Hoarseness is a relatively common complaint and needs to be treated only with high humidity. Granulomata are said to be sequelae of intubation but the incidence is low; prevention may be enhanced by avoiding tubes that are too snug and overinflated cuffs. The cuff should be inflated only enough to prevent leak; additional pressure will only enhance ischemia.

We have mentioned the possible use of tubes such as the Carlens tube for special situations in which endobronchial intubation is indicated. We do not propose to detail the technic for this tube in this manual. Endobronchial intubation inadvertently or deliberately with ordinary endotracheal catheters is possible by directing the bevel of the tube in the desired position to facilitate entrance of the tip into the preferred bronchus.

Obviously, tracheal intubation is a useful and beneficial procedure for maintenance of an airway; equally obviously, it is a technic that requires training and experience to make it safe, effective and nontraumatic. It is a procedure that *all* physicians should be familiar with so that they may be in a better position to establish and maintain an airway for resuscitative or long-term treatment when indicated. Because of the complications associated with it, however, it is obviously not a technic that should be used only to make it easier for the anesthetist.

CHAPTER SEVEN

Evaluation of Anesthetic Depth

IN THIS CHAPTER we outline ways in which the anesthetist may make a reasonably accurate estimate of not only the presence of "anesthesia" but also the extent of involvement of critical organs and systems within the body. Assessment of the presence and degree of "anesthesia" in the patient under conduction anesthesia is outlined in Chapter 22. What we have to say in this section will be pertinent only to the state known as "general anesthesia."

CONCEPTS OF THE STATE OF ANESTHESIA

There are several different definitions of the state of anesthesia. One of the more recent is the concept of MAC (minimal alveolar anesthetic concentration), proposed and refined by Eger.[1] This concept defines anesthesia as that state in which there is absence of movement (in 50% of patients) when a surgical incision is made. Delineation of the MAC producing that particular level of anesthesia and the impact of various factors such as age, narcotics and temperature on this concentration has been one of the more significant contributions to the understanding and practical application of inhalation anesthetic agents (Figs. 7-1, 7-2, 7-3). At present let us attempt to identify what we believe to be the state of "general anesthesia." What we put forward here will be reflected in our method of determining the patient's responses, which in turn reflect the degree of involvement of critical organs and systems by the anesthetic agent or agents—that is, the "depth of anesthesia." Our concept of anesthesia also will be reflected in our management of anesthesia.

We believe there are several components to the state of anesthesia. We believe that a complete state of anesthesia includes pain relief, relaxation, elimination of some reflexes and sedation-hypnosis. In the early days of anesthesia, these various elements were achieved by one agent, usually ether or chloroform. Now it is possible to satisfy these requirements more efficiently by use of several drugs each having relatively specific effects in optimal doses. For example, if relaxation is needed a muscle relaxant is indicated. If pain relief is needed (as manifested, for example, by movement of the patient in response to a stimulus), one needs to increase the concentration of an effective anesthetic agent or to add an agent such as a narcotic or another anesthetic agent. If undesired reflexes such as bradycardia and

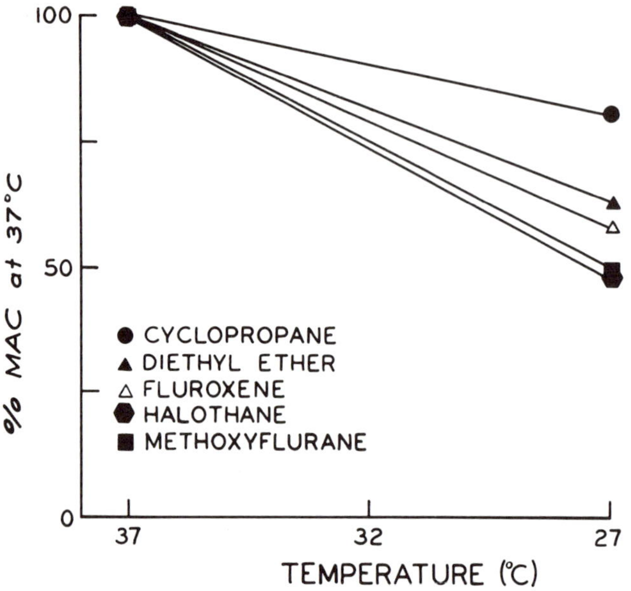

Fig. 7-1.—The *lines* represent the percentage decreases between 37 and 27° C of minimum alveolar concentration (MAC) of several agents. Cyclopropane, the least soluble agent, shows least decrease and the more soluble agents, halothane and methoxyflurane, show greater decreases. (From Regan, M. T., and Eger, E. I., II: Effect of hypothermia in dogs on anesthetizing and apneic doses of inhalation agents, Anesthesiology 28:689, 1967.)

hypotension from celiac reflex are encountered, specific drugs such as atropine can be used. The proper management of anesthesia includes attention to these different components. We do not believe that anesthesia is an "all or none" phenomenon. We do believe that the responses of the patient (depth of anesthesia) are on a continuum in proportion to the plasma concentration of the agent or agents to which the critical organs or systems are exposed. The number of molecules of anesthetic agent in the cells of these organs is related to the concentration in plasma to which they are exposed. We are aware that one of the more acceptable theories of narcosis states that "anesthesia" exists whenever a fairly precise number of molecules of any agent enters the cell. We prefer, in order to facilitate management of the practical state of anesthesia to fit the demands of surgery, to consider that "anesthesia" is a dynamic state with degrees of "depth" correlated to the plasma concentration of the agent.

We think that it is useful to consider that anesthesia may be "light" enough to relieve the patient of pain but leave him capable of responding to sound (e.g., voice command). We believe also that the anesthesia may be "deep" enough that profound muscle relaxation and pronounced respiratory and circulatory depression may exist. We accept the premise made by Eger that the responses of organs and organ systems vary with the particular agent used for anesthesia, but we believe that the state of anesthesia includes all responses. We do not restrict our definition of anesthesia to one response (movement in response to a skin incision in 50% of patients) although we

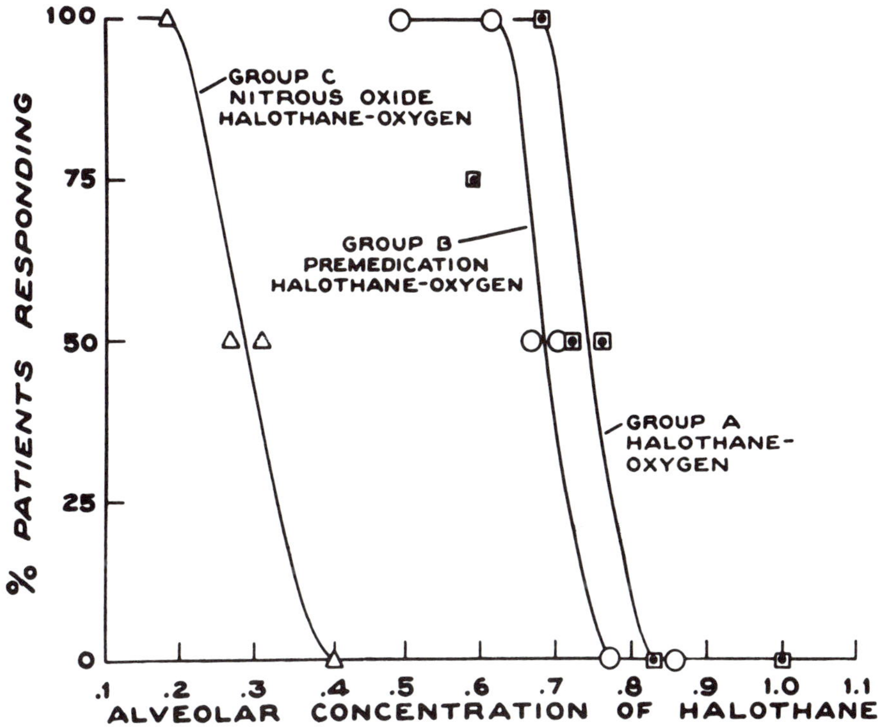

Fig. 7-2.—Determination of minimal alveolar anesthetic concentration (MAC) in groups of patients receiving either *halothane-oxygen, halothane-oxygen with morphine premedication* or *halothane-oxygen with nitrous oxide.* Note not only method of determination of MAC but also significant influence (lowering of MAC for halothane) of nitrous oxide, and impact of premedication (morphine) on decreasing of MAC for halothane. (From Saidman, L. J., and Eger, E. I., II: Effect of nitrous oxide and of narcotic premedication on the alveolar concentration of halothane required for anesthesia, Anesthesiology 25:302, 1964.)

recognize the usefulness of this approach in making comparisons among agents and in determining influence of such factors as temperature and narcotics. We believe, for example, that there can be one level of anesthesia at which there is no response by the patient to the grade of stimulus produced by a skin incision but at which there is a response to a more severe stimulus such as periosteal stripping. Our concept is fortified somewhat by the work of Melzack and Wall,[2] and of De Jong and associates.[3] They found that in the area of the first synaptic transmission of peripheral input (dorsal horn neurons)—the "gate" to further advance of the impulses centrally in the extralemniscal pathways—halothane and nitrous oxide depressed the spontaneous firing of the neurons and also reduced the response to cutaneous stimuli. This change was dependent on dose and time and somewhat selective in that nitrous oxide was more effective in blocking noxious stimuli than innocuous stimuli. In addition, De Jong and associates, and also Freund and coworkers, in taking the position that anesthetic "depth" is a function of the impact of anesthetics on the CNS, demonstrated the almost linear response of monosynaptic pathways to increasing concentrations of anesthetic agent[4,5]

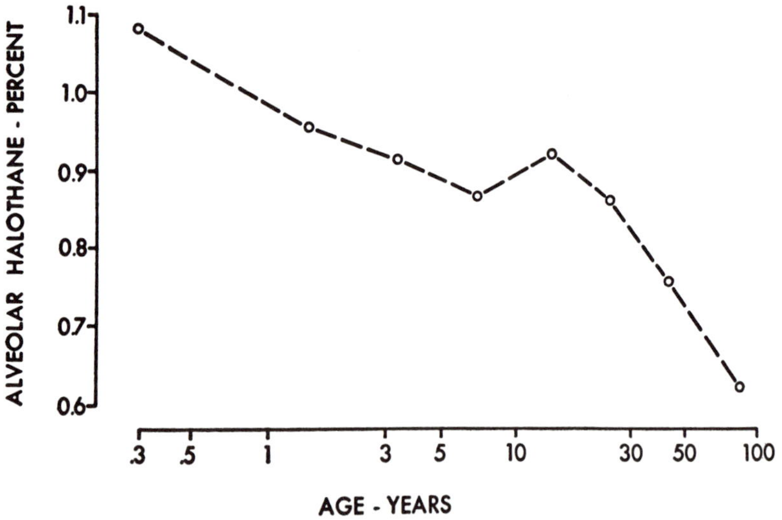

Fig. 7-3.—Relationship of mean alveolar halothane concentration and age. (From Gregory, Eger, E. I., II, and Munson, E. S.: The relationship between age and halothane requirement in man, Anesthesiology 30:488, 1969.)

and also the susceptibility of the H-reflex[5,6] to increasing concentrations of anesthetic agent (Figs. 7-4, 7-5, 7-6). This suggests to us that the state of anesthesia develops on a continuum and that exposure not only to different concentrations of agent but to different agents influences the responses to different types and degrees of stimuli. A satisfactory and adequate state of

Fig. 7-4.—Course of monosynaptic spike height (% of control) during exposure of one animal to several concentrations of halothane. Note rapid response to changes in halothane concentration, as represented by changes in spike height. (From De Jong, R. H., Freund, F. G., Robles, R. and Morikawa, K. I.: Anesthetic potency determined by depression of synaptic transmission, Anesthesiology 29:1139, 1968.)

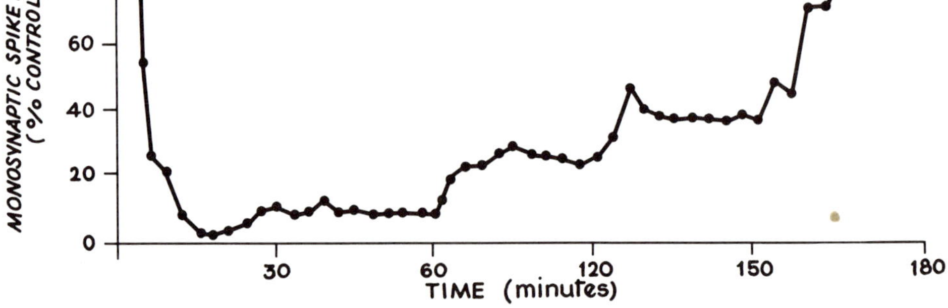

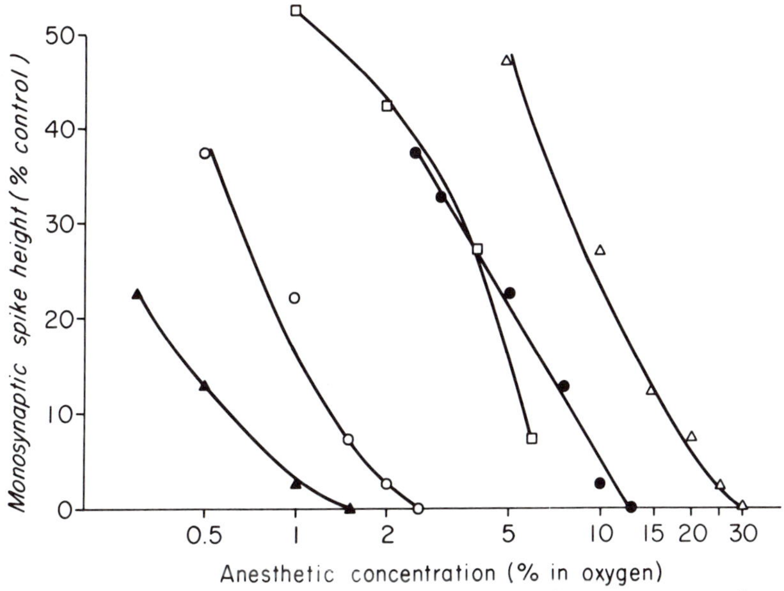

Fig. 7-5.—Mean monosynaptic spike heights plotted against inspired concentrations of different anesthetic agents on semi-log scale. Curves approach linearity but are not all parallel. (Key to symbols: ▲, methoxy-flurane; ○, halothane; ● ether; □ fluroxene; △ cyclopropane.) (From De Jong, R. H., Freund, F. G., Robles, R., and Morikawa, K. I.: Anesthetic potency determined by depression of synaptic transmission, Anesthesiology 29:1139, 1968.)

Fig. 7-6.—Schematic representation of neural arc involved in H-reflex and of M- and H- responses observed in oscilloscope. (From Freund, F. G., Martin, W. E., and Hornbein, T. F.: The H- reflex as a measure of anesthetic potency in man, Anesthesiology 30:642, 1969.)

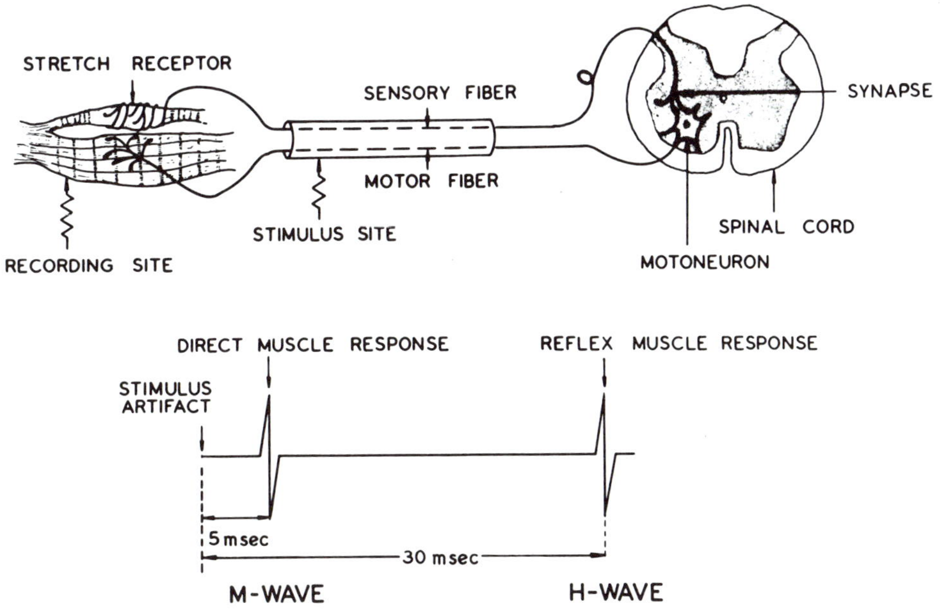

anesthesia exists also when it matches the input of stimuli in quantity and quality.

IMPORTANCE OF DETERMINING DEPTH OF ANESTHESIA

We urge that anesthetists give serious attention to "depth" of anesthesia because we make the assumption that, in any patient, only that level of anesthesia needed to meet the surgical requirements should be established. We hold the basic premise that the less the involvement of the patient's critical organs and systems (i.e., the lower the concentration of the agent, or the less "deep" the anesthesia), the less will be the damage to the patient, whether this be temporary or perhaps permanent. We emphasize, however, that we firmly believe in providing sufficient anesthesia to meet the surgical requirements. We believe that anesthesia that is "light" enough so that responses to surgical stimuli such as hypertension, tachycardia, recollection of stimuli, and increased muscle tension may result in unnecessary harm.

In the interests of both the patient and the convenience of the surgeon, it is useful to train oneself to observe the patient so closely that one can identify the changes in function of body organs and systems that reflect the impact of the different plasma concentrations of anesthetic agent. However useful the MAC concept may be, we are concerned that it has had a tendency to divert the attention of the anesthetist from close observation of the patient to unwise reliance on the presumed output of the gas machine. Dependence upon the MAC concept has led anesthetists to consider that anesthesia is being satisfactorily induced or maintained when the "MAC" (or multiples of it) for any agent in use is being metered from the machine in a high-flow system. Gas machines often do not deliver the concentration indicated by the flowmeters because of factors such as leaks, sticky flowmeters, cooling of the agent, and failure to cut in the valve to the vaporizer. The high-flow system (Chapter 11) is a critical part of the application of the MAC concept because only in such a system, after reasonable tissue equilibration, does alveolar concentration approximate the metered concentration. In low-flow (closed) systems, the concentrations metered by the machine do not approximate the MAC. In order to produce the MAC when the low-flow system is being used, the concentration delivered from the machine to the external circuit (soda lime canister, bag, and tubes) is appreciably higher (or lower) than the desired alveolar concentration, and it is difficult in the practical situation of clinical management of anesthesia to establish any reliable sort of ratio between concentration metered by the machine and the desired alveolar concentration. Consequently, it is essential that the anesthetist, even if he always limits his technic to that of the high-flow system, learn how to assess the various responses of the patient that give clues to the depth of anesthesia. All patients are not the same. In major surgical procedures the condition of most patients is not the same during or at the end as at the beginning. Furthermore, all surgeons are not the same, all surgical requirements are not the same, and all operating conditions are not the same. We submit that, if there are these many variables in an anesthetic situation, the anesthetist must learn to recognize and respond to those subtle as well as obvious changes that take place in the individual patient. Fortunately, many patients have responses that are peculiar to them. For example, some patients move a hand in response to a stimulus, other patients wrinkle an eyebrow, and other patients make more gross efforts such as leg movements; other patients respond by elevation of blood pressure, increase or decrease in pulse rate, perspiration, tearing, and pupillary changes, while still others have characteristic respiratory patterns.

ASSESSMENT OF DEPTH

On the basis of our belief that various levels do exist within the state of anesthesia, we therefore present what we believe to be useful means of assessing the patient's responses to an anesthetic agent. We recognize that these responses are not only peculiar in many respects to the agent used but also to the particular patient. We submit, as we have done repeatedly, that management of anesthesia is a matter of adjusting to the individual patient and to the individual situation. These signs that we shall present must be looked for in each patient. The signs are usually present but not seen by some anesthetists because they have not trained themselves to detect them. Looking for the signs and interpreting them focuses the attention of the anesthetist on the patient rather than on the apparatus. Apparatus is useful in providing information to support the assessment of the patient's responses and also in helping to train the anesthetist to correlate the signs with changes in vital organs and organ systems. For example, blood gas analysis can be useful not only in providing reliable data on the effect of the agent on the respiratory system but also in training the anesthetist to make better clinical judgments on the competency of the respiratory system. A most useful practice is to deliberately vary the anesthetic level in each patient from light to deep and vice versa early in the anesthesia in order to note the signs peculiar to that patient and to the agent used.

Our premise that there are different levels of anesthesia includes, of course, the concept that there is a state of no anesthesia. This lack of anesthesia is manifested by such signs as vocalization, swallowing, emesis, irregular and deep respiration (breath holding), excessive muscular movement, excessive stimulation of sympathetic system (sweating, tachycardia, and hypertension), and response (e.g., movement and pupil dilation) to pain. Pain may be caused by the skin incision, the use of towel clips or the movement of a sore joint. A few patients, especially children, play "possum" and manifest lack of anesthesia only by violent reaction to pain such as an incision. If anesthetists expose patients to the hazards of "crash induction" with thiopental and succinylcholine, lack of anesthesia may not be evident until the acute effect of the thiopental wears off. Persistent paralysis from the succinylcholine may then permit the nonanesthetized patient to show his unfortunate state only by dilation of the pupils or ineffectual efforts at movement.

Light Anesthesia

With progress from a lack of anesthesia to the first level of anesthesia or MAC, the activity described in the previous paragraph disappears. There is a practical need only in assessing light, moderate and deep levels of anesthesia. As the various bodily responses (or signs of anesthesia) are described, one must bear in mind that the purpose of anesthesia is to facilitate surgery and that the level of anesthesia is adjusted to provide optimum conditions for surgery within, of course, the limits of safety for the patient.

The MAC of an agent provides the minimal level or lightest level of agent used. However, there is a remarkable similarity in the basic signs with all agents and with all patients. Assuming a minimal dose of a preanesthetic narcotic and no relaxant, the patient in a light level of anesthesia shows no response to a pain stimulus equivalent to a skin incision, has progressed from irregular respiration to a more regular pattern of substantial tidal volume, and has lost his pharyngeal and laryngeal reflexes. Since, at this level, muscle relaxation from the agent itself is minimal, the signs reflect this and there is a tightness to the abdominal muscles. The recti stand out in tension, and the eyes are either roving or in a lateral position. The patient has lost his wink reflex; loss of this reflex is defined as the absence of active closure of the eyelid. The pupil no longer dilates in response to pain. With the return to this light level of anesthesia from a deeper level, the respiration often loses its "sine wave" pattern, with little or no inspiratory or expiratory pause and equivalent inspiratory and expiratory periods, to a somewhat less regular pattern. This latter pattern is often characterized by a pause at the end of inspiration (a sort of "hitch" in the inspiration), a relatively prolonged and "active" expiration (the patient seems to be actively or forcefully rather than passively expiring), and some unevenness or irregularity. Palpation of the abdomen shows that there is a tightening of the muscles during expiration; during expiration a depression can also be observed lateral to the recti due to contraction of the oblique muscles. If one is using the narcotic-nitrous oxide combination, the rate of respiration is usually faster than at lower levels of anesthesia. Such changes in respiration can be detected even with agents such as halothane and cyclopropane that tend to depress respiration more than fluoroxene.[6] Usually there is no depression of the arterial pressure at this level, even with such agents as halothane. The pulse rate often increases even with agents such as halothane and cyclopropane that ordinarily slow the pulse rate. One also sometimes sees tearing and sometimes perspiration.

Moderate Anesthesia

As anesthesia "deepens," respiration becomes faster and more regular and more shallow. The pattern loses the inspiratory "hitch" and the lengthened expiratory phase and the expiratory pause. With agents such as halothane, the blood pressure tends to be lower and the pulse rate slower. With agents such as ether, cyclopropane, and fluroxene, that tend to release catecholamines, there is minimal depression of the blood pressure and slowing of the pulse rate. Since muscle relaxation begins to be evident, the eyes now tend to be centrally placed and stationary, and abdominal and other muscle relaxation becomes apparent. The recti, which stood out prominently in the lighter levels, become less prominent and the creases along the lateral edge of the recti tend to meld into the flatter abdomen. Furthermore, the active expiratory effort of the recti which one felt in the lighter level, now begins to disappear.

Deep Anesthesia

As anesthesia deepens still further, the changes seen are, with all agents, a function of increasing depression of respiration and circulation. The depression of respiration is manifested by a decrease in tidal volume; usually there is a concurrent increase in rate. Hypotension occurs with all agents except that fluroxene, even at 12%, often does not produce hypotension. The signs of this level of anesthesia also reflect increasing muscle relaxation. Respiration is shallower and usually more rapid except in narcotic-nitrous oxide anesthesia in which it becomes slower but remains deep. With very deep anesthesia, the respirations are jerky or "gasping" in character and irregular in pattern.

There is irregularity of the respiratory pattern in both light and deep anesthesia. The distinguishing feature is the depth of respiration, which is minimal in deeper levels. Occasionally, even the expert can be misled by the appearance of the respiratory pattern. He may misinterpret irregular breathing as a sign of light anesthesia. If there is the slightest doubt as to whether the respiratory pattern, or any other sign, reflects light or deep anesthesia, the wisest and only move is to deliberately decrease the concentration of agent. As anesthesia deepens, in most patients there is a distinguishable change from an active intercostal movement to loss of intercostal contribution to the respiratory effort and an emphasis on diaphragmatic effort. This is manifested by a change from the normal movement of the thoracic cage with lifting of the chest on inspiration to a rocking movement in which there is an "out of phase" depression of the chest wall during inspiration and a flaring of the lower chest margins as the diaphragm exerts its pull in the absence of intercostal tone and activity. The anesthetist must, of course, be aware that a similar chest movement may be simulated by upper respiratory obstruction even without loss of intercostal activity. The pattern is simulated also by paralysis such as with muscle relaxants. The pulse rate often slows and the blood pressure falls. The heart tones become fainter and there is often a shift in emphasis on the first and second sound.[7] If hypercarbia is present from depressed respiration, cardiac irregularities may appear. At moderate levels of anesthesia, especially in the absence of narcotics, hypercarbia may maintain ventilation and, in a sense, obscure progression of depression due to the agent. The obvious terminal level of anesthesia is characterized by an exaggeration of the impact of the concentration of agent on respiratory effort and circulation. Respiration becomes minimal or absent and circulation deteriorates with ultimate disappearance of blood pressure and pulse.

PUPILLARY SIGNS.—We have said little about changes in the pupil because we believe that dilation or constriction of the pupil is limited in usefulness to assessing responses to concentrations of agent; they are influenced by premedicating drugs such as atropine and output of catecholamines by some agents. Usually the pupils dilate in very light anesthesia in response to pain, but they also dilate and become unresponsive to light in catastrophes such as cardiac arrest and have some usefulness in assessing the extent of brain damage.

ELECTROENCEPHALOGRAPHY.—The electroencephalagraph is not a reliable and practical method of assessing depth of anesthesia. With some agents, such as ether and thiopental, reasonably reliable and predictable changes in the brain wave pattern are associated with changes in depth. Such patterns, however, have not been established for many of the other commonly used agents. The EEG is affected by numerous other factors present during anesthesia such as Pa_{CO_2}, Pa_{O_2} and temperature. A further disadvantage is that the apparatus is expensive, bulky and subject to errors induced in the milieu of the operating room and special training is needed to enable one to interpret the wave changes.

RELATIVE VALUE OF RESPIRATION AND CIRCULATION IN ASSESSING DEPTH.—No one sign of anesthesia is infallible. One must observe all possible signs in each patient and then make the best clinical judgment possible as to the depth of anesthesia. Obviously, if there is any doubt, the only step is to decrease the concentration of agent and deliberately lighten the anesthesia until unequivocal signs are present, even to the extent of producing actual movements by the patient. Anesthetists are often hesitant to lighten anesthesia in such instances for fear of inconveniencing the surgeon or embarrassing themselves. We submit that if there is doubt about depth and if no effort is made to firmly establish the level by deliberate lightening to a point of certainty, there is then a possibility of severe depression and death due to unrecognized overdose. We submit also that though the surgeon may be upset by a temporary inconvenience, he is going to be even more upset if the patient dies because the anesthetist was afraid to test the level. We reiterate that it is valuable in the early phases of anesthesia deliberately to deepen and lighten the anesthesia to determine in each patient his peculiar responses to the agent at different concentrations. Generally, these responses in the individual patient are consistent.

Even though one must take into account all the possible clues to depth of anesthesia, there is a tendency to rely more upon one sign or set of signs for the usual assessment of depth. For us, the most useful sign is the respiratory pattern; we urge that each anesthetist learn to detect and interpret these changes. Since the advent of halothane, there has been a strong tendency to use circulatory responses as the common sign of depth. We are willing to accept that an increase in arterial pressure above normal (for an individual patient) and an increase in pulse rate often reflects lightening of anesthesia. We emphasize, however, that too often a return of the patient's blood pressure from a depressed level to his normal level should not always be interpreted as lightness requiring increase in inspired concentration; rather, it may represent simply a return to an acceptable normal level. Moreover, many patients adjust to high concentrations of anesthetic agents and the blood pressure returns toward "normal", even though the level of anesthesia is moderate to deep. We suspect that many anesthetists keep the blood pressure depressed in patients because they misinterpret the return to normal pressure as lightness and also because they do not train themselves to make other observations that could help them in their assessment of the patient's level of anesthesia. Furthermore, we are inclined not to use blood pressure and pulse as primary determinants of depth because the blood pressure is affected by many factors independent of the anesthetic agent; for example, position, hypovolemia, blood loss, "third-space" loss, intestinal manipulation, reflexes such as the carotid sinus and celiac plexus, Pa_{CO_2} and pH. We believe that respiration is a more sensitive indicator of changes in the concentration of an agent and that one can learn to assess changes in advance of those appearing elsewhere in organs and organ systems such as the circulation. We therefore urge that the anesthetist keep his eyes and ears on the patient, noting changes in the pattern of respiration, the depth of respiration and the presence or absence of intercostal movement, etc. In this matter of assessing response of patient to concentration of agent, we know of no substitute for close and constant contact with the patient and training oneself to the subtle but significant changes that take place.

In the case of a patient who has received relaxants, many anesthetists believe that it is not possible to assess the depth of anesthesia other than through observing changes in circulation. We submit that, except in unusual circumstances, it is not necessary to give relaxants in an amount that stops all respiratory activity to provide adequate working conditions for the surgeon. Assuming this is so, one then can still make reliable and useful observations about depth with the minimal respiratory effort present during relaxation. Although the depth of respiration does give some clue as to the level of anesthesia, one can make an assessment of the degree of depression of the respiratory centers and get a useful idea of anesthesia depth. A crude but practical method of determining anesthetic depth in the presence of controlled or artificial respiration (with or without relaxants) was developed years ago by Ralph Knight of the University of Minnesota. This method consists of stopping controlled or artificial respiration for 30 seconds and observing whether or not the patient makes a respiratory effort within that time. If the respiratory effort is made late in this period, anesthesia is probably at a satisfactory level. If no effort is made, the anesthesia is probably deeper than needed. If the effort is made early in the period, anesthesia probably is very light. Of course, this method of assessment depends not only upon absence of excessive relaxant but also on the degree of hyperventilation. If the Pa_{CO_2} is below that needed for initiating respiration, there will be a delay in response due to this factor rather than to the concentration of agent; blood gas analysis readily provides information that one can take into account. It is essential in using this method of assessment of depth to recognize that one is interested *only* in determining whether the respiratory centers are capable of initiating a respiratory effort; one is not interested in the amount of air moved but only in whether an effort is made to move air.

Thus, one looks only for a flicker of diaphragmatic movement in the presence of relaxant and not for a deep breath. The amount of air moved is a function of the amount of relaxant; the time at which a respiratory effort is made is a reflection of anesthetic depth as measured by depression of the respiratory centers.

In patients who are breathing spontaneously, another practical clue to depth of anesthesia is provided by manually overventilating the lungs of the patient for four or five breaths. If the patient resumes spontaneous respiration immediately, anesthesia is light; if resumption of spontaneous breathing is delayed, anesthesia may be moderate to deep.

Still another clue to depth of anesthesia in circumstances of controlled or artificial respiration comes from the observation of the tidal volume at a constant applied airway pressure. If the tidal volume decreases consistently, the change usually reflects a decrease in effectiveness of relaxant when used. If, however, the tidal volume changes erratically, this usually means a lightness of anesthesia. The change in tidal volume occurs because the patient is making respiratory efforts, some of which coincide with the inspiratory phase of the ventilator and some of which are out of phase.

ANALGESIA

The stage of analgesia appears prior to the development of anesthesia. It is a useful stage in which various minor and brief surgical procedures can be done; with practice, extended surgery can be done in very ill patients. Analgesia is characterized by relief of pain; yet, at the same time, the patient retains the ability to communicate and cooperate with surgeon and anesthetist. He retains also his protective pharyngeal and laryngeal reflexes and sufficient tone in the jaw muscles and tongue to maintain his airway. Patients are in the analgesic stage when they begin to respond somewhat thickly, complain of dizziness or lightheadedness and are slow in communicating. Constant contact with the patient is mandatory not only to ascertain the level of analgesia but also to maintain it. If the patient progresses into anesthesia, there will be loss of contact and some of the signs outlined for lack of anesthesia or very light anesthesia. If the patient comes out of the analgesia, response to pain is, or course, the prominent sign. Repetitive and minor changes in concentration of agent are needed. Agents with low solubility are more useful in achieving and maintaining the optimal concentration because changes can be effected more easily. Constant high-flow systems are useful also for the same reason. Attempts at producing intermittent analgesia, especially with agents of high solubility, by application of inhalers (such as proposed for urologic and obstetrical procedures) are often unsatisfactory because the optimum alveolar concentrations are difficult to achieve and maintain. The inhalers for self-administration of analgesia are hazardous because some patients progress into anesthesia with the concentrations delivered and may suffer from upper airway obstruction, emesis, and circulatory depression.

SUMMARY

We believe that it is important to be able to make judgments of anesthetic depth for reasons we have mentioned. We emphasize again that making these assessments makes it mandatory for the anesthetist to keep in close contact with the patient and we believe that to be a vital element in proper management of anesthesia. We believe also that it is helpful to be alert to the level of anesthesia not only to prevent the unfortunate results of anesthesia that is too deep but also to anticipate lightening anesthesia. If the anesthetist can detect lightening of anesthesia, he not only can prevent inconvenience to the surgeon and embarrassment to himself but he can save the patient from receiving unnecessarily high concentrations of the drug. Once the patient is light enough to respond to stimuli and move, higher concentrations and larger total amounts of anesthetic are required to restore satisfactory anesthesia. This is because, in light anesthesia, the circulation is speeded and this requires a higher input of agent to achieve necessary arterial and tissue concentrations. Redistribution of agent is also increased to nonessential areas of the body such as muscle tissue and fat, thereby lowering the concentration in the critical areas such as the brain.

Finally, by becoming adept in assessing levels of anesthesia, the anesthetist can avoid that nefarious practice of using relaxants to keep patients on the table while he frantically tries to catch up on the level of anesthesia.

REFERENCES

1. Eger, E. I., II, Saidman, L. J., and Brandstater, B.: Minimum alveolar anesthetic concentration: a standard of anesthetic potency, Anesthesiology 26:756, 1965.
2. Melzack, R., and Wall, P. D.: Pain mechanisms: a new theory, Science 150:971, 1965.
3. De Jong, R. H., Robles, R., and Morikawa, K. I.: Actions of halothane and nitrous oxide on dorsal horn neurons ("the spinal gate"), Anesthesiology 31:205, 1969.
4. De Jong, R. H., Freund, F. G., Robles, R., and Morikawa, K. I.: Anesthetic potency determined by depression of synaptic transmission, Anesthesiology 29:1139, 1968.
5. Freund, F. G., Martin, W. E., and Hornbein, T. F.: The H-reflex as a measure of anesthetic potency in man, Anesthesiology 30:642, 1969.
6. Munson, E. S., Larson, C. P., Jr., Babad, A. A., Regan, M. J., Buechel, D. R., and Eger, E. I., II: The effects of halothane, fluroxene and cyclopropane on ventilation: a comparative study in man, Anesthesiology 27:716, 1966.
7. Rence, W. G., Cullen, S. C., and Hamilton, W. K.: Observations on the heart sounds during anesthesia with cyclopropane or ether, Anesthesiology 17:26, 1956.

CHAPTER EIGHT

Position of the Patient

THE ANESTHETIST'S OBLIGATION in the matter of position of the patient, especially during the surgical procedure, is to help to ensure, if possible, that the position is compatible with the surgeon's needs and with the patient's needs for adequate ventilation and circulation and the absence of temporary or permanent neurologic deficit. Hopefully, with suitable communication, the needs of the patient can be the determinant factor and counter the exaggerated positions sometimes favored by surgeons for their personal convenience. If it is clearly established that a particular position is needed in the best interests of the patient as far as the successful completion of the operation is concerned, the anesthetist is obligated to make appropriate adjustments in anesthetic management to ensure proper ventilation and circulation and to help to avoid pressure points and positions that may induce neurologic deficits.

All who work in the operating room, including the anesthetist, must be alert to establishing and maintaining safety for the patient in the usual recumbent, prone or lateral positions. This means attending to such considerations as avoiding pressure on the elbows (which may lead to ulnar paralysis) and pressure or stretching of the brachial plexus, ensuring appropriate support of the chest and abdomen in prone position to facilitate ventilation and ascertaining that there is no unnecessary extension of neck, that the eyelids are closed and that no pressure is applied to the eyeballs. Placing a pillow under the knees of the patient in the supine position can facilitate abdominal wall relaxation; this not only enhances relaxation of the abdomen but also diminishes the likelihood of backache due to abnormal extension. Backache in patients after use of the supine position under spinal anesthesia or continued profound relaxation from relaxants can be minimized by placing a small pillow under the lumbar area during anesthesia. Backache is not uncommon in patients who have been placed in the full lithotomy position.

The anesthetist must be aware of the problems associated with the head-up or sitting position. Hypotension may be aggravated in this position and ventilation may be compromised, especially if the patient is flexed. If the surgical procedure involves the possibility of open veins, as in posterior approaches to the brain, air embolism must be anticipated.

The head-down or Trendelenburg position, especially in obese patients and usually in patients in whom the intestines are retracted with packs for pelvic surgery, often seriously impairs ventilation. One should be aware also that in the treatment of hypotension, one need only induce a head-down position of 5 to 10°; a greater degree does little to enhance venous return and does exaggerate the venous stagnation in the head. Elevating the legs is as effective in improving venous return as is the head-down position and less likely to impair ventilation.

Finally, one should always keep in mind the unfavorable impact of abrupt changes in position, especially in the deeply anesthetized patient or the patient under conduction anesthesia such as epidural or spinal. Such changes can produce severe changes in the competency of the circulation. Even such simple maneuvers as the abrupt lowering of the legs from a lithotomy position to the supine position can provoke severe hypotension in the patient whose circulation is of borderline competence. Wrapping of the legs with Ace bandages helps substantially to diminish stagnation of blood and lymph and perhaps helps to prevent development of thrombosis when the patient is in the sitting or head-up position.

CHAPTER NINE

The Recovery Period

THE RECOVERY PERIOD is one of the more critical and dangerous periods in the course of anesthetic management. Part of the danger is due to a natural tendency to relax and permit one's attention to flag and possibly be diverted from the patient following anesthesia and operation. There is a tendency to assume that once the operation and the acute process of anesthetic management are over, "anesthesia" for the patient is finished. This attitude is often evident in the common practice of diminishing one's attention to airway management after a mask or an endotracheal catheter has been removed. The erroneous assumption must be that, although the airway must be maintained for the active part of the anesthetic process, the patient is no longer anesthetized the moment the mask comes off the face or the endotracheal catheter is removed and can, therefore, take care of his own airway.

CHANGES IN PATIENTS REQUIRING CLOSE ATTENTION

Many patients suffer severe hypoxia, severe hypercarbia, and profound circulatory depression in the moments when dressings are being applied, anesthetic equipment is being disposed of, or the patient is being transferred to his room or recovery area and left in the care of others. This is the time when the patient is being shifted from a period of second-to-second observation to a period when observation is less intense and often by persons unfamiliar with recent changes in the patient and not able therefore to recognize or assess and treat further changes in the patient's condition. This is also the time, unfortunately, when the patient is in the process of returning to but is not yet at a state in which he can mobilize his protective reflexes and verbalize his problems. It is that period, then, during which there can be no diminution of attention by the anesthetist. It is also a period in which the anesthetist must assure himself that either the patient is in a state in which he can protect himself by means of intact reflexes or by communication or is in the care of someone competent to assess critical changes and take steps to correct problems. It is incumbent upon the anesthetist to inform those persons who are to continue observing and looking after the patient about past events, the current condition of the patient, and anticipated changes. If such persons are not sufficiently competent to properly care for the patient in whatever critical condition he may be, the anesthetist is obligated either to secure adequately trained personnel or remain with the patient.

The essential element of proper attention to the patient in the recovery phase of anesthesia is the recognition of the impact on the patient of a relatively abrupt change from a state of anesthesia to a state in which the patient is required to return to a state of self-care. There is an associated abrupt change often in inspired oxygen concentrations and in the Pa_{O_2}. It is therefore often wise to administer extra oxygen by whatever apparatus is convenient and effective under the circumstances. Usually, if the patient has been extubated, sufficient oxygenation can be maintained by use of a simple face mask or nasal prongs. If the patient remains intubated, it is convenient to attach a T-piece system (with humidification) to the endotracheal tube. It is necessary to verify the need for oxygenation or ventilation, or both, by arterial gas analysis. Added oxygen can mask hypoventilation and permit the development of profound hypercarbia and atelectasis.

There is often a change in the manner in which the airway is maintained; this is sometimes complicated by an impingement of the surgical procedure on the airway. Often it is advisable, if the patient is unresponsive and surgical manipulations or dressings impinge on the airway, to leave the endotracheal tube in place. If this is done, we recommend using a nasotracheal tube (except in infants) because it is more stable in position, avoids obstruction of the tube by the patient's clamping down on it during the awakening process and facilitates aspiration of secretions.

There is an abrupt change from care by the anesthetist of secretions, blood, vomitus and other substances in the airway to care by the patient of this material. Likewise, there is often an abrupt change in circulatory support by therapy such as the use of intravenous fluids and vasoactive agents. Also, an abrupt change in position often has a significant impact upon airway, ventilation and circulation.

All of these changes, especially in respiration and circulation, require that, frequently, repetitive measurement of vital signs be taken and recorded. Circulatory function can be assessed by simple methods such as use of the ordinary blood pressure cuff and stethoscope, but often measurement by transducer and oscilloscope is indicated, as well as ECG observations and blood-gas analysis.

With the discontinuance of anesthesia, especially with agents of low solubility, there is often an abrupt loss of analgesia and the patient begins to suffer pain. The reaction to pain is often manifested by excitement during the time when the patient is not yet oriented. Moreover, with the routine use of agents that are promptly eliminated, pain often returns while the patient is in the immediate recovery phase. Analgesic drugs, usually narcotics, are often necessary; however, they must be used cautiously to avoid depression of respiration and circulation in the patient who is still under the influence of anesthetic agents and of the effects of the operation. Cautiously, in this circumstance means, for example, the administration of only 2 to 3 mg of morphine (or equivalent doses of other narcotics). The intravenous route is also preferred to ensure prompt relief and immediate assessment of the effect of the narcotic. Patients who have received ketamine may respond in recovery to hallucinatory images. This reaction can be diminished by enforcing quiet in the area and by the administration of a barbiturate, diazepam or a similar sedative.

Since the introduction of recovery areas some years ago, there has been a tendency on the part of many anesthetists to pay less attention to bringing the patient to a state of orientation and stability with active protective reflexes while the patient is still in the operating room. Many anesthetists, because they have not trained themselves how to do it, are incapable of timing the discontinuance of an anesthetic in the operating room so that the patient either is responsive or has active protective reflexes. This inability of the anesthetist has been encouraged sometimes by surgeons who do not like the patient to be responsive during dressing applications or while in the operating room. Even if optimal facilities are available in the recovery area, we believe that it is in the best interests of the patient that the anesthetist should apply his knowledge of agents and technics and his familiarity with the surgical procedure, the surgeon, and the responses of the particular patient during anesthesia and surgery so that the patient can be brought to responsiveness in the operating room. Failing this ideal situation, the patient should, at least, be brought to a stage at which his protective reflexes are active and he is in as stable a physical state as possible. By so doing, one can significantly diminish the chances for acute and serious problems in the recovery area.

THE RECOVERY ROOM

The obvious demands of maintaining an operating schedule, the changes in patients brought about by major surgery and the recognition that recovery is a critical period for the patient have brought about the development of recovery rooms. It is not within the province of this book to elaborate upon the construction or maintenance of a recovery unit, but certain basic elements that ensure proper use of the recovery room in the interests of the patient are mentioned. The recovery unit should be located geographically close to the operating room area. This not only minimizes the time needed to transport patients in a critical period of recovery from anesthesia but also enhances the availability of anesthetist and surgeon. The unit should be a large open room with a central nurses' station. This facilitates observation of all patients and enhances mobility of patients and personnel. Movable curtains can isolate patients when needed but otherwise freedom of movement is mandatory. A convenient rule of thumb for the average surgical load is 1½ spaces in the recovery room for each operating room. Specially designed recovery carts should be used that permit easy access to the patient, tilting, and restraint where indicated. Fundamental equipment, such as suction, oxygen, blood pressure manometers and various oscillographs for ECG and arterial pressure measurement can be placed peripherally along the walls.

Basic Equipment for a Recovery Room

1. Equipment for assessment and treatment of respiratory inadequacy. Examples of such equipment are Ambu Bags, respirometers, face masks with

breathing tube extensions (for augmenting ventilation periodically), nasopharyngeal airways, oral airways, endotracheal tubes and laryngoscopes, respirators, apparatus for administering excess oxygen and access to blood-gas analysis facilities.

2. Equipment for assessment and treatment of heart and circulatory inadequacy. Examples of necessary equipment are ordinary arm cuffs and manometers for blood pressure measurement, transducers and oscillographs for direct arterial pressure measurement, drugs for raising (and lowering) the blood pressure, cardiotonic drugs, ECG apparatus, appropriate fluids and needles or catheters for fluid or blood replacement and a defibrillator.

3. Adequate suction apparatus.

4. Miscellaneous equipment for assessment and management of kidney function, such as measuring containers for urine output.

5. Temperature-measuring devices.

6. Carts (trolleys or gurneys) that facilitate access to patient, are stable, and permit tilting of the head up or down.

Overhead trolleys can be used conveniently for placement of IV bottles. Preferably access from the operating room area should be separate from the exit to private room or ward.

Personnel and Management

Obviously, personnel should be specially trained for work in the recovery room; this should include training for and participation in such special tasks as starting intravenous fluids, taking care of acute cardiac emergencies (fibrillation, etc.) and administering emergency drugs. We make no special plea for administrative responsibility except to say that anesthetists are usually more available around the clock than are surgeons, are usually better prepared to cope with acute processes that take place in the recovery room and are, of course, responsible for changes due to the anesthetic. Some person must be responsible for the training of personnel, for development of and alterations in the space and equipment, for discharge of patients from the recovery area and for adjudication of jurisdictional problems. If it is assumed that the recovery room is functioning primarily (and excepting emergencies) as a recovery area and not as an Intensive Care Unit (ICU), patients are discharged when the person in charge (usually the anesthetist) determines from observation of the patient and also judgment based upon objective data (as obtained, for example, through blood-gas analysis) that the patient is able to be properly cared for by personnel in the next area he can be transferred to. Obviously, therefore, it is necessary to know or to determine (or both) whether a patient should be transferred to the ICU, to a special area on the appropriate ward, to a single room with a special nurse, or to a single room or ward with only the ward type of nursing care available. It is often convenient and economical to locate the ICU adjacent to the recovery room. We do not believe that one space should function for both; we believe there should be a definite separation in function as well as in specific space.

CHAPTER TEN

Records

RECORDS are an indispensable part of the management of anesthesia. They are important primarily from the standpoint of graphically representing the patient's responses so that those responses can be analyzed and appropriate action anticipated or taken. Trends, which are better seen graphically, often are important in making the diagnosis of a problem and determining a course of action. For example, the abrupt onset of hypotension usually indicates a situation that differs from one associated with a gradual decline, and an increase or decrease in the trend in pulse rate gives an important clue to what is happening and what should be done. Records are important also with respect to the drugs used, the concentrations of anesthetic agent administered and the fluids given, not only in representing what is happening to the patient and what his needs are at the moment but also in predicting what his future needs may be. Thus, a record of the patient's needs for narcotic in a nitrous oxide-narcotic combination is a useful clue to the tolerance of the patient to such drugs and what doses of what drug might be indicated after operation. Records of these items are important also in establishing the relationship of factors such as the drugs and fluids given, operative events, and position changes to alterations occurring in the patient.

Records are important also in providing data for subsequent review and analysis so that agents, technics, fluid management, operative events, for example, may be assessed in the light of all the variables present and determinations made as to their effectiveness, hazards, and disadvantages.

The prevalence of litigation obviously makes records essential. This situation emphasizes that the complete record includes not only the record during anesthesia but notes of the preanesthetic visit to the patient, notes on the state of the patient in the recovery room, and appropriate notes on the patient's state on the days subsequent to anesthesia. Since courts accept only the written record and since the written record is the only reliable record of what transpired, the record must be legible, include all the pertinent material, be properly dated and timed and be appropriately signed.

Samples of anesthesia and recovery room records are illustrated in Figures 10-1 and 10-2. These are presented simply as samples, although years of use have established them as being practical and adequate. Necessary coding can be added to facilitate machine collection, sorting, and analysis of data. Those in private practice can, of course, add spaces to facilitate rec-

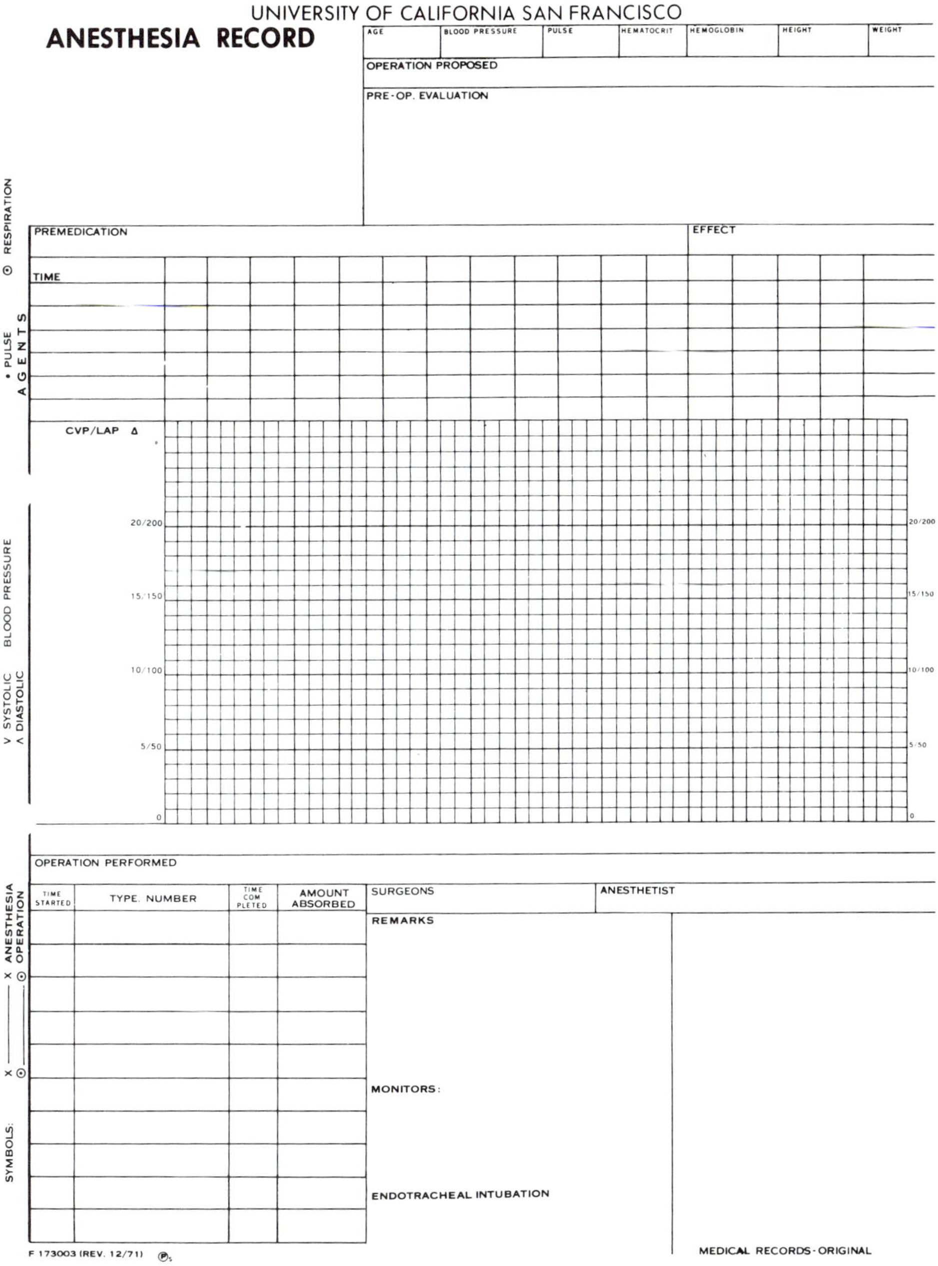

UNIVERSITY OF CALIFORNIA SAN FRANCISCO

ANESTHESIA RECORD

AGE	BLOOD PRESSURE	PULSE	HEMATOCRIT	HEMOGLOBIN	HEIGHT	WEIGHT

OPERATION PROPOSED

PRE-OP. EVALUATION

PREMEDICATION

EFFECT

TIME

⊙ RESPIRATION

• PULSE

AGENTS

CVP/LAP Δ

20/200

15/150

10/100

5/50

0

V SYSTOLIC

Λ DIASTOLIC

BLOOD PRESSURE

OPERATION PERFORMED

TIME STARTED	TYPE. NUMBER	TIME COMPLETED	AMOUNT ABSORBED

SURGEONS

ANESTHETIST

REMARKS

MONITORS:

ENDOTRACHEAL INTUBATION

SYMBOLS: X —— X ANESTHESIA ⊙ —— ⊙ OPERATION

F 173003 (REV. 12/71)

MEDICAL RECORDS-ORIGINAL

Fig. 10-1.—Sample anesthesia record.

ording data pertinent to considerations such as insurance, charges and payments. In general, we prefer as simple a record as is compatible with the keeping of pertinent data. Records can be so designed to make it possible to record all sorts of minutiae; there is, however, serious question about the value of this extent of record keeping in securing good patient care, and

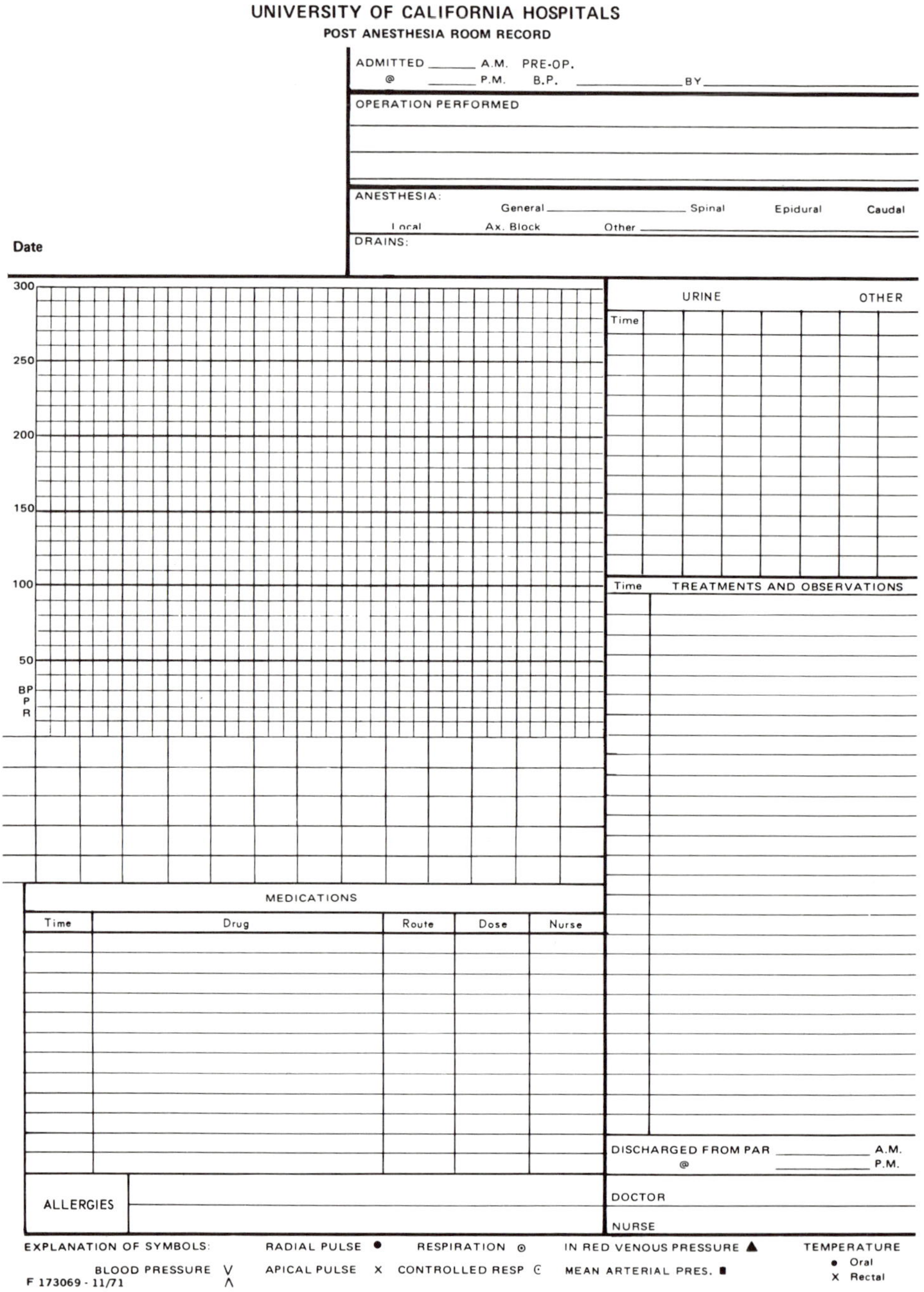
UNIVERSITY OF CALIFORNIA HOSPITALS
POST ANESTHESIA ROOM RECORD

ADMITTED ______ A.M. PRE-OP.
@ ______ P.M. B.P. ______ BY ______

OPERATION PERFORMED

ANESTHESIA: General ______ Spinal Epidural Caudal
Local Ax. Block Other ______

DRAINS:

Date

300 250 200 150 100 50 BP P R

URINE OTHER
Time

Time TREATMENTS AND OBSERVATIONS

MEDICATIONS

Time	Drug	Route	Dose	Nurse

ALLERGIES

DISCHARGED FROM PAR ______ A.M.
@ ______ P.M.

DOCTOR

NURSE

EXPLANATION OF SYMBOLS: RADIAL PULSE ● RESPIRATION ⊙ IN RED VENOUS PRESSURE ▲ TEMPERATURE
BLOOD PRESSURE V Λ APICAL PULSE X CONTROLLED RESP Ͼ MEAN ARTERIAL PRES. ■ ● Oral X Rectal

F 173069 - 11/71

Fig. 10-2.—Sample postanesthesia (recovery room) record. *(Continued.)*

there is an inverse relationship between the amount of data to be recorded and the validity of the data.

We do make a plea for keeping the record current. All too often the record is made up 15 to 30 minutes after the anesthesia has been started and

Patient Name ______________________ Unit Number ______________________

Time	No.	SOLUTION	ml GIVEN	ml in BOTTLE	TOTAL ml

Time	TREATMENTS AND OBSERVATIONS (continued)

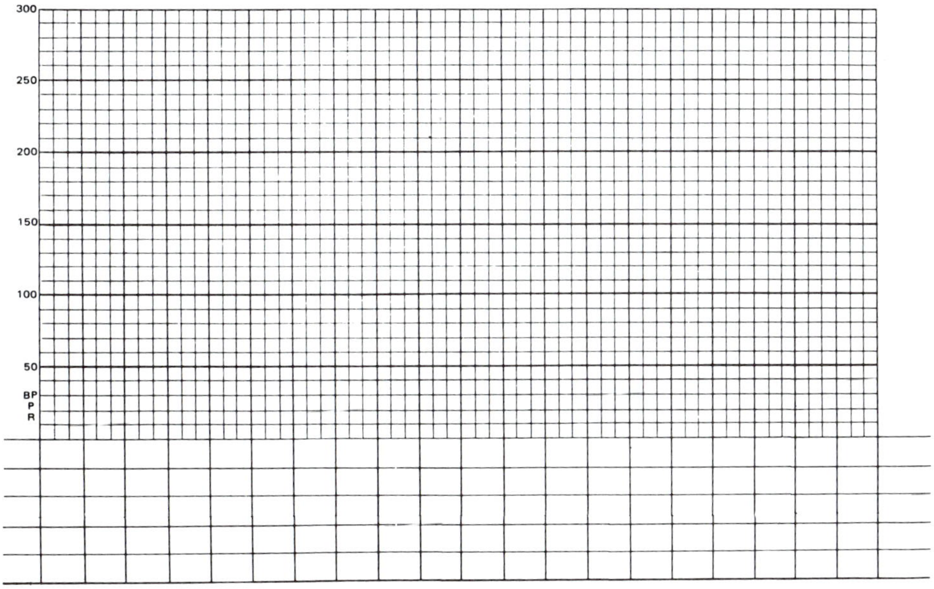

Fig. 10-2 (cont.).—Back of sample of postanesthesia (recovery room) record form.

maintained. The excuse is that the attention of the anesthetist in this critical period should be directed to the patient and not to the record. It is difficult to quarrel with this point of view, but we have serious doubts about the accuracy of the record made *ex post facto*. One's memory during the acute stress of induction and the business of starting intravenous infusions, changing the patient's position, ensuring adequate anesthesia for beginning of the operation, establishing the equipment in the proper situation, among other procedures, is often faulty, especially in regard to the relationship of what was done, what drugs were given and the responses of the patient. We submit that it is entirely possible, except in unusual circumstances, to learn to keep a current record. If the record is to have any meaning and to accurately reflect what happened, it must be a current one and not reconstructed several minutes later. Keeping such a record often encourages or forces the anesthetist to make observations that he might not make otherwise, and this can provide useful information about the responses of the patient. Keeping the record current often emphasizes the amount of drug given, the rate at which concentrations of agent were increased (or decreased), the time during which the drugs were given, the rate and degree of response of the patient and so on. One often finds that one's sense of time is distorted, and recording helps to keep the timing more accurate. Most anesthesia machines have adequate space for a record during induction—unless one uses up the space unnecessarily with an elaborate and space-consuming array of equipment such as syringes, drugs, laryngoscope and endotracheal catheters.

PART 3

Technical Aspects

CHAPTER ELEVEN

The Anesthetic Machine

ETHER, CHLOROFORM AND NITROUS OXIDE were the first anesthetic agents given by inhalation. At room temperature ether and chloroform are liquids with a high vapor pressure. These properties, combined with their potency, permitted their use as anesthetics with simple equipment. A piece of cloth can be impregnated with liquid ether or chloroform and held close to the patient's nose and mouth. Their vapors, though diluted by room air, are potent enough to produce anesthesia without serious diminution of the tension of inspired oxygen (O_2).

Nitrous oxide (N_2O), however, is a gas at room temperature and has such low potency that high concentrations must be inhaled to produce effective anesthesia. The first anesthetic machines were designed and used to store and administer N_2O. Early models that limited dilution of N_2O by air progressed to those that provided total exclusion of air and provided for addition of O_2. These latter machines permitted use of higher N_2O concentrations and the maintenance of an O_2 tension compatible with life.

Modern anesthetic machines are designed to provide controllable flows of gases and vapors of volatile liquids which are accurately measured in volumes per unit of time into systems that deliver the mixture to the patient. There are two distinct components of an anesthetic machine: the part concerned with preparation of the gas mixture and the system concerned with delivery of the mixture to the patient.

PREPARATION OF THE GAS MIXTURE

Packaging and Delivery of Gases

Oxygen, carbon dioxide and the anesthetic gases nitrous oxide, cyclopropane and ethylene are stored in cylinders. The high pressures of the compressed gases (as high as 2000 lbs per square inch (p.s.i.)) and the explosive properties of some of the gases (cyclopropane and ethylene) make use of these agents potentially hazardous. Through the cooperation of the Interstate Commerce Commission, fire underwriters and national anesthesia and hospital associations, safety standards for the storage and handling of cylinders of compressed gases have been formulated.

All cylinders of gases used on anesthetic machines are "pin indexed" to prevent interchange of cylinders in the yokes on gas machines that hold the cylinders. Two metal pins on the yoke fit into two corresponding holes in the valve casing on the tank. The positions of the pins and holes are specific for each gas. Other safety standards include provision for the elimination of contaminants and color coding of cylinders.

Many hospitals pipe O_2 from a central source throughout the building. Nitrous oxide also is often piped to operating rooms from a central supply of large cylinders. Pressure tubing is used to connect wall outlets to the anesthetic machines. The coupling systems at wall outlets and machines are designed to prevent accidental interchange of N_2O and O_2. If the anesthetic machine uses gas delivered from cylinders, it is necessary to include in the system between the cylinder and the metering device a reducing valve, so that the gas pressure in the cylinder can be reduced to a constant value. If the gases are delivered from a central piping system, the reducing valve usually is located at the central source and the line pressure is kept at approximately 50 p.s.i.

Anesthetic machines have pressure gauges to determine the gas pressure in the cylinders. The pressure does not reflect the volume available; the latter depends on the critical and the ambient temperature of the gas. The critical temperature is that temperature above which a gas cannot be liquefied by pressure. The ambient (room) temperature in the operating rooms is above the critical temperature of O_2. Therefore, the gas in an O_2 cylinder is not liquefied by the pressure in the cylinder and the volume available is directly proportional to the pressure. When the pressure gauge registers 900 p.s.i., half as much gas is available as was available at 1800 p.s.i. The precise volume depends on the size of the cylinder, for example, 165 gallons of O_2 in an *E* cylinder at 1800 p.s.i.

At room temperature N_2O, cyclopropane, and CO_2 are below their critical temperature. Freshly filled cylinders of these gases contain liquid N_2O, cyclopropane and CO_2. The cylinder pressure does not reflect the volume of gas available. As gas is withdrawn from the cylinder it is replaced by an equal volume vaporized from the liquid without change in pressure until all the liquid is exhausted. Only at that stage does the cylinder contain compressed gas whose pressure is directly proportional to the amount of gas in the cylinder. This amount is small in the case of cyclopropane, which liquefies at 75 p.s.i. (approximately 5 atmospheres). For example, when all the liquid in a cyclopropane cylinder is vaporized the gas content is only 5 times the volume capacity of the cylinder. Obviously, greater volumes of the gases that liquefy at room temperature can be stored in cylinders; for example, 420 gallons of N_2O can be stored in an *E* cylinder at 750 p.s.i. as opposed to 165 gallons of O_2 in an *E* cylinder at 1800 p.s.i.

Anesthetic machines have check valves that prevent retrograde flow from the machine to cylinders or to the central piping system. This avoids transfilling of tanks, the exposure of connecting hoses to the high pressure of gas cylinders and the leakage of gases through inlet ports that are not connected to cylinders or gas hoses.

Valves delivering gas to metering devices function in the same manner as water faucets, allowing greater flows as the size of an aperture is increased. The flow at any setting remains constant as long as the drop in gas pressure across the aperture remains constant.

The flow of gases is measured by flowmeters. Many types have been used, but most modern machines use rotameters. The measuring unit includes a vertical glass tube through which the gas flow is directed upward. The bore of the tube is tapered so that the cross-sectional area increases from entry to delivery. A "float" or "bobbin" rotates and is held suspended in the tube by the gas flow. Its point of suspension is constant for any particular flow rate. The scale is calibrated by the manufacturer with known flows of the same gas that the flowmeter is to measure. The components are not interchangeable with other sets and are accurate for only a gas with a density and frictional characteristics that are the same as those of the gas with which it was calibrated.

A manifold gathers the various gases that have passed through their appropriate flowmeters. To ensure against accidental decrease in O_2 concentration, O_2 must be the last gas added in the manifold. Leakages in apparatus proximal to the point of O_2 inflow then cannot diminish the O_2 content and leakages distal to that point result in loss of volume without qualitative change in the mixture.

From the manifold, the gas mixture (the total flow rate and composition of which is known) is delivered to an outlet port. For emergency purposes, provision is made for delivery to the outlet port of a large volume of O_2 through an O_2 "flush" valve that bypasses the flowmeters and manifold.

Vaporizers

The modern anesthetic machine is not complete without a means for administering vapors of the volatile liquid anesthetics in accurate and controllable flows. The rate of vaporization depends on a liquid's vapor pressure, which in turn is a function of its temperature. As a result, constant temperature is a requisite for constant rate of vaporization and predictable output from a vaporizer. Vaporization of a liquid requires energy in the form of heat; this is the latent heat of vaporization. Unless otherwise provided, this heat is obtained from the liquid itself, and thus its temperature is lowered. Consequently, anesthetic vaporizers are made of materials such as copper, which conduct heat from the room air to liquid to offset heat loss during vaporization.

The output of vaporizers is controlled by passing known volumes of O_2 in fine bubbles through the liquid. The surface area of the gas-liquid interface increases as the bubble size diminishes. The increased interface accelerates the equilibrium of gas tensions or, in other words, the saturation of gas with vapor of the liquid. When saturated, the gas mixture emerging from the vaporizer consists of O_2 and vapor of the volatile liquid in a proportion dictated by the vapor pressure of the liquid. For example, at room temperature (20° C) the vapor pressure of halothane is 240 mm Hg. If the total gas pressure of the mixture is 760 mm Hg (ambient atmosphere pressure), the O_2 exerts a pressure of 520 mm Hg and the halothane 240 mm Hg. In this

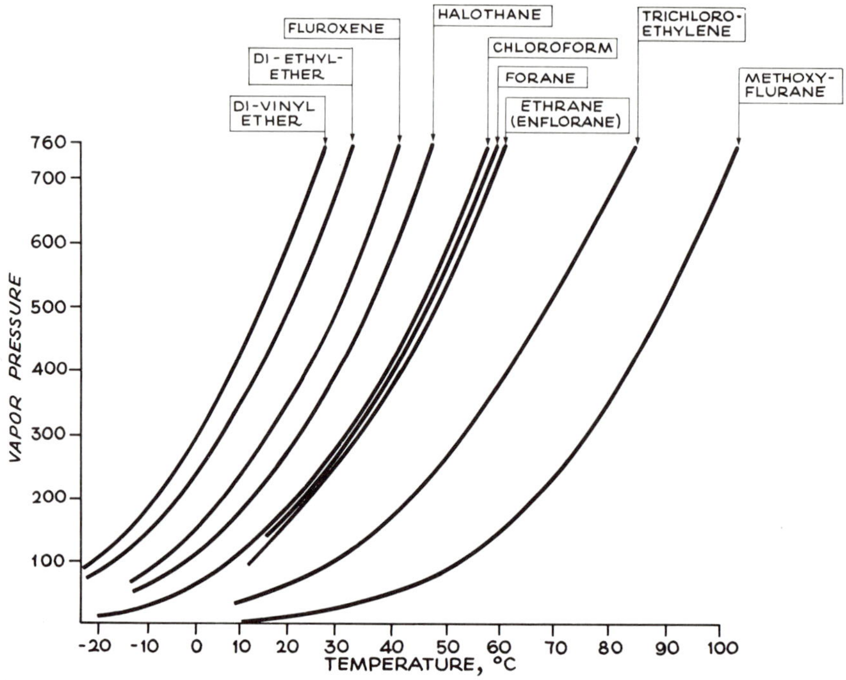

Fig. 11-1.—Vapor pressure curves for inhalation anesthestic agents at different temperatures.

mixture, therefore, there are 520 molecules of oxygen for every 240 molecules of halothane, or approximately a proportion of 2:1. Consequently, 100 cc of O_2 passed through a halothane vaporizer acquire 50 cc of halothane vapor, and 100 cc of O_2 passed through an ether vaporizer acquire approximately 140 cc of ether (vapor pressure, 480 mm Hg) to emerge as 240 cc of O_2-ether mixture.

Graphs depicting the vapor pressure of the various anesthetic liquids are available (Fig. 11-1). By knowing the vapor pressure, the flow rate of O_2 through the vaporizer, and the total flow rate delivered from the outlet port of the gas machine to the delivery system of the machine (to be outlined later), one can calculate the percentage of anesthetic vapor in the mixture delivered from the outlet port. For example, if one delivers a total flow of 5 liters (3 liters N_2O and 2 liters O_2), 100 ml of O_2 through the vaporizer will pick up 50 ml of halothane. The 50 ml of halothane carried in 5000 ml results in a 1% halothane mixture. If 100 ml of O_2 picks up 140 ml of ether, the 140 ml of ether in a 5000 ml total flow results in a 3% mixture. If the total flow is decreased, the percentage of anesthetic is increased, provided the flow through the vaporizer is the same. Conversely, if the total flow is increased the percentage is decreased. It is evident that efficient vaporizers at known and constant temperatures can deliver controllable flows of the vapor of a volatile liquid. However, one must be quite aware that many factors may influence the output of the vaporizer and change the resultant presumed percentage concentration of anesthetic vapor. For example, there may be a leak in the vaporizer such that the vapor is vented into the operating room rather than to the outlet port; also, if the amount of liquid in the vaporizer is low, there may be insufficient opportunity for saturation of the O_2. With high flows through the vaporizer, there may be a significant decrease in the temperature of the liquid and a resultant decrease in the vapor pressure. Finally, most machines have a valve that directs the output of the vaporizer into the outlet port of the machine. If the anesthetist fails to open this valve, the output of the vaporizer is shunted into the room and not to the delivery system of the machine (and the patient).

Some vaporizers (e.g., Fluotec and Pentec) are placed in the outflow line of total gas flow. These vaporizers are designed so that within certain temperature and flow ranges, the output of the vaporizer is reasonably constant and the valve controlling the vaporizer can be calibrated in terms of percentage of vapor. These devices are convenient but they do have disadvantages. The percentage output is not predictable in low-flow or closed systems (to be described) because the flow rates are below those for which the vaporizer is calibrated. They are susceptible to inconstancy of flow when impurities in the liquids (or preservatives) "gum" up the fine ports within the apparatus. Also, for some unknown reason, they are often limited in output and this prevents the delivery, when needed, of higher concentrations.

DELIVERY OF THE GAS MIXTURE TO THE PATIENT

Systems for Control of Carbon Dioxide and Management of Rebreathing

To achieve efficient use of anesthetic gas and vapor and to avoid dilution of the anesthetic mixture and associated decrease in the O_2 concentration, it is necessary to exclude room air. This can be done in a simple

Fig. 11-2.—Elements of modified Ayre's T-piece.

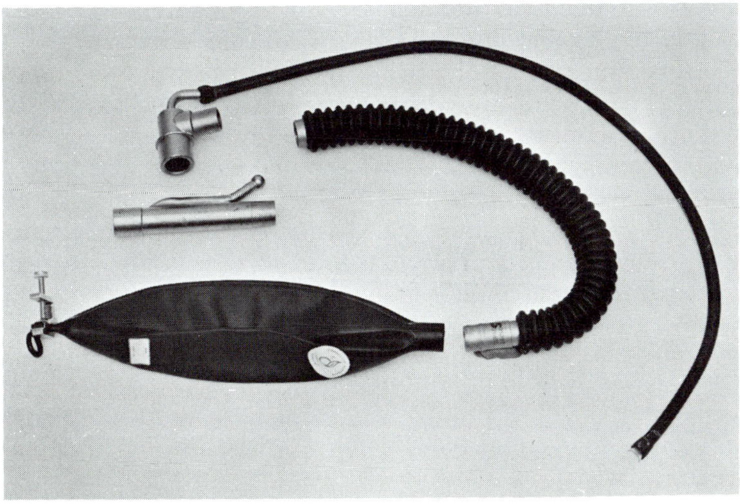

rebreathing bag and mask (or endotracheal tube) system. However, as will be described in the section on closed and high-flow systems, this must of necessity be a wasteful high-flow system because no provision is made for absorption of exhaled CO_2. Nonrebreathing can be facilitated either by a variety of nonrebreathing valves (e.g., Leigh, Stephen-Slater, and Ruben valves) that vent each expiration from the apparatus or by valveless systems that depend on high-flow volumes to "wash out" the CO_2 (e.g., Ayre's T-piece and its modification) (Fig. 11-2). The flow rate necessary (to avoid accumulation of CO_2 in a system using nonrebreathing valves is equal to the minute volume of the patient's respiration. The flow necessary in the Ayre's T-piece (or its modifications) is equal to approximately twice the minute volume. As a result, the latter system is practical only in infants and small children. Any high-flow system exposes the respiratory tract of the patient to the dessicating effect of dry inspired gases unless they are humidified.

Economy, humidification, exclusion of room air and control of concentrations are achieved by use of a circle filter system. The essential parts of this system are 1) a reservoir bag, 2) two flexible hoses, 3) two unidirectional valves, 4) a canister containing a CO_2 absorber and 5) an overflow ("pop-off") valve.

Inspiratory flow rates during quiet respiration measure 20 to 30 liters/min and can reach hundreds of liters/min during rapid respiration. The reservoir bag maintains an available volume to satisfy the inspiratory flow rates, which are much greater than the flows delivered by anesthetic machines. Failure to satisfy this demand is a form of respiratory obstruction. The reservoir bag serves two other purposes: it can be compressed manually to exert a positive airway pressure for assisted or controlled respiration and its movements supply an observer with information concerning the rate, character and rhythm of the patient's respiration.

The two tubes ("elephant tubes") through which the patient moves anesthetic mixture (and O_2) to and from the reservoir bag are made flexible for convenience in handling and for prevention of obstruction by kinking. Their length and diameter are a matter of convenience. Unidirectional valves are situated so that one tube serves for inhalation and the other for exhalation. This arrangement eliminates dead space by preventing the inhalation of exhaled gases until they have passed through the CO_2 absorber and have had their O_2 content replenished. This arrangement accounts for the "circle" label of this system. Incompetence or absence of a valve permits respiration back and forth in one tube. The volume of this rebreathing is dead space or wasted respiration. Valves that do not open and close easily introduce resistance to flow. This is a form of respiratory obstruction that increases the work of breathing.

The canister containing the CO_2 absorbent can be located anywhere in the system, providing exhaled gases pass through it before they are inhaled. The canister capacity when filled with absorbent should allow gas space for at least one tidal volume. Canisters with double this capacity ("jumbo" canisters) are in common use for reasons of economy. One-half of their content of absorbent can be used to exhaustion and replaced without loss of efficiency.

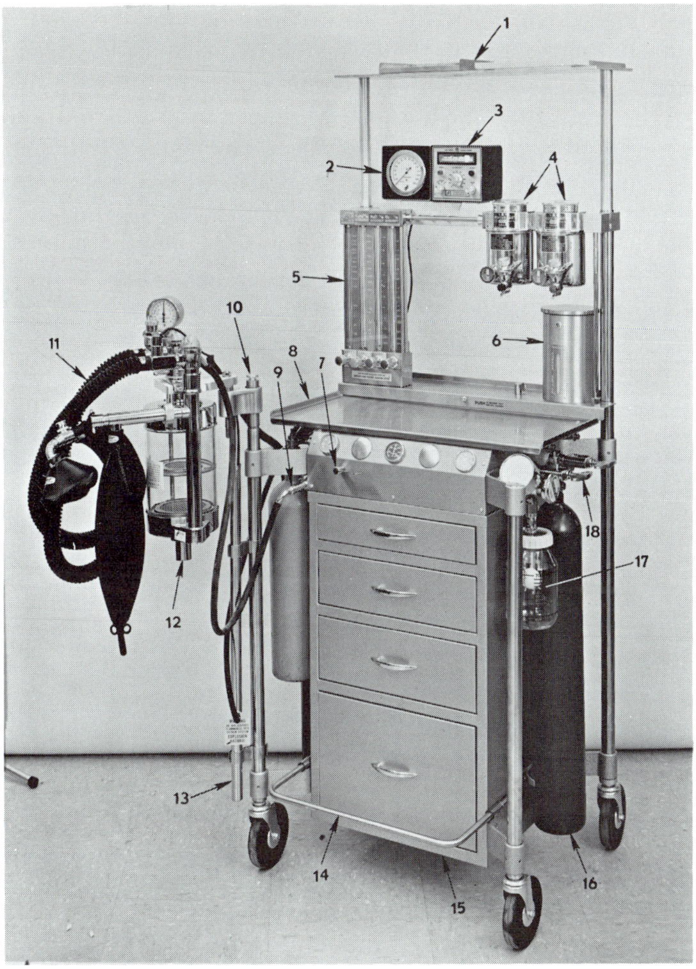

Fig. 11-3.—Standard anesthesia machine. *1*, electrical instrument shelf; *2*, blood pressure gauge; *3*, $0_2\%$ monitor; *4*, vaporizers; *5*, flowmeters; *6*, copper kettle vaporizer; *7*, 0_2 flush valve; *8*, table; *9*, common gas outlet; *10*, telescoping pole; *11*, circle breathing circuit; *12*, CO_2 absorber; *13*, gas evacuation system; *14*, foot rest; *15*, drawers and cabinets; *16*, gas cylinders; *17*, suction set; and *18*, yokes.

CO_2 absorbent consists of porous granules of hydroxides of sodium, calcium or barium or combinations of them. They are chemical bases whose OH^- ion combines with the H^+ ion of acids. The CO_2 of exhaled breath dissolves in water and combines with it to form carbonic acid, H_2CO_3. The water for this reaction is found in the water vapor of exhaled breath and in the absorbent granules. Carbonic acid reacts with the bases to form a salt (carbonate) and water and to produce heat:

$$H_2CO_3 \pm Ca(OH)_2 \rightarrow CaCO_3 \pm 2H_2O \pm \text{heat}$$

When this reaction has used up all the base, the absorbent granules have been changed to a salt and are hard and gritty. Any carbonic acid on their surface cannot be neutralized and it changes the color of indicators, such as ethyl violet, to give visual evidence of the absorbent's exhaustion.

The overflow valve ("pop-off" valve) may be situated anywhere in the circle system. Its placement in the exhalation side of the system saves needless use of absorbent for CO_2 that is to be vented. The overflow valve is a device permitting gas to flow out of the system by overcoming a resistance that can be varied at will. The valve is necessary because when flows of gas and vapor above those providing just the amount of gas or vapor taken up by body tissues or consumed (O_2) are introduced into the external breathing system (bag, tubing and canister), some provision must be made for venting the excess gas and vapor. The valve resistance to outflow can be increased during manual compression of the reservoir bag (for assisted or controlled ventilation) to minimize loss of volume before adequate airway pressure is obtained.

Inflow of anesthetic mixture is usually located on the inhalation side of the system, to allow changes in the inhaled mixture with least delay.

High-flow and Low-flow (Closed) Systems

The anesthetic machine (Fig. 11-3) with its reasonably precise metering of gases and vapors, together with the circle system permit use of a low-flow or closed system. This is possible not only because the low flow of gas and vapor can be metered but also because the canister absorbs exhaled CO_2. The closed system is that system in which all the CO_2 is dealt with by the absorbent (rather than by a high-flow of gases and venting to atmosphere) and in which only that anesthetic gas or vapor and oxygen necessary for uptake in the body and metabolism are provided. For example, after the initial high uptake of anesthetic agent (depending on its solubility and diffusibility) and equilibration with vessel-rich tissues (Chapter 15), input of anesthetic gas and O_2 can be decreased to only that volume that is required for equilibration in the vessel-poor tissues (fat) and consumption of O_2. This means, for example, that if N_2O is used, the input of this gas can be reduced to approximately 400 ml/min. As the tissues become saturated over ensuing minutes and hours, the input of N_2O can be decreased fairly quickly from 400 ml/min to 200 ml/min and ultimately turned off completely. It means also that, for example, halothane input can be reduced to an O_2 flow through the vaporizer of as little as 20 to 30 ml/min (10 to 15 ml of halothane) and, again, as saturation is attained, the input can be stopped. O_2 need be supplied only as needed to meet the metabolic needs of the patient. In the average healthy adult in a moderate level of anesthesia, the O_2 input can be expected to be in the range of 150 to 250 ml/min. These low inputs are possible because the patient rebreathes the same anesthetic mixture over and over in the circle system, CO_2 being removed by the absorbent and O_2 being supplied as needed. If one uses N_2O in the closed system, it is mandatory that one use an O_2 analyzer to monitor the O_2 concentration. This is necessary because one cannot depend upon the accuracy of meters at low flows, and one can detect the changes in uptake of N_2O and the use of O_2 only by changes in the concentration of O_2 evident in the analyzer. If one uses N_2O in a closed system the method is as follows: Assuming a tightly closed system, one observes both the size of the rebreathing bag and the analyzer. If the rebreathing bag increases in size, one may be delivering too much of either N_2O or O_2. If too much N_2O is being delivered, the O_2 concentration shown on the analyzer will decrease. If too much O_2 is being delivered, the O_2 concentration will increase. If the two gases are being delivered in excess of the amount being taken up or consumed but in an appropriate balance, the O_2 concentration will not change and the bag will simply overfill. If the bag decreases in size, either too little O_2 or too little N_2O is being delivered. If too little O_2 is being delivered, the O_2 concentration will decrease. If too little N_2O is being delivered, the O_2 concentration will decrease. If too little of both gases is being delivered but in appropriate percentage the analyzer will show no change in O_2 concentration but the bag will continue to diminish in size. If the two gases are being delivered in the proper percentage and in the proper amount, the bag will remain at a constant size and the analyzer will show a constant O_2 percentage. The system is then "in balance."

If an anesthetic agent is used only with O_2 (i.e., no N_2O), an O_2 analyzer is not necessary because an excess of O_2 is always present in the mixture. The input of anesthetic agent is dictated by the needs of the patient for lighter or deeper anesthesia. The input of O_2 is determined by a change in the size of the breathing bag; if it overfills, too much O_2 is being delivered. If it decreases in size, too little O_2 is being delivered.

Analyzers for specific volatile agents such as halothane and fluoroxene are now available and reasonably inexpensive. Insertion of one of these in the external circuit provides constant measurement of the anesthetic concentration. These are not mandatory (as is the oxygen analyzer) when using the closed system, but they are useful and should encourage the use of the closed system.

The closed system is advantageous from several standpoints: (1) high humidity can be maintained, which means that there is less drying of the respiratory tract; (2) the cost of gases can be significantly decreased; (3) subliminal inhalation of agents (especially fluorinated drugs) by operating room personnel can be eliminated (thus decreasing perhaps the incidence of liver disease, abortions and acne) and (4) inflammable or explosive agents can be used safely and effectively. Changes in concentration of anesthetic vapor within the closed system ordinarily take place more slowly than in the high-flow system because the inflow of gases into the system is substantially less than the minute volume of the patient. This can be interpreted as an advantage because increases in depth of anesthesia take place more slowly and thus more deliberate observation is permitted. On the other hand, decreases in the concentration may take place more slowly and this might be considered a disadvantage. However, an abrupt decrease in concentration can be effected by venting the bag and filling the system with O_2 repetitively, if necessary. There is no known contraindication nor an increased hazard to use of the closed system with potent agents such as halothane. Use of the closed system demands that the anesthetist pay more attention to the patient than to presumed outputs from the machine for assessment of anesthetic effect. This can hardly be counted as a hazard.

High-flow systems are systems in which the input of anesthetic mixture exceeds the amount necessary for uptake and metabolism. The description of uptake and distribution of anesthetic gas and vapor (Chapter 15) will help one to understand the fundamentals of the high-flow system. Usually the high-flow system approximates the *minute volume* of the patient's respiration (5 liters/minute). Lower flows than this permit one to approach but not attain the advantages of the closed system. Higher flows facilitate, at the onset of anesthesia, the input of sufficient gas to accommodate for rapid uptake, diffusion and distribution of agent. This is particularly true of N_2O, which is relatively less soluble than other agents but highly diffusible. The principal advantage of the high-flow system is the ability to predict alveolar concentration from delivered (or metered) concentration of agent. This is possible because the flow approximates the minute volume and there is essentially a total exchange of gas every minute between lung and the external system of bag, canister, and tubing. The disadvantages are (1) drying of respiratory tract, (2) wasting of anesthetic gas, (3) venting of toxic agents into the room and subsequent exposure of personnel, (4) inadaptability to inflammable or explosive agents and (5) the assumption that all patients respond to the prescribed concentration offered.

In recent years, especially since the introduction of halothane, the high-flow system has prevailed. It is time to reconsider the advantages of the closed system.

Before starting any anesthetic procedure, the anesthetist must check his anesthetic machine. First, the anesthetist confirms the gas sources by connecting the machine to the wall outlets, noting the pressures of the gas cylinders and the level of the fluid in the vaporizers. Next, the anesthetist fills the reservoir bag of the circle filter system with O_2 and compresses it manually while the outlet of the system is occluded. By this maneuver the anesthetist checks the connections to the circle system and locates leaks that might prevent exertion of positive airway pressure. The color of the absorbent should be noted. Then, the anesthetist inspects the accessory equipment, such as inhaler masks and their connectors and head straps. Some anesthetists also apply the mask to their own faces and breathe, in and out, one or two breaths of oxygen. In this manner they may detect any unexpected resistance in the circuit. Checking output of the machine by inhalation prevents the accidental inhalation by the patient of an excessive concentration of agent such as might occur with an undetected "wide open" meter for gas or vapor. Finally, the anesthetist can check the output of vaporizers. We doubt that the highly unlikely toxic effects to the anesthetist outweigh the advantages of inadvertent exposure of the patient to dangerously high concentrations.

All physicians and all who work in operating rooms, recovery rooms and emergency areas should know enough about anesthetic machines to use them for emergency resuscitation with oxygen.

CHAPTER TWELVE

Technics of Arterial Puncture and Venipuncture

VENIPUNCTURE

THE ESTABLISHMENT of an intravenous line in association with anesthesia of all types is common and almost ludicrous in some circumstances. For example, there is reasonable doubt that an "intravenous" is a requirement for a patient having a simple rib biopsy under regional block or for administration of thiopental and N_2O for a simple D and C. Establishment of a relatively permanent intravenous line may cause appreciable discomfort and also some hazard of phlebitis, embolism and infection of the blood stream.

It is important to realize that often it is not necessary to establish the intravenous line before induction of anesthesia. Many patients are subjected to discomfort, the benefit of premedication is lost and a much less desirable state for induction of anesthesia is produced if one persists in trying to set up an intravenous infusion when veins are difficult to find or to enter successfully. At the time of arrival in the operating room, many patients have veins that are collapsed because of fear or cold and are difficult to find. In such circumstances, one can either find a small vein with a fine needle and introduce thiopental or other drugs to facilitate induction or induce anesthesia by mask. In children, in whom the incidence of postanesthetic hallucination is less frequent, ketamine may be used intramuscularly to induce sleep and facilitate placement of an intravenous line. After induction by any of these technics, the veins are often much more prominent and a permanent large-bore needle or catheter can be introduced easily.

Selection of Vein

A discussion of some of the practical aspects of venipuncture will help to make this useful, common (but sometimes overused) and potentially difficult technic successful, stable and minimally discomfiting to the patient. Figure 12-1 shows the superficial and deep veins most accessible for introduction of intravenous medication. The sites most often used for establishing long-term intravenous lines are those on the dorsum of the hand and the forearm. Antecubital veins and those just anterior to the medial malleolus of the tibia at the ankle are used less frequently. The antecubital vein is an

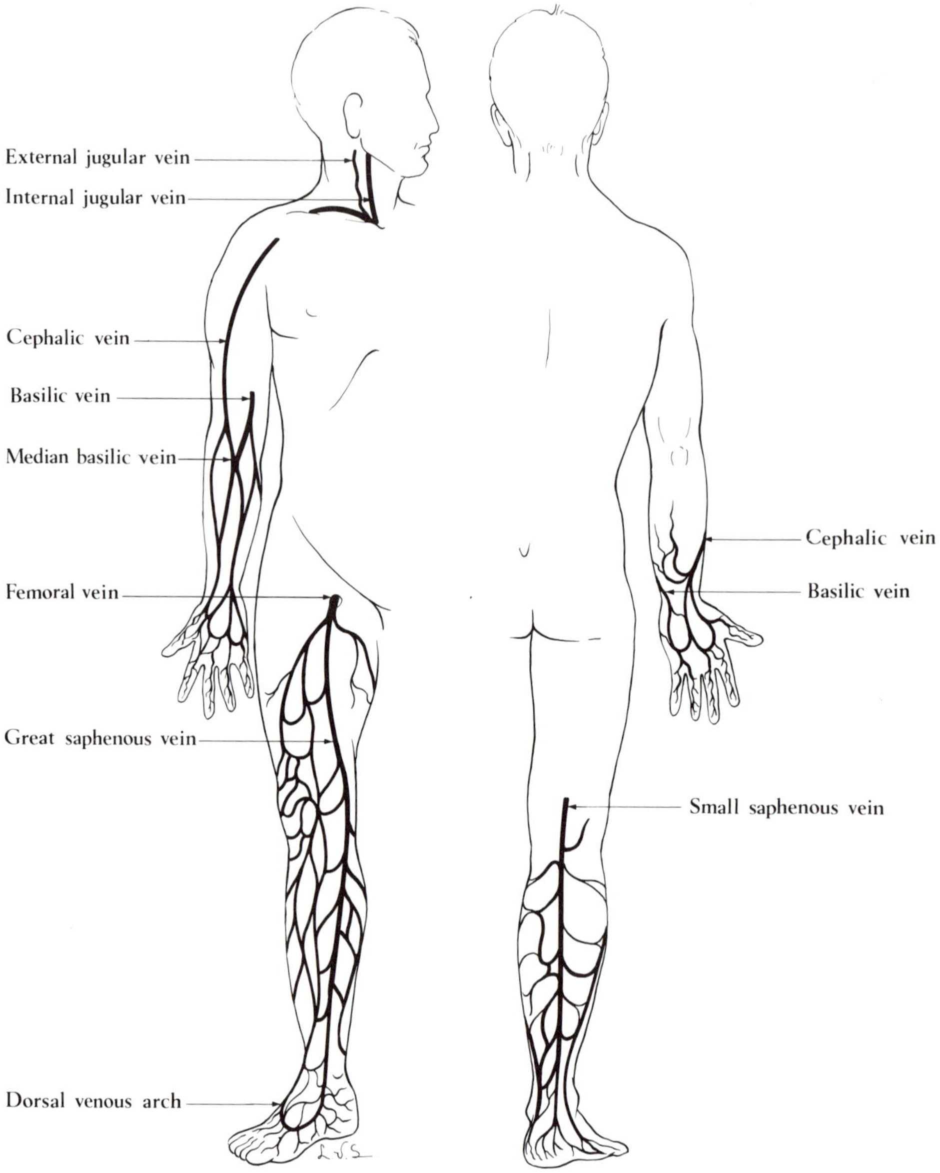

Fig. 12-1.—Location and course of veins most accessible for venipuncture.

uncomfortable site for the patient and should be left for intermittent sampling. Use of the veins of ankle and foot is now limited to infants and small children. The frequency of phlebitis at this site in adults precludes its use except in circumstances in which other sites are not available.

Veins which are most easily seen and which have reasonably straight courses are more suitable for venipuncture than those that are deeply situated and those that are tortuous or have many branches. While veins are often much more readily identified and more prominent after anesthesia has

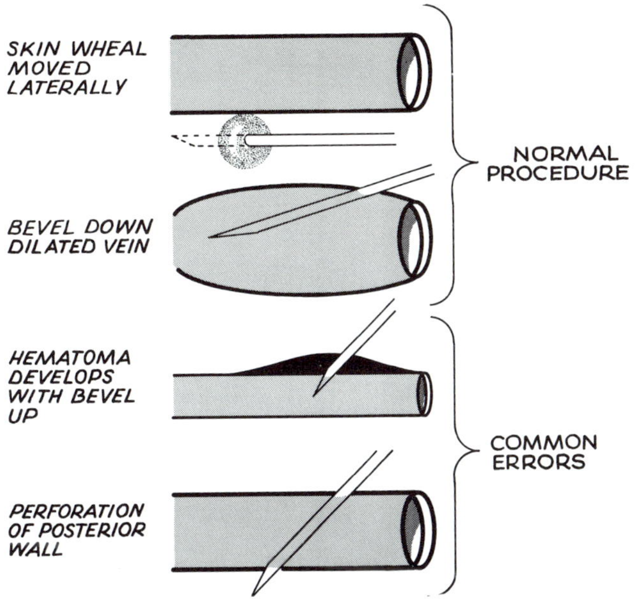

Fig. 12-2.—Technical aspects of venipuncture.

been established, one can increase the visibility and availability of veins by other methods. One of these is to place the extremity in a dependent position with a tourniquet around the limb. Another is to gently snap or pat the skin over the vein, which becomes dilated because of this counterirritant action. Still another method is to apply hot moist towels over the area selected for venipuncture, the heat helping to dilate the veins. In more difficult situations, one may increase visibility and accessibility by inserting a small needle in a small vein and injecting saline distal to a tourniquet.

Entry into Vein

To increase one's chances of successful and stable venipuncture, one should first identify the vein that is most easily seen and one that has a straight course long enough to permit one to insert a substantial length of needle or catheter. It is imperative that the needle be inserted in the direction of the vein; many unsuccessful attempts at venipuncture are due to the improper alignment of needle and vein so that the needle enters the vein at an angle and goes through the vein rather than along its natural course within the lumen. The tourniquet should be placed approximately 5 cm above the point of insertion of the needle. This ensures dilation of that particular vein and also helps to fix the vein. One should be careful to apply only that pressure needed to cause venous obstruction; pressure should not produce arterial closure. If one desires, the injection site may be infiltrated with a minimal amount of local anesthetic solution. The optimal site of entry of skin is away from the vein (Fig. 12-2). This diminishes the chances for accidental through-and-through penetration of the vein and subsequent

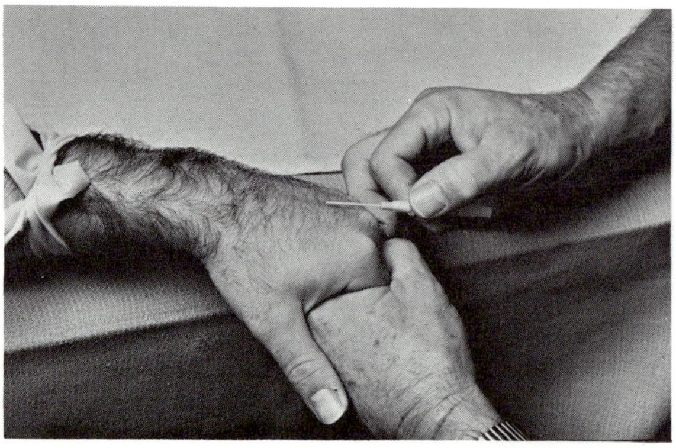

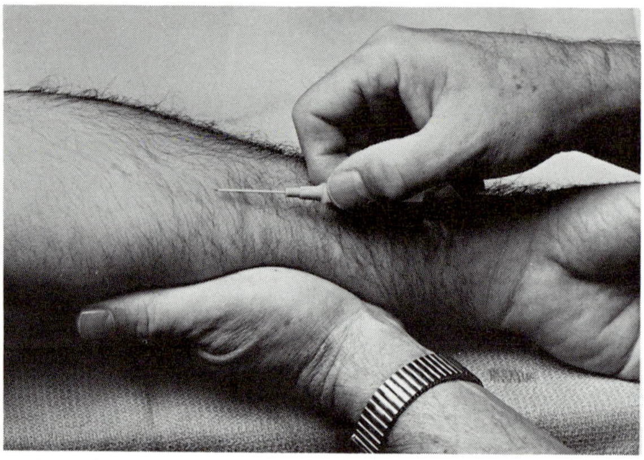

Fig. 12-3 (top).—Placement of tourniquet and fixation of hand for insertion of needle in vein on back of hand. Tourniquet is close to vein to be used and hand is flexed at knuckles, fingers of fixing hand being below plane of insertion of needle.

Fig. 12-4 (bottom).—Position of fixing hand to stabilize arm and immobilize forearm veins.

hematoma formation. The optimal site of entry into the vein itself is that point along the vein that permits one to place the needle or catheter under direct observation, to insert the needle or catheter into the vein for a desirable distance and to position the needle or catheter flat against the skin to secure it.

After the site of entry has been determined, the needle or catheter (with or without the attached syringe) is grasped in the one hand while the other hand is used to fix the vein so that it does not buckle on attempts to enter it. Fixing the vein is an important part of the technic; more venipunctures are unsuccessful (due to failure of entry, rupture of the vein, etc.) because the vein is not properly fixed than because of any other factor. It is essential also that the hand and/or the thumb used for fixing the vein be kept in place until the vein is entered and the needle or catheter advanced. It is bad practice to release the traction on the vein and to attempt to insert needle or catheter while palpating the vein. These relationships are better seen than felt. If one is using a vein on the back of the hand, the vein may be fixed by placing the thumb distal to the knuckle of the fingers of the hand and then applying pressure and traction with it (Fig. 12-3). Grasping the arm by the free hand will help to fix veins of the forearm (Fig. 12-4).

The needle or catheter is then introduced into the skin away from the vein and brought over the vein prior to puncture of the vein itself. The common practice is to have the bevel of the needle up. This, of course, is an acceptable practice and perhaps facilitates entry into the vein. However, we prefer to have the bevel facing down. If the bevel is inserted face up, the needle should be turned 180° after the vein has been entered so that the bevel is down when the needle is advanced. By entering the vein with the bevel down, there is less possibility of puncturing the vein wall that is furthermost from the skin and less likelihood of leak from part of the bevel being out of the vein (see Fig. 12-2). Furthermore, it is easy to see the dimple produced in the vein ahead of the needle in the bevel-down technic just before the needle enters the vein and one can easily identify the relationship of needle and vein. Establishing the relationship of the needle to the vein (above, below or to the side) is also critical to successful entry; this can be done by gently elevating the point of the needle to determine where it is in relation to the vein. Finally, the bevel-down relationship facilitates securing the needle flat against the skin. In the bevel-up position, the point may be either just inside the vein (and perhaps partly out) or inserted in such a manner that the bevel impinges on the anterior wall and becomes occluded; these positions of the bevel and needle force one to support the hub of the needle on padding with a resultant highly unstable position from which the needle is usually easily displaced.

The needle or catheter should be advanced sufficiently within the vein to ensure that it will not come out the insertion site. It is not necessary to insert needles and catheters to the hub. In the first place, no needle should ever be introduced to the hub because a needle may break at the hub, leaving nothing to grasp in order to retrieve the needle or catheter. In the second place, many successful punctures are ruined by unnecessarily advancing the needle or catheter to its full length; the needle or catheter then often pierces the vein wall either where there are no branches (usually if the vein is inadequately fixed), or at a branching point, or the needle or catheter impinges on a valve or a junction point (causing difficulty either in removing blood or in the free introduction of fluid). Once the needle or catheter has been introduced and advanced, it should be secured, preferably flat against the skin with appropriate taping. If under the circumstances of the site of placement there is a tendency for the needle or catheter tip to impinge upon the anterior wall of the vein and bulge the skin, that portion should also be taped (as well as the hub) to prevent the point from puncturing the vein.

Types of Needles and Needle-Catheter Combinations

There are numerous acceptable combinations of needle and plastic catheter that permit introduction of a guide needle either inside or outside a plastic catheter and withdrawal of the needle guide, the catheter being left

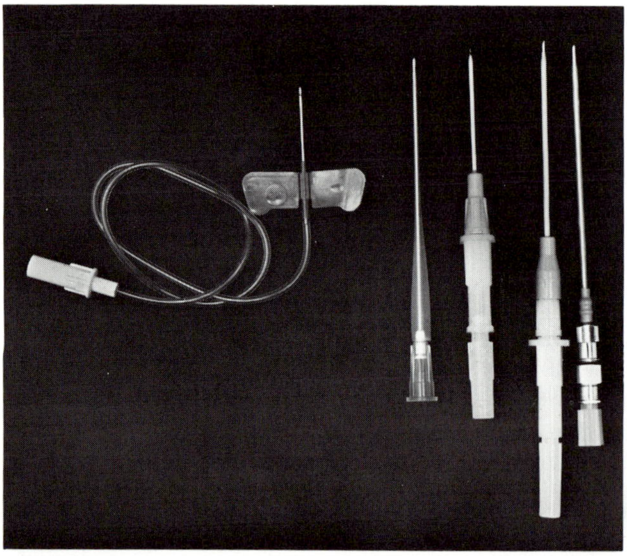

Fig. 12-5.—Examples of needle-catheter combinations and scalp vein needle.

in place (Fig. 12-5). These devices are useful in that the remaining catheter is less easily displaced than an indwelling needle. They do have drawbacks in that there is a higher incidence of phlebitis and some reaction to the catheter substance itself. The incidence of phlebitis and infection can be lessened by meticulous attention to asepsis on introduction of the needle or catheter and prevention of contamination by appropriate dressing. Application of an antibiotic ointment, such as neomycin ointment, at the puncture site may be effective in reducing local infection and phlebitis.

Sometimes it is either not possible to establish an intravenous line by needle or it is believed that a more stable long-term arrangement can be ensured by exposing the vein and inserting a catheter under direct vision. This "cut down" technic is simple but, of course, precludes the use of that particular vein again. A small incision is made where a suitable vein has been identified or at a site where a suitable vein can be expected to be found. The incision is then spread with an appropriate instrument deep enough to expose the vein. When a vein has been exposed and identified, the forceps used for spreading the tissue are inserted under the vein so that a loop of ligature can be brought back under the vein. By cutting the loop end one is left with two strands. After the vein has been cleaned, the more distal strand is tied around the vein and the ends are left long. The more proximal strand is gathered in the fingers of one hand and traction applied with both strands so as to lift the vein out of the incision. A small pointed knife blade is then inserted across the top half of the vein so as to open a slit while the posterior (deeper) portion of the vein is left intact. The cannula is then introduced and advanced to the desired distance. The upper strand is then tied around vein and cannula and the wound closed and dressed.

Scalp vein needles are now made in several sizes and their use is no longer limited to infants (see Fig. 12-5). They are useful needles for pur-

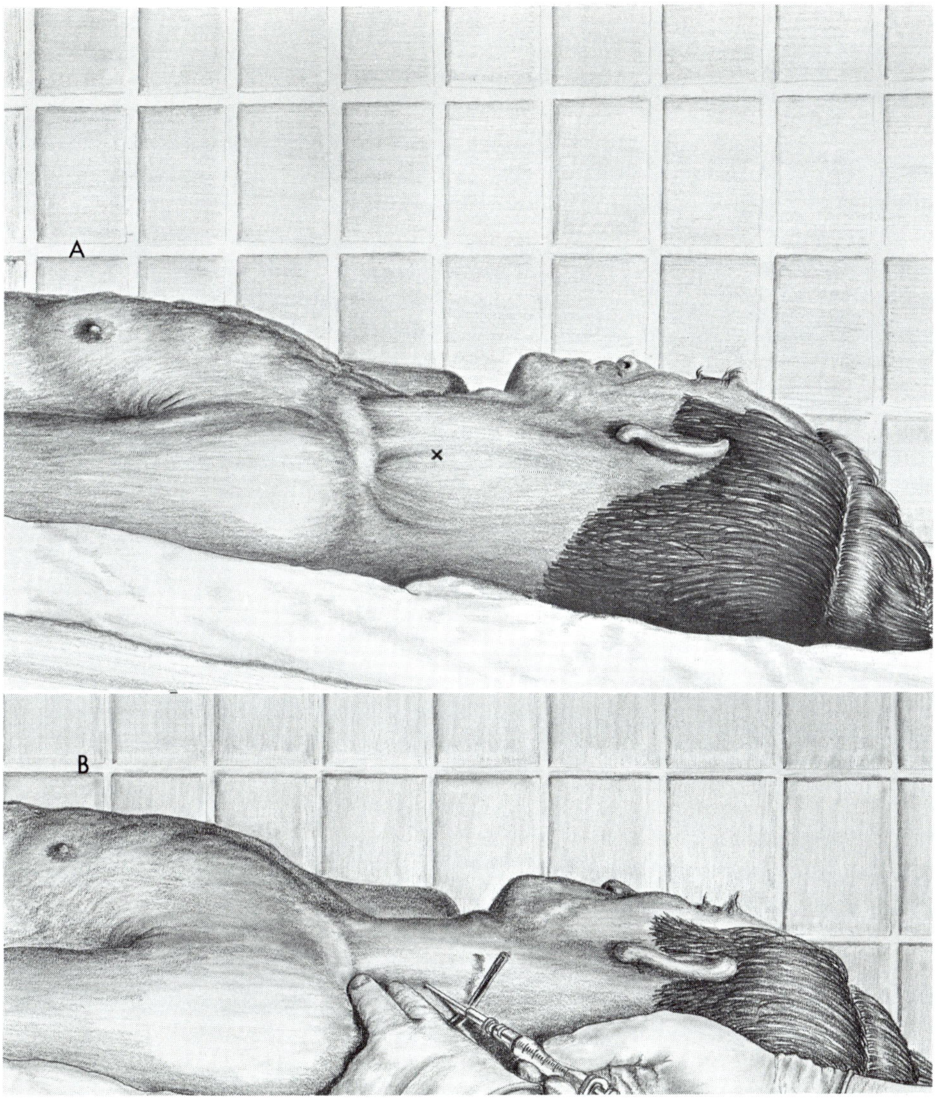

Fig. 12-6.—Technic of entry into internal jugular vein. **A**, correct position of head and neck for placement of a needle; note point for insertion of needle (*X*) and its relationships to border of the sternocleidomastoid muscle and clavicle. **B**, palpation of internal jugular vein with left hand while needle with syringe attached is directed toward internal jugular vein; note planes of needle and syringe in relation to that of neck, head and table. (From Jernigan, W. R., Gardner, W. C., Mahr, M. M., *et al.*: Use of the internal jugular vein for placement of central venous catheter, Surg. Gynecol. Obstet. 130:520, 1970.)

poses of induction of anesthesia. They are also applicable to relatively long-term use (several days) if a site can be found (such as the back of the hand) where stabilization is possible. They are useful also in that the butterfly flap on the hub facilitates fixation. Generally, as with other standard needles, they cause less irritation and phlebitis than indwelling catheters.

Establishment of a Central Venous Pressure Line

One of the more useful intravenous lines is the central venous pressure (CVP) line. The advantages and problems of this technic are discussed in Chapters 5 and 20. Usually the plastic catheter is introduced through an antecubital vein and advanced until the tip is either in the vena cava at its junction with the atrium or in the atrium itself. The catheter tip can be located in several ways. One way is to accept the established fact that in most adult patients the distance between insertion in the antecubital space and the vena cava or atrium ranges from 40 to 60 cm. Catheters are available with inserting needles of large bore through which catheters, with or without indwelling guide wires, can be inserted. Some of these devices have the catheter and bracing wire incorporated into one package that includes a spool for storing the catheter (see Fig. 5-2). The spool can be unwound to introduce the catheter; the spool then can be disconnected so that only the catheter with connecting links and needle are left in place. Another way to determine the site of the tip is to connect the catheter to a strain gauge and an oscillograph calibrated to venous pressures. One advances the catheter to the point at which the ventricular tracing appears and then retracts it to the point indicated by the tracing of the atrium. One can also use either radiopaque catheters or inject radiopaque material through the catheter to determine placement of the tip. Placement of the tip of the CVP line can be done by interpretation of a rather typical ECG tracing when the tip reaches the atrium. However, this technic enhances the possibility of electrical stimulation of the heart if grounding is improper and, in our opinion, this hazard eliminates the technic.

The subclavian vein may be used also for venipuncture for either sampling of blood or for long-term placement of an intravenous line. The technic is of limited and questionable value not only because an intravenous line can usually be established elsewhere with less difficulty but also because the technic is tricky, substantial experience is needed to ensure a reasonable incidence of success and there is an appreciable incidence of pneumothorax and hemorrhage.

The *internal* jugular vein, however, offers a satisfactory and safe approach to the establishment of a CVP line. The advantages to this approach are the direct line to the superior vena cava and atrium (especially on the right side), lack of pneumothorax, minimal bleeding, the large caliber of vein, limited opportunity for occlusion of catheter, fixation of the vein facilitating entrance and accommodation of a large-bore catheter. The technic of entry into the internal jugular vein (Fig. 12-6) is as follows:

With the patient's head turned sharply to the left (although the reverse side may be used), the point of entrance of the needle is defined by outlining the posterior border of the sternocleidomastoid muscle and marking a point two fingerbreadths above the clavicle along that border. This point of entry often is slightly below the apex of the triangle made by the posterior border of the muscle and the external jugular vein. The patient is placed in a slight head-down position to minimize aspiration of air and to dilate the vein. The needle or needle-catheter combination is then introduced through the skin of the neck and directed medially and caudad toward the suprasternal notch. The needle is kept close to the posterior aspect of the muscle until it enters the vein. The catheter is then introduced through the needle and the tip placed in the superior vena cava or atrium as has just been defined.

ARTERIAL PUNCTURE

Determination of arterial pressure by means of indwelling needles or catheters is now common and useful practice. Stable oscillographs with simplified calibration and operation are available and permit second-to-second observation of both systolic and diastolic pressures as well as mean pressure. Either needles (such as the scalp vein needle) or the combination of needle and catheter used for intravenous lines can be inserted into an artery. For purposes incident to management of anesthesia (as opposed to the needs of cardiac surgery or angiography, when the femoral artery is often used), either the brachial artery or the radial artery at the wrist is used. The radial artery is preferred because it is more accessible. It is wise to apply the Weber test to ensure patency of the ulnar artery prior to establishing a long-term radial artery line. This is done by blanching the skin of the hand by pressure on both radial and ulnar arteries and then releasing the pressure on the ulnar alone. Return of color to the hand gives reasonable assurance of a functioning ulnar artery.

Identification and fixation of the radial artery can be facilitated by extreme extension of the hand at the wrist and fixing the hand and wrist in the palm-up position with padding and tape (Fig. 12-7). Usually a wheal of local anesthetic solution is raised, and then the needle or combination of needle and catheter is inserted over the artery while the free finger of the other

Fig. 12-7.—Position of hand and wrist for insertion of needle in radial artery. Note hyperextension of wrist and fixation of arm, wrist and hand on short padded board.

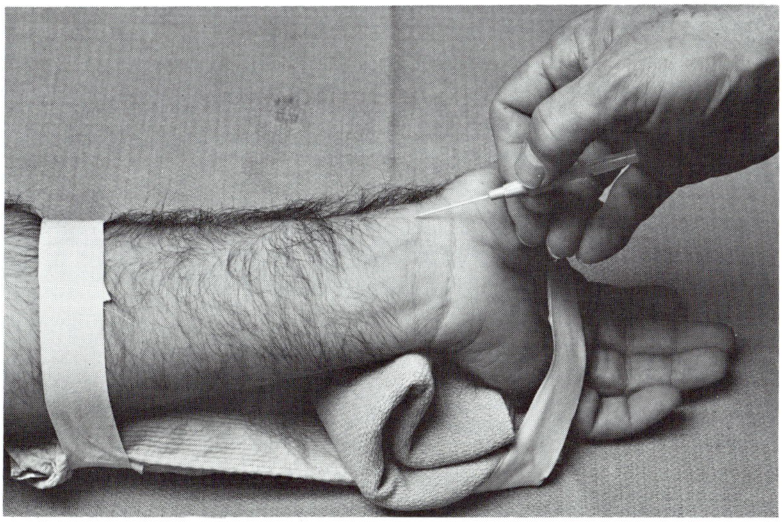

hand identifies and secures the artery as firmly as possible. The needle is inserted directly over the artery and relatively straight into it. If the outflow of arterial blood continues after puncture is made, the needle or needle and catheter can then be depressed and advanced into the artery to a point at which there is undamped oscillation on the oscillograph. Often the needle goes through the artery. If such is the case the needle is withdrawn until blood again flows freely and the needle is advanced to the optimum position. If a catheter is used, the needle insert is withdrawn before the catheter is withdrawn so that when the catheter tip reenters the artery it can be advanced without the needle insert. The needle or catheter is then fixed in position. If penetration is unsuccessful and there is a hematoma, pressure must be applied to stop the bleeding. Pressure must be applied also when the needle or catheter is removed. The same technic for entry is used but the needle can usually be a small one (25 gauge) if arterial blood is needed only for intermittent sampling as for gas analysis. Arterial puncture is no longer a major procedure and, with the proper technic, there is a minimum of continued spasm or interruption with subsequent impaired or absent circulation distal to the puncture site. A profound vagal response (bradycardia and hypotension) may occur in a few patients. This can be corrected easily with the intravenous administration of atropine and the temporary inhalation of excess oxygen.

PART 4

Pharmacology of Anesthetic Drugs

CHAPTER THIRTEEN

Drugs Used for Premedication

PREMEDICANT DRUGS are those drugs which are administered in the preoperative period and which may be regarded as important, valuable and integral parts of the total anesthetic management. In selecting what premedicant drugs to give, the anesthetist should have a knowledge of the basic actions of the various drugs. The objectives of premedication are outlined in Chapter 3.

SEDATIVE-HYPNOTICS

Drugs whose major action is to produce sedation or sleep are classified as sedative-hypnotics. Included among them are the so-called tranquilizers because most of the evidence suggests that their effects do not differ appreciably from those of the traditional drugs in this category. In appropriate doses, these drugs produce drowsiness or sleep from which the patient can be easily aroused. The diminished awareness of surrounding activities tends to allay anxiety. The drugs should not interfere with normal mentation, motor ability or coordination. If given in excessive doses or to patients in pain, sedative-hypnotics may produce restlessness, disorientation, confusion and complete loss of cooperation. In premedicant doses, they do not usually produce any appreciable depression of respiration or circulation. However, when used in combination with other premedicant drugs such as the opiates, the net effect will be greater sedation than that produced by the same dose of sedative used alone. If one anticipates that the patient may experience pain in the preoperative period, these drugs should be avoided or used only in combination with an analgesic.

The most important toxic effects of these drugs are associated with gross overdose, which causes profound central nervous system depression or prolonged administration causing physical dependence. A profound overdose is a medical emergency; it requires tracheal intubation to prevent aspiration of gastric contents and ventilatory and circulatory support during the period of unconsciousness. Sedative-hypnotics can produce allergic reactions, usually involving the skin, and may have additive effects when used in combination with antihypertensive (reserpine, alpha methyldopa) or antihistaminic drugs as well as the opiates. With more prolonged administration, some sedative-hypnotics are capable of stimulating or inhibiting the action of liver enzymes that are responsible for the metabolic degradation of many drugs including the barbiturates themselves, diphenylhydantoin (Dilantin) and warfarin (Coumadin). The significance of these changes in the management of anesthesia is not clear, except perhaps in relation to the avoidance of these drugs in patients with porphyria. Apparently the barbiturates can induce a hepatic enzyme, hepatic synthetase, to increase the synthesis of body porphyrins and precipitate acute porphyria.

The sedative-hypnotics are either weak acids (e.g., barbiturates) or weak bases (e.g., diazepam) and exist mostly in the unionized state in the body. Consequently, they readily cross body barriers (blood-brain or placental), the rates of transfer being primarily dependent on lipid solubility. The short-acting barbiturates (e.g., pentobarbital, secobarbital) are readily absorbed from the stomach and hence can be given orally as well as parenterally. Diazepam is absorbed from the small intestine and colon, and this, of course, delays its onset of action; as a premedicant, therefore, this drug is usually given intramuscularly.

The sedative-hypnotics are readily distributed throughout the body and it is the distribution in tissues such as muscle and fat, which effectively remove these drugs from the central nervous system, that largely accounts for the termination of the sedative effects of these drugs. The sedative-hypnotics are metabolized primarily in the liver at a rate of 1 to 3% per hour and are excreted in changed form in the urine. Except for barbiturates that are resistant to metabolic degradation (barbital and phenobarbital), the duration of action of the sedative-hypnotics is not likely to be appreciably altered by impaired renal function.

Sedative-hypnotics have been used for many years in the treatment of convulsions due to overdoses of local anesthetics. Recent studies by De Jong and Heavner have shown that these drugs, given as premedicants, double the dose of lidocaine required to produce seizures in cats.[2] Because these drugs are effective in raising the seizure threshold to local anesthetics, their use would seem advisable when injections of large doses of local anesthetics are anticipated. Diazepam would seem to be the preferable agent because of its lesser respiratory, circulatory and sedative effects.

NARCOTICS

Contraindications

Just as there are indications for the use of opiates (see Chapter 3), so their pharmacologic actions mitigate against their indiscriminate use in some circumstances. These circumstances include the following:

1) *Moderate to severe respiratory insufficiency.* Although the opiates are potent respiratory depressants, they produce almost no detectable respiratory changes when given in premedicant doses to healthy men. This is not necessarily the case, however, in patients with respiratory disease, in whom opiates given as premedicants may abolish the existing compensatory responses to the disease and lead to respiratory failure. If opiates are deemed necessary, they should be given only while the anesthetist is present and can observe the patient for adverse responses.

TABLE 13-1.—COMMONLY USED NARCOTICS

GENERIC NAME	PROPRIETARY NAME	DOSE (MG) EQUIVALENT TO MORPHINE 10 MG/70 KG BODY WEIGHT	DURATION OF ACTION (HR)
Morphine		10	4-6
Meperidine	Demerol	100	3-4
Pentazocine	Talwin	45	3-4
Alphaprodine	Nisentil	40	1
Fentanyl	Sublimaze	0.2	0.5

2) *Moderate to severe hypovolemia.* The opiates are good smooth muscle dilators; dilation of veins in the presence of hypovolemia may precipitate profound shock. This is especially likely to occur if there is a sudden shift in the patient's body position (e.g., from supine to sitting or lateral decubitus).

3) *Increased intracranial pressure.* Patients with increased intracranial pressure are prone to neurologic abnormalities such as drowsiness or confusion. The sudden onset of coma is a surgical emergency necessitating rapid intraventricular drainage. The administration of opiates may harm these patients in one of two ways. First, by their sedative effects, the opiates may render a somnolent patient comatose; the resulting situation thereby falsely mimics the true surgical emergency. Second, the opiates may impair ventilation sufficiently to cause CO_2 retention and increased cerebral blood flow; the increased flow, in turn, will increase intracranial pressure and may precipitate a sudden coma.

4) *Evaluation of neurologic status in the immediate postoperative period.* The best example of the situation in which postoperative neurologic evaluation is desired is observation of the patient undergoing extracranial carotid surgery for cerebrovascular occlusive disease. The operation requires that there be a temporary occlusion of a portion of the blood supply to the brain. Should a neurologic deficit result, it is highly desirable to be able to detect it as soon as possible in the postoperative period so that treatment for focal cerebral ischemia can be started. Any drugs causing prolonged postoperative central nervous system depression are contraindicated under these circumstances.

5) *Anesthesia with potent inhalation anesthetics for operations in which spontaneous ventilation is desired.* Most inhalation anesthetics (excluding nitrous oxide) depress ventilation by decreasing tidal volume. As a compensatory response, respiratory frequency increases to maintain a more normal minute ventilation and CO_2 excretion. Opiates prevent or lessen the frequency responses without providing any compensatory increases in tidal volume. Hence the combination of opiates and potent inhalation anesthetics (halothane, fluroxene and cyclopropane) may cause profound respiratory depression, hypercapnia and respiratory acidosis if these patients are allowed to breathe spontaneously.

6) *History of biliary colic.* Both morphine and meperidine can precipitate biliary tract spasm and biliary colic in patients susceptible to this disease. Other potent opiates should probably be avoided in such patients.

Narcotic-Nitrous Oxide Combinations

Selection of the best opiate for premedication depends mostly on the desired duration of action. A number of narcotics are available; Table 13-1 lists only those in common clinical practice. Except for dosage and duration of action, the pharmacologic effects of the various narcotics listed are similar.

Anesthetists have individual preferences for morphine or meperidine but there is little sound evidence favoring one over the other. At equianalgesic doses, both drugs produce approximately the same amount of respiratory or circulatory depression. However, it is now clear with the popular reintroduction of the nitrous oxide-narcotic technic that morphine has significantly less impact on mentation and responsiveness than either meperidine or fentanyl. As increasing doses of the latter drugs are given to the awake patient, his responsiveness gradually decreases. The lack of responsiveness correlates well in most patients with the concurrent level of analgesia and general depression. Not so with morphine—patients given morphine in doses producing analgesia and general depression equivalent to that of meperidine and fentanyl maintain contact with their surroundings. As a result, it is more difficult to establish an end point or to determine the appropriate doses of morphine. Furthermore, this lack of development of nonresponsiveness causes potentially hazardous problems in the postanesthetic period. The patient given morphine awakens promptly and seems well oriented in the immediate postanesthetic period in the presence of surgical stimuli. As a result, the anesthetist and others are deluded into believing that the associated depression, especially of respiration, is similarly minimal. However, in the absence of stimuli, profound respiratory depression, even to apnea, develops. This is in contrast to the slower and concomitant return of responsiveness and general depression (especially respiration) with meperidine and fentanyl. Patients given large doses of morphine as a part of nitrous oxide anesthesia or as an anesthetic for cardiac surgery should be watched very closely, maintained on artificial ventilation or given repeated doses of narcotic antagonists for as long as 24 hours. One must also keep in mind that very small doses of narcotic for pain relief must be given. The traditional dose given to a patient with a significant amount of retained morphine may precipitate profound depression.

One adverse effect of opiate premedication is that of emesis. The opiates are potent emetics and can cause persistent nausea and vomiting that is discomforting to both patient and anesthetist. A history of such an episode should preclude the use of opiates or should cause the anesthetist to substitute an analgesic such as pentazocine, which is not an opiate. Use of antiemetics with opiates is sometimes helpful. For example, the combination of fentanyl and droperidol (Innovar) is seldom associated with nausea because of the potent antiemetic action of the latter drug.

For operations of 2 hours or less, the ultrashort-acting drug, fentanyl, or the short-acting drug, alphaprodine, is most appropriate. For longer operations, meperidine or morphine is more suitable. Should accidental overdose occur, depression can be reversed with a narcotic antagonist, preferably naloxone.

When used as anesthetics or adjuvants to nitrous oxide, the narcotics are given intravenously in repeated small doses (e.g., 25 to 50 mg of meperidine or its equivalent) until surgical anesthesia is obtained. Given intravenously, the onset of action is within a few minutes and noticeable depression of central nervous system function occurs. With each incremental dose, the patient becomes more drowsy and less aware or interested in the surroundings. The addition of nitrous oxide (60 to 70%) with or without a small dose of thiopental (50 to 100 mg) renders the patient unconscious and preparations for operation can begin. Additional small doses of narcotic (10 to 25 mg of meperidine or its equivalent) will usually be needed prior to the surgical incision and at periodic intervals (30 to 60 min) thereafter. Administration of additional doses should be avoided during the last hour of the operation to lessen the possibility of central nervous system depression in the early postoperative period. Small doses of thiopental (25 to 50 mg) or subanesthetic concentrations of halothane (0.1 to 0.3%) or fluroxene (0.3 to 0.6%) can be substituted as needed.

Actions of Narcotics

The mechanism whereby the narcotics depress central nervous system function is not known. Preliminary evidence, however, suggests that the analgesic action of morphine is mediated through the release of catecholamines within the central nervous system. Drugs such as reserpine or phenoxybenzamine, which deplete the brain of catecholamines, may also antagonize the analgesic actions of morphine.

RESPIRATORY ACTIONS.—All narcotics depress ventilation, the magnitude of the depression being as great or greater than morphine at equianalgesic doses. Respiratory frequency is usually decreased with increasing doses, an effect that can be used as a sign of increasing depth of anesthesia. Correlation of respiratory depression (as measured by slowing of rate) and general depression (analgesia and sedation-hypnosis) is usually good so that, in most patients, when the respiratory rate approaches 10 per min, the general depression is satisfactory for anesthesia in combination with nitrous oxide. Some patients, however, respond differently from those in whom the response is an average one. Some patients, for example, show an abnormal depression of the respiratory rate in relation to the general depression; other patients show minimal depression of the respiratory rate with satisfactory general depression. As a result, the respiratory rate is not always a reliable measure of general depression. The tidal volume may be unchanged, increased or decreased when nitrous oxide is included, but the net effect is invariably a decrease in alveolar ventilation and an increase in Pa_{CO_2}. The narcotics also depress the ventilatory responses to inhaled CO_2. Mild increases in Pa_{CO_2} (< 50 torr) are rarely of concern but greater increases may necessitate the use of controlled ventilation and partial reversal of the narcotic effect with an antagonist such as naloxone. For patients with a more profound slowing of respiratory rate in relation to the general depression, it is possible to restore a satisfactory rate with small doses of naloxone or other narcotic antagonist. We emphasize that the doses must be small (e.g., 0.05

mg of naloxone). This ability of narcotics to produce different effects such as respiratory depression, circulatory depression and mental obtundation leads us and others to believe that the narcotics have separate components to their actions, and that these can be reversed separately by the antagonists.

CIRCULATORY ACTIONS.—The effects of opiates on the circulation depend upon the net balance between their direct actions on peripheral vasculature and their indirect actions via the sympathetic nervous system. The narcotics decrease peripheral vascular resistance and increase peripheral blood flow; probably this effect is primarily mediated through a direct action on smooth muscle, but vasodilation from histamine release cannot be excluded. If the blood volume is inadequate or if the patient's posture permits pooling of blood in the extremities (e.g., if the patient is in the sitting position) severe hypotension may occur. Because the narcotics stimulate the release of endogenous catecholamines, there are increases in cardiac contractility, stroke index, central venous pressure and pulmonary arterial pressure. The net result is usually a maintenance or increase in blood pressure; this makes the narcotic-nitrous oxide technic a favorite one for use in patients with circulatory instability and accounts for its frequent selection for anesthesia in patients undergoing open heart operations. In the elderly or debilitated, however, in whom sympathetic nervous system responsiveness may be lacking, circulatory support may be lacking. Circulatory depression from opiates can usually be reversed by fluid administration and small doses of vasopressors (e.g., ephedrine, 25 to 50 mg intravenously).

OTHER ACTIONS.—Other complications of narcotics that have not been mentioned include loss of smooth muscle tone to the bowel and bladder, which causes constipation and urinary retention, and release of ADH, which causes a decrease in urine formation. For the most part, the narcotics undergo metabolism in the liver, primarily N-demethylation, before being excreted in the urine. Hence, these drugs should be given more cautiously in patients with liver disease. Contraindications to the use of narcotics during anesthesia are essentially the same as for the use of these drugs as premedicants.

ANTICHOLINERGIC DRUGS

Anticholinergics antagonize the actions of acetylcholine. The two that are commonly used as premedicants are atropine and scopolamine.[3] These drugs are alkaloids of the belladonna plant, atropine being a racemic mixture of *d*- and *l*-hyoscyamine and scopolamine being *l*-hyoscine. Because *d*-hyoscyamine is inactive, atropine is only one half as potent as its *l* isomer.

The mechanism whereby the belladonna alkaloids inhibit the actions of acetylcholine is not known. However, the antagonism is selective in that it primarily affects structures innervated by postganglionic cholinergic nerves. Because these are the same nerves that are stimulated by the alkaloid, muscarine, the belladonna alkaloids are also known as antimuscarinic agents. Only when given in very large doses do the belladonna alkaloids exert any effects on autonomic ganglia or at skeletal neuromuscular junctions.

The postganglionic parasympathetic junctions are not equally sensitive to the belladonna alkaloids. Small doses block salivary, bronchial and sweat secretions; slightly larger doses produce pupillary dilatation, loss of accommodation and a lessening of vagal tone to the heart; large doses inhibit parasympathetic control of the bladder and gastrointestinal tract, causing urinary retention and loss of motility of the gut.

Since the belladonna alkaloids are not equipotent in their actions, the choice of drug depends upon the effects desired. Atropine is the more potent blocker of vagal tone to the heart. If, for example, the belladonna is being given primarily to prevent bradycardia during tracheal or esophageal intubation, then atropine is the preferred drug. If the belladonna is being given to diminish oropharyngeal secretions or to cause sedation and amnesia, then scopolamine is the better agent.

Both atropine and scopolamine are poorly absorbed from the stomach and must be given by subcutaneous or intramuscular injection to provide reliable absorption. Maximum effects occur within 20 to 30 minutes and wane within an hour. Because of the short duration of action, timing of the drug administration is critical. Generally the drugs are given 30 to 45 minutes prior to the anticipated start of anesthesia. Both drugs are partially altered by the liver and excreted, in both altered and unaltered forms, in the urine.

The toxic effects of an overdose of belladonna include fever, skin flushing, tachycardia and development of a poikilothermic state. Treatment consists of controlling body temperature and preventing acidosis or heart failure. Pyridostigmine (10 mg) also may be helpful as a reversal drug.

Contraindications to the use of atropine and scopolamine are few. These drugs should probably be avoided or used in low doses in febrile patients, especially children. Patients with Down's syndrome hyperreact to atropine, developing profound increases in heart rate.[4] The reason for this is not known but the observation suggests that the dose should be reduced to one half of that which would ordinarily be administered. It is often stated that atropine or scopolamine should not be used in patients with asthma, bronchitis or obstructive airway disease because of the danger of producing inspissation of secretions and bronchopneumonia; there is no evidence to substantiate this and it is our belief that these drugs can be used safely in such patients. Likewise, glaucoma is not a contraindication to the use of either atropine or scopolamine because premedicant doses cause insignificant ocular effects.

REFERENCES

1. Way, W. L., and Trevor, A. J.: Sedative-hypnotics, Anesthesiology 34:170, 1971.
2. DeJong, R. H., and Heavner, J. E.: Local anesthetic seizure prevention: diazepam vs. pentobarbital, Anesthesiology 36:449, 1972.
3. Eger, E. I., II: Atropine, scopolamine and related compounds, Anesthesiology 23:365, 1962.
4. Harris, W. S., and Goodman, R. M.: Hyperreactivity to atropine in Down's syndrome, N. Eng. J. Med. 279:407, 1968.

CHAPTER FOURTEEN

Inhalation Anesthetics

WITHIN THE LAST 20 YEARS, there has been a great increase in the number of new anesthetics that have been developed. Initially, the primary motivation to develop new anesthetics was to eliminate the problem of flammability. The mainstays of anesthesia formerly were diethyl ether and cyclopropane, both agents being highly flammable. The first breakthrough came in 1956 with the introduction of halothane, a fluorinated hydrocarbon. Except for its sometimes adverse cardiovascular effects, halothane appeared to be the ideal anesthetic. Because of the instant success and popularity of halothane among physicians and patients, rival pharmaceutical companies attempted to develop even better inhalation anesthetics. Hence the development of methoxyflurane, enflurane (Ēthrane) and, most recently, isofluorane (Forane). Primary emphasis was placed on finding anesthetic drugs that had a potency equal to or greater than that of halothane but with less depression of circulatory or respiratory function.

Throughout this developmental phase, it was assumed that if excessive depression of the organ systems (e.g., heart, lungs and kidneys) could be avoided during anesthesia, then patients would recover quickly and completely when the anesthetic was discontinued. That the inhalation anesthetics could have delayed or long-term adverse effects was not taken into account for several reasons. First, the exposure to these agents was short, only a matter of hours. Second, it was generally thought that the inhalation anesthetics, unlike intravenous anesthetics, were chemically inert in the body; that is, there was no biotransformation and they were excreted via the lungs in exactly the same amount and form as had been inhaled. Third, although there were scattered reports of serious postoperative complications (i.e., hepatic or renal failure) after the use of these drugs, these complications were usually ascribed to the severity of the patient's illness or to the use of drugs known to produce these changes. We know now that these presumptions are incorrect. Severe toxicity can occur despite brief exposure. The inhalation anesthetics are not chemically inert, but rather undergo metabolism in varying degrees to other compounds, some of which may have adverse effects. Finally, controlled studies, which excluded other diseases or drugs as being the probable causative factors for postoperative toxicity, revealed that the inhalation anesthetics were the likely culprits.

HALOTHANE (FLUOTHANE)

Halothane is a fluorinated hydrocarbon, its structural formula being 2-bromo, 2-chloro, 1:1:1-trifluoroethane. The drug is packaged in amber-colored bottles and contains 0.01% thymol to inhibit decomposition to volatile acids with prolonged exposure to light. The drug has a sweet, nonirritating odor, is nonflammable and nonexplosive and is compatible with soda lime. The physical properties of this agent are shown in Table 14-1.

Halothane can be administered by the open-drop technic or by injection of minute quantities of liquid into the inspired gas line. However, because of the potency of this agent, the preferred method of administration is by means of a calibrated, out-of-circle vaporizer. Two types of vaporizers are commonly used: the copper kettle or Vernitrol,* in which a side flow of oxygen is used as the carrier gas, and the Fluotec† vaporizer, which has temperature compensation and uses a portion of the total gas delivery for carrying the halothane vapor. Halothane may be used alone or in combination with nitrous oxide. Concentrations for induction will vary from 2 to 6%; maintenance concentrations average 1% with nitrous oxide (60 to 70%) or 1.5% without nitrous oxide. The minimum alveolar anesthetic concentration (MAC) for halothane is shown in Table 14-2.

Most, but not all, of the halothane inhaled is excreted by the lungs. About 12 to 20% of that inhaled is excreted in the urine as nonvolatile metabolites, primarily bromide ion and trifluoroacetic acid. The intermediary compound is thought to be trifluoroethanol; this compound is the most toxic of the metabolites thus far identified. Most of the metabolism seems to occur in the liver, since induction of liver enzyme systems has been observed in animals and men exposed to halothane repeatedly. Whether hepatic enzyme induction occurs in anesthetists and operating room personnel from prolonged or repeated exposure to halothane is not clear. However, because halothane does appear to produce adverse effects on the liver in some patients, it is advisable for anesthetists to limit the exposure of such patients to halothane. This can be done by decreasing the general use of halothane, restricting its use to operations for which it has distinct advantages over other anesthetics. Exposure also of operating room personnel can

TABLE 14-1.—PHYSICAL PROPERTIES OF INHALATION ANESTHETICS

PHYSICAL PROPERTY	HALOTHANE	FLUROXENE	METHOXYFLURANE	ENFLURANE	DIETHYL ETHER	CYCLOPROPANE	NITROUS OXIDE
Molecular weight	198	126	165	185	74	42	44
Boiling point (°C)	50.2	43.2	104.7	57	35	−33	−89
Specific gravity	1.86	1.13	1.4	1.5			
Vapor pressure at 20°C (torr)	242	282	20	175	440		
Flammability	None	>4%	>4%	No	Yes	Yes	No

*Vernitrol—Ohio Medical Products, Madison, Wisconsin.
†Fluotec—Fraser-Sweatman Inc., Lancaster, New York.

be lessened by using the closed system or by removing the gases exhausted from the anesthetic circuit by suction.

Adverse Effects

The adverse effects of halothane can be divided into those occurring in the operative period and those occurring in the postoperative period. In the operative period, the most commonly observed adverse effects are those of depression of respiration and circulation (Chapters 19 and 20). Halothane is an excellent uterine relaxant that may be advantageous when version and extraction or manual exploration of the uterine cavity for retained placenta are required. However, uterine atony is hazardous to patients undergoing therapeutic suction abortion; uterine blood loss during this procedure is significantly greater during halothane anesthesia than during anesthesia with nitrous oxide, thiopental and meperidine.[2]

HALOTHANE AND HEPATIC FAILURE.—The most serious adverse effect in the postoperative period is hepatic failure. It is now generally accepted that halothane can affect the liver, although it took more than 10 years of extensive use of the drug and a national study[3] to accumulate sufficient data to document the causal relationship. Current evidence suggests that the incidence of hepatitis following halothane anesthesia is about 1 in 10,000 and that fulminant hepatic necrosis and death occurs in 1 in 40,000 patients receiving halothane anesthetics.

Because of the widespread concern about the possible hepatotoxicity of halothane, a national study of the problem was undertaken in 1963 by a joint committee of the National Academy of Sciences and the National Research Council.[3] A collaborative retrospective study of the incidence of fatal hepatic necrosis occurring within 6 weeks of anesthesia comprised 856,515 anesthetics in 34 cooperating institutions. Several major conclusions were reached, including the following:

1) Fatal postoperative massive hepatic necrosis is rare.
2) The incidence of fatal hepatic necrosis was significantly higher for cyclopropane and nitrous oxide-barbiturate anesthesia than for halothane.
3) Halothane is a safe anesthetic, the overall mortality rate being 1.87%, compared to a rate of 1.93% for all anesthetics.

The mechanism whereby halothane causes hepatitis is not known. The prevailing view is that halothane is not a direct toxin, like chloroform or carbon tetrachloride, but rather that the toxicity is the result of a sensitization reaction. The characteristic features of hepatotoxins such as chloroform are as follows: they invariably produce liver damage if administered in an adequate dose; the lesions are readily reproducible in most animal species; the severity of the injury is directly related to the dose; and the lesions are characteristic and readily distinguishable on histologic examination. Halothane hepatitis seems to show none of these characteristics. Rather, halothane hepatitis occurs only in selected individuals, in females more often than males, and only after more than one exposure to the agent. The clinical and histologic evidence favors a delayed sensitization reaction. Clinically, fever, arthralgia and eosinophilia commonly accompany the hepatitis, suggesting an allergic-like reaction. The latent period, the time between exposure and the onset of hepatitis is extremely variable in halothane hepatitis, in contrast to the features of toxic hepatitis. Even more convincing evidence is the study by Klatskin and Kimberg, who exposed an anesthetist suspected to be halothane-sensitive to 0.1% halothane for 5 minutes.[4] This brief exposure provoked an acute hepatitis that was documented clinically, biochemically and histologically. Moreover, in patients suspected of having halothane hepatitis, active but transient histiocytic granulomas that are confined principally to the periportal areas have been observed.[5] These granulomas are similar to those seen in other types of allergic or hypersensitivity reactions.

Patients with presumed halothane hepatitis frequently develop low titers of antibodies to mitochondria, which suggests that halothane or one of its metabolites has combined with mitochondria, rendering them antigenic. The antimitochondrial antibodies tend to disappear with recovery from the disease. Stimulation of lymphocytes by halothane, as measured by incorporation of tritiated thymidine into the deoxyribonucleic acid of lymphocytes, occurs in most patients with presumed halothane hepatitis but not in healthy controls, patients with hepatic disease or in patients who were exposed to halothane but did not develop liver damage.[6] The lymphocyte stimulation or sensitization appears to be temporary. The test may prove to be valuable for diagnosis of halothane hepatitis.

In summary, it would appear that halothane can cause hepatitis and acute hepatic necrosis, probably by means of a delayed sensitization reaction. However, we do not know that the cause is the same in all patients and, in some patients, it may be due to a toxic metabolite of halothane. To minimize the occurrence of halothane hepatitis, we recommend that the drug be avoided in patients having a history of unexplained fever, jaundice or eosinophilia (or all of these) following a previous operation. Unexplained temperature elevation alone, however, should not contraindicate subsequent use of halothane.

Although not usually possible, it is highly desirable to ascertain the prior anesthetic experience of such patients to determine whether halothane had been used. In general, we also tend to avoid the repeated administration of halothane in the same patient over short intervals (i.e., less than 3 months) and in patients with known liver disease. We recognize that the rationale for avoiding use of halothane in patients with acute or chronic cirrhosis is unsound, because if halothane hepatitis is an allergic disease, patients with cirrhosis are no more susceptible than the general population. Even so, if hepatitis should occur in these patients, it would be difficult not to incriminate halothane. Our practice is to avoid the almost universal tendency these days to think first of halothane as the agent of choice. Rather, we prefer to use halothane only when other solutions to the anesthetic problem, such as the use of regional anesthesia, spinal or epidural anesthesia, nitrous oxide-narcotic combinations, nitrous oxide combined with spinal or epidural anesthesia (single-dose or continuous anesthesia) and flammable agents such as cyclopropane or ether, have been considered.

Recognized authorities in the field advise that halothane should be avoided in patients with allergic histories (e.g., asthma and hay fever). There is, however, no sound evidence that patients with general allergies are more susceptible to halothane hepatitis and we have continued its use, where necessary or indicated, in such patients. Finally, it would seem unwise to substitute other halogenated hydrocarbon anesthetics (methoxyflurane or fluroxene) for halothane in patients who have a suspected history of halothane hepatitis. Reports of hepatitis from these agents also can be found.

A less serious complication following the use of halothane is intense shivering. It occurs in the early postoperative period and is self-limiting in an hour or so. It is thought to be caused by the accidental total body cooling that occurs commonly in patients anesthetized in cool operating rooms. Apparently the temperature regulating mechanisms in the brain detect the loss of heat and attempt recovery by inducing shivering and increasing heat production. No specific drug therapy seems indicated in these patients.

FLUROXENE (FLUROMAR)

Fluroxene is fluorinated ether (trifluoroethyl vinyl ether); its physical properties are shown in Table 14-1. The compound is packaged in brown bottles and contains 0.01% N-phenyl-1-naphthylamine to prevent polymerization and hydrolysis to acetaldehyde and trifluoroethanol in the presence of light and moisture.

Although developed prior to halothane, the drug has never gained widespread acceptance. Because of its flammability, its mild ethereal odor and its penchant for producing postoperative nausea and vomiting, it is regarded by many anesthetists as having no distinct advantages over diethyl ether. Its advocates would argue to the contrary. In concentrations of 4% or less, the drug is not flammable; except for induction, this concentration is quite adequate for surgical anesthesia when combined with nitrous oxide. The odor of fluroxene is not as unpleasant as diethyl ether and, in fact, it can be difficult to distinguish fluroxene by odor from halothane. The tendency to produce nausea and vomiting is real and has been estimated to occur in about 50% of patients receiving the drug. Unlike ether, however, the distress does not usually persist for more than 1 or 2 hours after operation, and most patients are relatively amnesic to its occurrence.

Because its vapor pressure is similar to that of halothane, the drug may be vaporized in the same type of vaporizers used for halothane (copper kettle, Vernitrol or Fluotec) and delivered via a standard circle or nonrebreathing system. Fluroxene is used almost invariably with 50 to 70% nitrous oxide; the necessary concentrations are 4 to 8% for induction and 2 to 4% for maintenance. Muscle relaxation is not profound but is usually adequate for endotracheal intubation, so that muscle relaxants are not always needed. Fluroxene is a stimulant of salivary secretions; therefore, atropine or scopolamine are essential premedicants.

The principal advantages of fluroxene are those of a rapid induction and recovery and minimal effects on respiration and circulation (see Chapters 19 and 20). Like halothane, fluroxene undergoes biotransformation, probably in the liver. About 12 to 15% of the drug is excreted in the urine as nonvolatile metabolites (probably trifluoroethanol glucuronide and trifluoroacetic acid). Fluroxene is not a suitable substitute for halothane in patients thought to be candidates for halothane hepatitis. As use of the drug increases, reports of hepatic necrosis are beginning to appear[7]—primarily because of the concern about hepatitis associated with halogenated agents. Whether these are primary drug effects or drug interactions is not clear.

METHOXYFLURANE (PENTHRANE)

Methoxyflurane is a halogenated ether, its formula being 2,2 dichloro-1,1 difluoroethyl methyl ether. Its physical properties are shown in Table 14-1. It is packaged in opaque bottles and contains 0.01% butylated hydroxytoluene (an antioxidant) to enhance stability during storage. The odor of methoxyflurane is sweet, often being likened to that of Juicy Fruit gum.

Methoxyflurane is the most potent of the known inhalation anesthetics; this is its principal advantage. Concentrations as low as 0.2 to 0.4% are adequate to maintain surgical anesthesia. However, because potency is directly related to solubility, methoxyflurane is the most soluble of the inhalation anesthetics. Herein is one of the three major disadvantages of this drug. Because of its extreme solubility in all body tissues, induction of and recovery from anesthesia are quite slow. As a result, methoxyflurane is rarely used for induction of inhalation anesthesia; rather, anesthesia is usually induced with thiopental, or other short-acting barbiturates, and the use of nitrous oxide (50 to 70%) is essential. Usually, repeated small doses of thiopental (25 to 50 mg) are needed to prevent patient movement during the first 15 to 30 minutes of induction. Muscle relaxants are generally required for endotracheal intubation. Because of its low vapor pressure, the maximal deliverable concentration is 3%. This concentration is used during the first 5 to 10 minutes of induction. Methoxyflurane may be vaporized from a copper kettle, Vernitrol or a vaporizer (Pentec) specially designed for the use of this agent.

Recovery from anesthesia, like induction, is slow because of the solubility. The anesthetist therefore must anticipate the conclusion of the operation well in advance (45 minutes to 1 hour) to avoid a period of prolonged anesthetic depression and unconsciousness in the recovery room. Such advanced predictions are not easily made, even by experienced anesthetists. Because of the long induction and recovery times, this drug is relatively unsuitable for operations that have anticipated durations of less than 2 hours.

Like halothane, methoxyflurane is a potent depressant of both respiration and circulation (see Chapters 19 and 20). More important, though, are its adverse effects on the liver and kidneys. There are several case reports of acute hepatitis and fatal hepatic necrosis following methoxyflurane administration. Because the clinical syndrome, biochemical changes and histologic lesions are indistinguishable from those produced by halothane, the mechanism may be one of a delayed sensitization reaction.[8, 9] Hence methoxyflurane is not a suitable substitute for halothane in patients suspected of being susceptible to anesthetic hepatitis.

METHOXYFLURANE AND RENAL FAILURE.—Unlike other inhalation anesthetics, methoxyflurane has also been shown to be a potent nephrotoxin.[10,11,12] The results of studies in rats and of prospective studies in man suggest the following:

1. Methoxyflurane is directly toxic to the kidneys. Consequently, the incidence of the disease will relate directly to the dose and duration of administration.

2. The onset of the disease usually occurs within 24 hours of administration but may be delayed for 2 or 3 days postoperatively.

3. The disease is characterized by polyuria, hypernatremia, an increased serum concentration of urea nitrogen and serum hyperosmolality. The inappropriate diuresis (from 4 to 7 liters/day) may result in profound dehydration and weight loss. The kidney loses its ability to concentrate or dilute urine, as evidenced by a relatively fixed specific gravity (1.010) and loss of responsivity to Pitressin or fluid administration.

4. The course of the disease varies from complete recovery in 10 to 20 days to prolonged impairment of renal function and, occasionally, death.

5. The probable cause of the disease is the effect of metabolites of methoxyflurane. Biotransformation begins immediately after methoxyflurane enters the body. Less than 40% of the drug is excreted unchanged; the remainder either undergoes cleavage at the ether linkage to form CO_2, fluoride ion, and dichloroacetic acid or undergoes dechlorination and oxidation to methoxydifluoroacetic acid.[13] The two acids may undergo further degradation to oxalic acid. Both the fluoride ions and the oxalic acid appear to be toxic to the kidneys. Patients with this disease show increased concentrations of inorganic fluoride in their serum.[11] Fluoride injections into rats cause a polyuric renal failure similar to that seen in man.[12]

6. Histologic examination of the kidneys shows degenerative changes in the convoluted tubules with dilation, pyknosis of cell nuclei and slough of necrotic tubular epithelial cells.[12] Oxalic acid crystals may be seen in the lumen of tubules. Electron microscopy shows mitochondrial swelling, degeneration and rupture.

Because of the clearly documented nephrotoxic property of methoxyflurane, we believe that the drug should not be used in routine clinical care. Our reasoning is as follows: First, there are no surgical procedures for which methoxyflurane is clearly the ideal anesthetic agent to the exclusion of all other drugs or technics; methoxyflurane has no properties that are of special value in anesthesia and surgery. Second, because anesthetic drugs are available in such an adequate number and variety, one should never have to use methoxyflurane for lack of a suitable drug. Third, although the manufacturer of methoxyflurane advises use of the drug in its lowest effective dose and for periods not exceeding 4 hours, there is no guarantee that subcellular toxic changes may not occur even if these precautions are heeded. We do not know whether such changes occur or whether they may result in renal failure at a later time. Fourth, because the clinical manifestations of the disease are subtle in onset and the patient may become seriously ill before the polyuric nephropathy is diagnosed, failure of diagnosis or misdiagnosis places the patient at increased risk of death. Finally, there is no specific treatment for the disease except that of supportive care and careful regulation of fluid intake and electrolyte balance.

Studies of the renal effects of this drug should continue but until more is known about the drug and its short- and long-term effects on the kidney, we urge that it not be used in routine clinical care.

ENFLURANE (ĒTHRANE)

Enflurane is now available for general use. Because of limited clinical use, the data available for the other fluorinated agents are not yet available for this drug. However, it is apparent from laboratory and clinical investigation that it is an effective agent with a MAC value of 1.68. Its solubility is similar to that of halothane and, as a result, induction and recovery are reasonably rapid. The drug has a musty odor but it is well tolerated on inhalation. It produces respiratory depression. Circulatory depression (hypotension) seems to be as frequent and as profound as with halothane. Its principal advantage is said to be due to a more stable molecule; this presumably should result in less biotransformation and therefore less toxicity. However, because during the metabolism of enflurane an inorganic fluoride ion is released in a way that makes it similar to methoxyflurane, it is possible that enflurane may cause nephrotoxicity. A complication peculiar to this drug is the production of abnormal EEG changes with occasional overt muscle twitchings and convulsions. This effect seems to be more prevalent when administration is associated with hyperventilation. Obviously, determination of the role of this drug in clinical practice as a nonexplosive agent must await extensive use. To date its advantages seem to be limited.

ISOFLURANE (FORANE)

At the present time, isoflurane is still controlled as an experimental agent. Its development is another of the efforts to secure a nonflammable agent with a minimum of adverse organ effects such as hypotension and liver toxicity. Laboratory and clinical investigations seem to indicate that the drug has promise in the areas desired but its role in clinical use also awaits extensive clinical application.

As with enflurane, the attempt was made to obtain the beneficial effects of diethyl ether while eliminating its disadvantages.

DIETHYL ETHER

Ether is a colorless liquid having the physical properties shown in Table 14-1. It contains 3% ethanol and is packaged in copper-lined cans to retard oxidation. Exposed to air, it forms peroxides and acetaldehyde.

Ether is rarely used today because of its flammability, disagreeable odor and tendency to produce protracted nausea and vomiting. Its major advantages are respiratory and circulatory support and its ability to produce excellent muscular relaxation. Only small amounts of ether undergo biodegradation in the body, making it a safe anesthetic from this point of view.

TABLE 14-2.—MINIMUM ALVEOLAR ANESTHETIC CONCENTRATIONS (MAC) OF INHALATION ANESTHETICS

AGENT	MAC (%)
Halothane	0.76
Fluroxene	3.40
Methoxyflurane	0.16
N_2O	101.00
Cyclopropane	9.20
Ether	1.92
Isoflurane	1.25
Enflurane	1.68

CYCLOPROPANE

Cyclopropane (trimethane) is a cyclical hydrocarbon whose physical properties are shown in Table 14-1. It is packaged in steel cylinders (sometimes colored orange) at a pressure of 75 p.s.i. It has a characteristic "gastric" odor that is mildly irritating and provokes the formation of copious amounts of salivary secretions. Atropine or scopolamine therefore are essential premedicants.

Cyclopropane is a complete anesthetic in that it will provide surgical anesthesia. Concentrations for induction vary from 20 to 50% and for maintenance from 10 to 20%. The MAC for cyclopropane is 9.2 (Table 14-2). Muscle relaxation with cyclopropane is poor and muscle relaxants are usually necessary when relaxation is desired.

The major advantages of cyclopropane are its rapid rates of induction and recovery and the support of blood pressure, which occurs as a result of its ability to liberate endogenous catecholamines. Except for its flammability, cyclopropane is almost an ideal agent. The drug is flammable at all clinical concentrations and precautions must be taken to avoid static charges in the operating room. Use of conductive flooring and grounding of all objects minimizes the hazards of static charges. Use of the electrosurgical cautery is prohibited during cyclopropane anesthesia. Finally, to minimize the amount of cyclopropane circulating in the room, the drug is always given in a closed-circle system, maintenance flows consisting of just the amount of oxygen and cyclopropane necessary to balance uptake. These precautions, together with adequate ventilation and humidification of the operating room, will prevent the occurrence of explosions. Indeed, the incidence of explosions with cyclopropane, even when it was used frequently, was less than the incidence of toxicity owing to sensitization or biotransformation of halogenated agents. Probably the primary reason for the profound decrease in use of cyclopropane is the widespread use of the electrocautery.

NITROUS OXIDE

Nitrous oxide (nitrogen monoxide, N_2O) is the oldest known inhalation anesthetic, having been prepared by Priestley in 1776 and recognized for its anesthetic properties by Humphry Davy in 1799. Despite its early recognition, another 50 years passed before it became widely recognized for its anesthetic properties.

N_2O is an odorless gas which is marketed in color-coded (blue) cylinders as a liquid under pressure of about 750 p.s.i. It is usually administered in concentrations of 50 to 70% at flow rates (per minute) that vary from 7 liters during induction to 2 or 3 liters during maintenance of anesthesia. The drug can be given in a closed system by matching anesthetic inflow to uptake, but to do this precisely and safely requires the use of an oxygen analyzer to ensure that the inspired O_2 concentration is acceptable.

The principal disadvantage of N_2O is its relative lack of potency. Almost invariably, other anesthetics must be used with nitrous oxide to achieve surgical levels of anesthesia. Among those that can be used include thiobarbiturates, opiates, more potent inhalation anesthetics and agents producing conduction anesthesia. Muscle relaxants also must be used if muscle relaxation is needed. However, the need for supplemental agents is not meant to imply that the contribution of N_2O to the total anesthetic management is insignificant. Indeed, it is not! N_2O serves at least two valuable purposes. First, it provides good analgesia, as evidenced by the fact that when N_2O is administered in concentrations of 50 to 60% it decreases the anesthetic requirement for halothane or fluroxene by 50 to 60%. Second, because of its low blood solubility, the onset of analgesia and amnesia from N_2O is rapid, which thereby compensates for the lack of these properties among most other anesthetics. To gain maximal effectiveness from N_2O, it should be administered at high flows (7 or 8 liters/m) for the first 10 minutes with careful attention to leaks in the anesthetic system (e.g., around a mask) that cause dilution of N_2O by room air. The initial high flow is needed for two reasons. First, it is necessary to compensate for the high diffusibility of N_2O and its rapid disappearance, therefore, from the lung. Second, it is necessary to permit more rapid denitrogenation and thus a lung full of N_2O and oxygen rather than N_2O, nitrogen and O_2.

N_2O depresses respiration and circulation approximately in proportion to its potency as an anesthetic (see Chapters 19 and 20). It is devoid of muscle relaxing properties. It also has little, if any, effects on uterine tone or contractility; hence its widespread popularity and usage as a supplemental anesthetic for obstetrics. Although there is no evidence that N_2O undergoes any significant degree of biotransformation in man, it is by no means biologically inert.[14] The drug has been shown to cause enzyme induction, bone marrow depression and teratogenic effects with prolonged administration (hours to days).

As testimony to its lack of toxicity, the contraindications to the use of N_2O are few and these relate mostly to its ability to cause hypoxemia. When inhaled in high concentrations (60 to 70%), it may cause hypoxemia in a manner similar to that produced by nitrogen in room air. Obviously, hypoxemia is inevitable if an erroneously high concentration is administered. Less apparent are cases of blood or tissue hypoxemia that occur because of unsuspected hypoventilation or ventilation-perfusion abnormalities in the lungs or because of a sudden unexpected depression of circulation from whatever cause. In our opinion, use of N_2O should be questioned when the pulmonary function is known to be abnormal or when sudden respiratory or circulatory depression may occur. Without frequently repeated blood-gas analysis, hypoxemia is extremely difficult to detect in unconscious or anesthetized patients. Because of this, it is prudent to avoid the use of N_2O and to rely on other, more potent, drugs when hypoxemia is of potential occurrence.

Diffusion hypoxia is a complication that in modern anesthetic practices is unique to N_2O. It occurs at the termination of N_2O/O_2 anesthesia if the patient is allowed to breathe room air. Although N_2O and nitrogen are both relatively insoluble in blood, nitrogen is only about 1/30th as soluble as N_2O. Consequently, at the end of anesthesia with N_2O, molecules of N_2O pass from the blood into alveolar gas spaces in a volume that is 30 times the volume of nitrogen taken up into the pulmonary blood. The net result is a dilution of alveolar O_2 and arterial hypoxemia. The decreases in Pa_{O_2} range from 5 to 15 torr, but may be much greater if pulmonary (airway obstruction) or circulatory (shunting) disorders occur. The problem can be obviated by administering 100% O_2 for 1 to 2 minutes at the end of anesthesia before the patient is allowed to breathe room air.

REFERENCES

1. Black, G. W.: A review of the pharmacology of halothane, Br. J. Anaesth. 37:688, 1965.
2. Cullen, B. F., Margolis, A. J., and Eger, E. I.: The effects of anesthesia and pulmonary ventilation on blood loss during elective therapeutic abortion. Anesthesiology 32:108, 1970.
3. Subcommittee on the National Halothane Study of the Committee on Anesthesia, National Academy of Sciences—National Research Council. Summary of the National Halothane Study: possible association between halothane anesthesia and postoperative hepatic necrosis, J.A.M.A. 197:775, 1966.
4. Klatskin, G., and Kimberg, D. V.: Recurrent hepatitis attributable to halothane sensitization in an anesthetist, N. Eng. J. Med. 280:515, 1969.
5. Dordal, E., Glagou, S., Orlando, R. A., and Platz, C.: Fatal halothane hepatitis with transient granulomas, N. Eng. J. Med. 283:357, 1970.
6. Paronetto, F., and Popper, H.: Lymphocyte stimulation induced by halothane in patients with hepatitis following exposure to halothane, N. Eng. J. Med. 283:277, 1970.
7. Reynolds, E. S., Brown, B. R., Jr., and Vandam, L. D.: Massive hepatic necrosis after fluroxene anesthesia—a case of drug interaction?, N. Eng. J. Med. 286:530, 1972.
8. Klein, N. C., and Jeffries, G. H.: Hepatotoxicity after methoxyflurane administration, J.A.M.A. 197:207, 1966.
9. Brenner, A. I., and Kaplan, M. M.: Recurrent hepatitis due to methoxyflurane anesthesia, N. Eng. J. Med. 284:961, 1971.
10. Crandell, W. B., Pappas, S. G., and Macdonald, A.: Nephrotoxicity associated with methoxyflurane anesthesia, Anesthesiology 27:591, 1966.
11. Mazze, R. I., Trudell, J. R., and Cousins, M. J.: Methoxyflurane metabolism and renal dysfunction: clinical correlations in man, Anesthesiology 35:247, 1971.
12. Mazze, R. I., Cousins, M. J., and Kosek, J. D.: Dose-related methoxyflurane nephrotoxicity in rats, Anesthesiology 36:571, 1972.
13. Holaday, D. A., Rudofsky, S., and Trenhaft, P. S.: The metabolic degradation of methoxyflurane in man, Anesthesiology 33:579, 1970.
14. Cohen, E. N.: Metabolism of volatile anesthetics, Anesthesiology 35:193, 1971.

CHAPTER FIFTEEN

Uptake and Distribution of Inhalation Anesthetics

THE PRIMARY OBJECTIVE of clinical anesthesia is to obtain a tension in the brain of appropriate drugs sufficient to induce anesthesia. With present technics, however, inhalation anesthetics cannot be presented directly to the brain; rather, they must be administered through the lungs to arterial blood and thence to the brain. By obtaining and holding the desired tension of anesthetic gases in the alveoli, one can in time attain the same tension in arterial blood and brain and thereby achieve an anesthetic state.

The movement of molecules from inspired gas to brain and other tissues is called uptake. When uptake is complete, the brain and other tissues are then in equilibrium with the concentration of gas in the lungs; movement in and out of lung (or blood) is equal. Many factors influence the uptake of anesthetic drugs.

FACTORS INFLUENCING UPTAKE OF ANESTHETIC DRUGS

Pulmonary Ventilation

The first step in uptake is pulmonary ventilation, which transfers molecules from the inspired gas to the lungs. The greater the ventilation, the more rapidly will the alveolar tension of an anesthetic reach the inspired tension. It is not total minute ventilation but rather the "effective," or alveolar, ventilation that determines uptake. Only alveoli that are in direct communication with pulmonary capillary blood can contribute molecules to arterial blood. Hence, the greater the wasted ventilation fraction (dead space) of total ventilation, the greater the delay in achieving the desired arterial anesthetic tension. Also, any decrease in ventilation as a result of factors such as partial or complete airway obstruction, excessive premedicant depression or partial paralysis limits the rate of development of an alveolar tension of anesthetic gases and thereby delays induction. Conversely, any increase in ventilation that is the result, for example, of excitement or positive pressure breathing increases the rate at which the alveolar tension reaches that being inspired.

Another pulmonary factor to be considered is the volume of gas in the

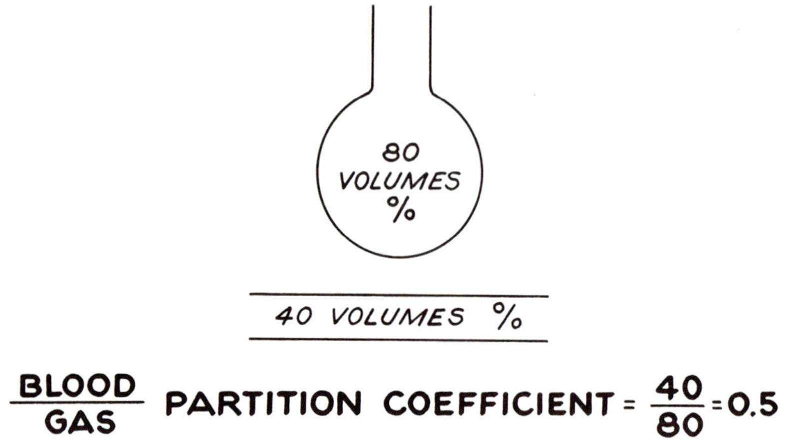

Fig. 15-1.—Theoretical blood-gas partition coefficient for nitrous oxide. Alveolus contains nitrous oxide 80 vol% while adjacent pulmonary capillary, at equilibrium, contains 40 vol%. This gives blood-gas partition coefficient of 0.5; in reality, ratio is 37.6/80 = 0.47 (Table 15-1). [From Eger, E. I., II: in Gray, T. C., and Nunn, J. F. (eds.): *Inhalational Anesthesia: Pharmacokinetics in General Anaesthesia* (3rd ed.; London: Butterworths, 1971).]

lungs diluting the inspired anesthetic gas. This volume is the functional residual capacity (FRC); that is, the lung volume at resting end-expiration. The larger this diluent volume, the slower the rate at which the alveolar tension reaches the inspired tension. For example, induction may be delayed in patients with chronic obstructive lung disease in part because of large FRC values. The reverse might be true for patients with restrictive lung disease and small FRC values.

Classic experiments in denitrogenation of the lungs have shown that if alveolar ventilation and FRC are normal, oxygen tension in the lungs reaches inspired tension (pure oxygen) in about 3 minutes. The same would be true for anesthetic gases; that is, the tension of anesthetic gas in the lungs would quickly reach that being inspired except that, unlike oxygen (which has a low, fixed [at rest] rate of loss from lungs to blood), there is a variable loss of molecules of anesthetic gas from lungs to blood. The loss is great at the start of anesthesia and gradually diminishes as inhalation of gas continues. The major factors that regulate the rate of loss of molecules of anesthetic gas from lungs to blood (i.e., uptake) include solubility, cardiac output (and hence pulmonary circulation) and tension of anesthetic gas in mixed venous blood.

Solubility

Solubility of anesthetic gas in blood and tissues is one of the primary factors influencing the development of anesthetic tension in the lung. All anesthetic gases are soluble to some extent in blood. As anesthetic gas molecules reach the alveoli, a proportion thereof—depending upon their solubility—move into the pulmonary capillary blood and are carried away to

TABLE 15-1.—PARTITION COEFFICIENTS OF SOME INHALATION ANESTHETIC AGENTS (AT 37 C) IN ORDER OF INCREASING BLOOD SOLUBILITY

ANESTHETIC GAS	PARTITION COEFFICIENT: BLOOD/GAS	OIL/GAS	TISSUE/BLOOD	VENOUS CLEARANCE RATES IN ONE PASSAGE THROUGH LUNGS %(a)
Ethylene	0.14	1.3	1 (Brain, heart)	84
Cyclopropane	0.42	12	1 (Brain)	66
Nitrous oxide	0.47	1.4	1 (Brain, heart)	63
Fluroxene (Fluormar)	1.4	48	1.4 (Brain)	36
Isoflurane (Forane)	1.4	98		36
Enflurane (Ēthrane)	1.9	98		30
Halothane (Fluothane)	2.3	224	2.6 (Brain)	26
Diethyl ether	12	65	1 (Brain)	7
Methoxyflurane (Penthrane)	13	970	2 (Brain)	6

(a) Venous clearance rates are calculated values.[1]

the tissues. If the loss of molecules of anesthetic gas into the blood equals that being inhaled, the alveolar anesthetic tension cannot increase, and so neither can arterial blood and brain tensions. The greater the solubility of an inhalation anesthetic in blood, the greater its uptake into blood, the slower the rate of rise of the alveolar tension of anesthetic to that being inspired and the slower the induction of the anesthetic state.

Anesthetic solubility may be expressed several ways but, for our purposes, the most useful expression is as a ratio of the concentration of anesthetic between two phases at equilibrium. This concentration ratio is called a *partition coefficient.* For example, if the alveolar concentration of nitrous oxide is 80 vol.% and this were in equilibrium with a pulmonary blood concentration of 40 vol.%, the blood/gas partition coefficient would be 0.5 (Fig. 15-1). Partition coefficients of anesthetic gases are conventionally blood/gas or tissue/blood ratios. The *Ostwald solubility coefficient* is the same as a partition coefficient when 1) a gas phase exists and 2) the anesthetic gas is at 1 atmosphere pressure.

Solubility coefficients for some of the commonly used inhalation anesthetics are shown in Table 15-1. These can be divided into three general groups according to their solubility in blood: 1) the relatively insoluble agents, ethylene, nitrous oxide and cyclopropane; 2) the moderately soluble agents, fluroxene, isoflurane (Forane), enflurane (Ēthrane) and halothane; and 3) the highly soluble anesthetics, diethyl ether and methoxyflurane (Penthrane). From this information and the knowledge that solubility in blood determines in large part how much anesthetic is taken up into the blood from the lungs, we can predict that induction of anesthesia will be most rapid with nitrous oxide or cyclopropane, slower with agents such as halothane and prolonged with methoxyflurane.

Anesthetic gases differ as well in their solubility in fat. Using oil as a representative of body fat, solubility may be extremely low (e.g., with nitrous oxide), moderate (e.g., with halothane), or high (e.g., with methoxyflurane). Anesthetic gases having a high fat solubility also have a high solubility in tissues such as brain that contain a large amount of fat. For example, both halothane and methoxyflurane have brain/blood partition coefficients exceeding 2 (see Table 15-1). Tissue solubility affects uptake by serving as a reservoir for anesthetic gas. The greater the tissue solubility, the greater the amount of anesthetic that is removed from arterial blood traversing tissues. As a result, less anesthetic is contained in mixed venous blood returning to the lungs; therefore, more anesthetic is taken up from the alveoli as the blood traverses the lungs, thereby delaying the rise in alveolar tensions. Fortunately, from the standpoint of induction of anesthesia, the brain is a member of the vessel-rich group of tissues (e.g., heart, kidneys, and viscera) that receives 75% of the cardiac output, despite constituting only 6% of the body mass. As a result, the time required for equilibration with the alveolar concentration is less for these tissues than for tissues having a much lower blood supply (e.g., fat).

Solubility in blood and other tissues affects not only the rate of induction of anesthesia but also the rate of recovery from anesthesia. During recovery from anesthesia, when the inspired concentration of anesthetic gas is low or zero, the alveolar concentration of anesthetic gas is determined by the balance between the amount of anesthetic gas released by blood into the alveoli and the amount removed from the alveoli by pulmonary ventilation. The greater the solubility in blood and tissue of an anesthetic, the greater the reservoir of anesthetic gas available to be excreted by ventilation and the longer the recovery period. The amount of anesthetic cleared from mixed venous blood during a single passage through the lungs will vary from a predicted high value of 84% with ethylene to a low value of 6% with methoxyflurane (see Table 15-1).

Values for anesthetic solubility for any agent will vary somewhat, depending on the composition and temperature of the tissue into which the anesthetic is being dissolved. For example, anesthetic solubility in blood will increase when the blood contains abnormally large amounts of protein or lipids; this is especially true for the more fat-soluble agents. Solubility for all anesthetic agents increases as body temperature decreases; hypothermia enlarges the reservoir for anesthetic drugs and thus delays induction or recovery from any agent. Hyperthermia would have the opposite effect but, except in rare instances, the temperature increase is too small to be of practical importance.

Anesthetic gases are soluble in varying amounts not only in body tissues but also in anesthetic apparatus, especially the rubber used for conductive tubing and reservoir bag, in direct proportion to solubility in lipids. Rubber goods saturated with anesthetic gas may delay recovery by maintaining an unexpectedly elevated inspired concentration when the inflow concentration is zero. Anesthetists can avoid this problem by using apparatus made of plastics which have a very low anesthetic solubility or by substituting fresh rubber goods at the conclusion of anesthesia.

Cardiac Output

Changes in cardiac output affect the rate of induction of anesthesia in just the reverse manner to changes in pulmonary ventilation. As ventilation is increased, more molecules of anesthetic gas are deposited per minute into the lungs and the more rapid is the increase in alveolar and brain anesthetic concentrations. In contrast, an increase in cardiac output delays development of an alveolar anesthetic gas concentration by rapidly carrying away those molecules deposited in the pulmonary capillary blood. As a result, the higher the cardiac output, the lower the alveolar concentration and the slower the induction of anesthesia; for example, during excitement, induction with inhalation drugs may be prolonged. A low cardiac output may have the reverse effect because, although each unit of blood passing slowly through the lung may take up more molecules, the total amount of blood passing through the lungs is decreased and the total uptake is diminished. As a result, alveolar concentration increases more rapidly and the greater gradient between alveoli and blood augments the input of molecules of anesthetic gas into blood from lung, thus reversing the initial lower uptake. It is especially important for the anesthetist to remember this when inducing anesthesia in patients in shock or those suffering from low cardiac output. Induction will be unexpectedly rapid and anesthetic overdose is a real hazard.

Venous Anesthetic Concentration

Another factor that influences uptake, and hence the rate of induction of or recovery from anesthesia, is the difference in anesthetic tension between alveolar gas and venous blood (P_A-P_V). Early in induction of anesthesia, arterial blood deposits most of its anesthetic gas into tissues and venous blood returns to the lungs with a low anesthetic gas tension. With time, however, tissues remove lesser amounts of anesthetic gas from arterial blood and venous gas tension increases. When this venous blood having a higher anesthetic gas tension reaches the lungs, the gradient between lung and blood is diminished and less anesthetic is transferred from lungs to blood.

COMPENSATORY MEASURES INFLUENCING UPTAKE

The anesthetist can influence anesthetic uptake and so alter the rate of induction or recovery in several ways. These include regulation of the inspired concentration, the inflow volume, the effective ventilation, or the cardiac output.

Concentration Effect

Induction with an inhalation agent may be expedited by increasing the inspired concentration of the agent. Regardless of the agent, the higher the inspired concentration, the more rapid the approach of the alveolar concentration to that being inspired. The effectiveness of increasing concentration, however, varies with the agent. Increasing the inspired concentration is most effective with agents such as diethyl ether, which has a low solubility but must be given in relatively high concentration. Increasing the concentration is less effective with agents such as nitrous oxide, which has a low solubility but must be given in high concentration. Increasing the concentration is least effective with agents such as halothane, which has a high solubility[1] but needs only low concentrations to produce anesthesia. The phenomenon whereby the higher the inspired concentration, the more rapid the increase in the alveolar concentration and hence induction of anesthesia, is called the concentration effect.[2]

The concentration effect can influence the rate of induction of more than one anesthetic at a time. If two anesthetic gases are administered simultaneously, one in high concentration (e.g., N_2O 70%) and one in low concentration (e.g., halothane 0.5%), the rapid uptake of nitrous oxide will not only cause its own concentration to increase but also that of halothane, thereby hastening the rate of rise in the alveolar halothane concentration. This is called the second gas effect.[2]

Flow Rates

The rate of induction also can be hastened by using a high flow rate of anesthetic gases. The higher the inflow volume, the more rapidly the anesthetic system is depleted of nonanesthetic gases, including those being exhaled by the patient. Use of high-flow rates (7 liter/min or more) is particularly important for achieving rapid induction with agents of low solubility (e.g., nitrous oxide). However, the greatest benefits of high flows are attained in the first 10 minutes and little is gained in continuing them beyond that time. Use of high inflow volumes has little application to drugs of high solubility.

Ventilation

Although augmenting ventilation hastens induction, the effect is much greater for the more soluble than for the less soluble anesthetics. Augmenting ventilation does hasten induction with nitrous oxide or cyclopropane but the effect is short-lived. After 10 to 20 minutes, changes in ventilation have little influence on anesthetic depth with nitrous oxide, if one ignores any changes in cerebral blood flow that the ventilatory changes may have induced. Induction (or recovery) with soluble agents is appreciably enhanced by augmenting ventilation. The combination of controlled ventilation and use of a high inspired anesthetic concentration may rapidly result in anesthetic overdose and death. It is therefore extremely important to reduce the inspired concentration of soluble agents when ventilation is augmented or controlled. The input of anesthetic gases is increased also with controlled or augmented ventilation in gas machines that do not have check valves to prevent transmission of increased pressure in the anesthetic system to the liquid anesthetic in vaporizers.

Cardiac Output

Manipulation of cardiac output by such maneuvers as changes in body position, fluid infusion, and vasopressor therapy can alter rates of induction and anesthetic depth. As with changes in ventilation, changes in cardiac output affect the uptake of soluble agents much more than that of the insoluble ones. A potentially lethal situation exists when soluble agents are given in high concentrations to patients who have a low cardiac output, who have air hunger and hyperventilation or who, because of compensatory vasoconstriction, have minimal flow to organs other than the brain and heart. In general, under these circumstances the insoluble agents such as nitrous oxide or cyclopropane are less apt to cause sudden anesthetic overdose. If more soluble agents are used, the anesthetist must be alert to early signs of anesthetic overdose and be prepared to decrease the inspired concentration.

Ventilation-Blood Flow Ratios

Ventilation-blood flow abnormalities in the lungs are common in patients undergoing general anesthesia and surgery, and may influence anesthetic uptake and rate of induction or recovery. This abnormality has a greater impact on the uptake of insoluble than on that of soluble anesthetics. For soluble agents, the areas having normal ventilation-blood flow relationships can compensate for the abnormal areas, and total uptake is little changed from normal. However, no such compensation can occur with insoluble agents and, consequently, induction or recovery may be unusually prolonged.

REFERENCES

1. Larson, C. P., Eger, E. I., II, and Severinghaus, J. W.: The solubility of halothane in blood and tissue homogenates, Anesthesiology 23:349, 1962.
2. Eger, E. I., II: Inhalational Anesthesia, in Gray, T. C., and Nunn, J. F. (eds.): *Pharmacokinetics in General Anaesthesia* (3d ed.; London: Butterworths, 1971), pp. 439-464.

CHAPTER SIXTEEN

Intravenous Anesthetics

THIOPENTAL

THIOPENTAL is a representative of a group of ultrashort-acting barbiturates that can be injected intravenously for induction and maintenance of anesthesia. Thiopental is the sulfur analogue of sodium pentobarbital. *Thiamylal*, the sulfur analogue of sodium secobarbital, and *methohexital*, an oxybarbiturate, are the other commonly used members of this class of compounds; they resemble thiopental in most of their pharmacologic properties.

Thiopental is packaged in bottles as a pale yellow powder, to which sterile distilled water is added to yield the 2.5% solution that is used in anesthesia. Thiopental is strongly alkaline (pH, 10 to 11) because sodium carbonate (6 mg/gm) is added to prevent the precipitation of the insoluble barbituric acid radical upon exposure to atmospheric carbon dioxide. The alkaline pH is beneficial in that it makes the solution bacteriostatic, but it also makes it incompatible with acid solutions. Thiopental must be given separately from drugs such as meperidine, morphine or ephedrine to prevent precipitation in the intravenous line.

For induction of anesthesia the usual dose of thiopental ranges from 2 to 3 mg/kg body weight. Some anesthetists precede this dose with a test dose (25 to 75 mg) and wait 1 minute to determine the pharmacologic effect. As we have already emphasized, such a dose is that recommended for the "average" healthy patient. The anesthetist always must adjust this dose to patients who are not "average"; for example, the debilitated, the aged, patients who have had prior heavy premedication or those who have received large doses of narcotic associated with nitrous oxide-narcotic anesthesia. The susceptibility of a patient's cardiovascular system to depression by thiopental may be gauged by measuring the arm-to-tongue circulation time and changes in blood pressure. In the absence of narcotic or other major respiratory depression, the patient characteristically takes two to three deep breaths just prior to becoming unconscious. As a result, it is not necessary to ask the patient to count or to repetitively inquire if he is asleep. For maintenance of anesthesia, thiopental is used with nitrous oxide for procedures of short duration (less than 30 minutes). Muscle relaxation from thiopental is poor and muscle relaxants are used as needed.

Thiopental has a rapid onset of action, producing unconsciousness within 1 to 2 minutes. Recovery from a single intravenous injection is equally rapid because of redistribution of thiopental from the brain to other organs such as muscle, the blood flow and total mass of which are both large. Prolonged administration, however, leads to drug accumulation in all tissue compartments and these depots cause excessive drowsiness or unconsciousness in the postoperative period. Thiopental is metabolized almost completely, the primary site being the liver. The rate of metabolism averages 10 to 15% of the injected dose per hour; this contributes in part to hastening the rate of emergence from the drug.

Thiopental is a potent depressant of both respiration and circulation and should be given cautiously to patients with disorders of either of these systems. Patients may become apneic, and ventilatory support or preoxygenation may be advisable. Coughing, sneezing and laryngospasm—especially in patients with a history of allergies—sometimes are associated with the administration of thiopental; probably these are due to the lack of depression (perhaps potentiation) of pharyngeal and laryngeal reflexes. If it occurs, one should suspect minimal contamination of the upper airway with mucus, gastric content, gum or some other foreign material. By increasing the dose or following the drug with succinylcholine one can usually stop the irritation and its manifestations. Although reports of allergic reactions to thiopental are rare, hypersensitivity can occur.

The adverse effect of thiopental and similar agents on the heart and circulation is, unfortunately, often discounted. There is ample evidence to demonstrate that thiopental can profoundly depress myocardial function, even when given in "usual doses." There is evidence also that, especially in the patient with impaired cardiac function and hypovolemia (i.e., fluid and blood loss), the "usual" doses of thiopental can result in cardiac arrest.

Thiopental readily crosses the placental barrier, and maternal and fetal blood levels reach equilibrium within 3 minutes of injection. Therefore, unless delivery can be accomplished within 1 or 2 minutes, it should be delayed for as long as is feasible after an injection of thiopental.

Because of its alkalinity, thiopental is irritating to tissues. An extravascular injection of a small volume is of no concern, but a large volume, depending on the site of injection and local vascularity, may cause extensive necrosis. Intra-arterial injections should also be avoided because the drug can cause pain distal to the injection site, arterial spasm, loss of pulse and, occasionally, loss of parts of an extremity. Should this occur, immediate therapy is indicated; it includes stopping the injection and injecting a solution of local anesthetic (up to 5 ml of 1% lidocaine) or papaverine (40 to 80 mg) into the artery (through the same needle). Additional therapy may include sympathetic blockade (stellate or brachial plexus block) to relieve pain, lessen the spasm and increase the collateral circulation and also systemic heparinization to prevent thrombosis.

Occasionally, patients manifest generalized shivering after a thiopental anesthetic. The cause for this is not known but is thought to be loss of body heat or increased sensitivity to cold. Treatment is symptomatic but, if the shaking becomes excessive, it may be controlled effectively with methylphenidate (10 mg) or chlorpromazine (5 to 10 mg).

In summary, the use of thiopental is contraindicated in patients with hypersensitivity to barbiturates, who give a history of porphyria or who are are in status asthmaticus. Its use should be questioned in patients with severe cardiovascular or respiratory disorders or who are in shock. Resuscitation equipment must be immediately available whenever use of this drug is anticipated.

CHAPTER SEVENTEEN

Dissociative Anesthetic Agents

NEUROLEPTIC DRUGS

NEUROLEPTIC ANESTHESIA, as the name implies, is anesthesia with neuroleptic drugs. The neuroleptic state is characterized by two features: 1) complete disinterest and detachment from the environment (dissociative anesthesia) *without* loss of consciousness or ability to communicate with others; and 2) loss of desire to move or change the body position. In its extreme form, the patient may forget to breathe or move his respiratory muscles.

The drug that is commonly used to produce neurolepsis is droperidol. It may be used alone, as in the treatment for nausea and emesis, but usually it is combined with fentanyl in the preparation known as Innovar. "Neuroleptic anesthesia," however, is due to the droperidol and not to the fentanyl. Fentanyl is a narcotic and behaves like a narcotic; when used with nitrous oxide, its contribution to the nitrous oxide-narcotic anesthesia is the same as that of any other narcotic. There is, in fact, little significant difference between "neuroleptic anesthesia" and the usual nitrous oxide-narcotic anesthesia except for the addition of small amounts of droperidol. What particular element droperidol adds to anesthesia achieved with nitrous oxide other than decreasing the frequency of nausea, is difficult to specify.

Droperidol has additional pharmacologic actions worthy of note. It is an alpha-adrenergic blocking drug and hence can cause peripheral vasodilation and hypotension. It is a potent antiemetic, thereby lessening the incidence of nausea and vomiting when used in combination with opiates. Its duration of action is from 6 to 12 hours, which is in contrast to that of fentanyl (30 minutes to 1 hour). Rarely, droperidol may cause behavioral disturbances such as mild, fleeting hallucinations or extrapyramidal seizures. Usually these require only supportive treatment.

The combination of fentanyl and droperidol (Innovar) is useful for premedication, for induction of anesthesia and as a supplement to regional anesthesia. For premedication, the dose of Innovar ranges from 0.5 to 2 ml intramuscularly; the same dose range is applicable to its use for supplementing regional anesthesia. As an adjunct to general anesthesia with nitrous oxide, Innovar is usually given in increments of 1 to 2 ml every 5 minutes until anesthesia is achieved. We find it inadvisable to continue the combination of fentanyl and droperidol for maintenance of nitrous oxide-narcotic anesthesia because the droperidol accumulates within the body and produces prolonged postanesthetic confusion and exaggerated dissociative responses. If given too rapidly, Innovar may cause rigidity of the muscles, especially of the chest and abdomen, which makes assisted or controlled ventilation impossible. Muscle rigidity, which is probably caused by fentanyl, can be reversed by a narcotic antagonist such as naloxone or by a muscle relaxant (succinylcholine or *d*-tubocurarine).

KETAMINE (KETALAR)

Ketamine is another recently introduced dissociative anesthetic agent. Ketamine is a phencyclidine derivative; this family of compounds has both depressant and stimulatory effects on the central nervous system. Ketamine is prepared in concentrations of 10, 50 and 100 mg/ml; it has an acid pH (3.5 to 5.5) and so cannot be mixed with barbiturates. Given intravenously in doses of 1 to 2 mg/kg, the onset of action is rapid (less than 1 minute) and the duration of action is from 5 to 10 minutes. Ketamine also can be given intramuscularly; the usual dose is 5 to 10 mg/kg, the onset of action is within 5 minutes, and the duration of action ranges from 15 to 30 minutes.

Although ketamine, like droperidol, is classified as a dissociative anesthetic, the two drugs differ in several respects. First, ketamine is a total anesthetic; that is, it produces complete amnesia and analgesia. Supplementation by nitrous oxide and a narcotic, although possible, is not as essential with ketamine as it is with droperidol. Second, the pattern of sleep produced by ketamine is somewhat different from that produced by any other currently used agents. The eyelids usually do not close, nystagmus and generalized hypertonus commonly occur and slight involuntary and purposeless movements may be observed. Increasing the dose of ketamine usually does not abolish these movements and, if they are troublesome, other drugs such as nitrous oxide may have to be administered. Because of the hypertonus, muscle tone in the oropharynx is maintained and airway obstruction from relaxation of soft tissues is an infrequent occurrence. The metabolic disposition of ketamine in man is not known, but studies in rats suggest that most of the drug is biodegraded in the liver and excreted in the urine.

Ketamine usually causes increases in both systolic and diastolic blood pressures, the average increases being about 25% of the resting values. Apparently the rise in blood pressure is due to an increase in both minute volume and in stroke work index and heart rate, the latter usually increasing to about 20% above normal. Peripheral vascular resistance either remains unchanged or decreases. The increased cardiac output and pressor responses from ketamine are thought to be due to liberation of endogenous catecholamines. This property diminishes the hypotension that might be seen in patients with either hypovolemia or shock who require anesthesia.

Respiration usually is not depressed by ketamine and arterial blood-gas values usually remain within normal ranges. Ketamine is a potent sialagogue, an effect that can be difficult to prevent or treat with atropine or scopolamine. It is also a potent cerebral vasodilator, increasing both cerebral blood flow and intracranial pressure. Because of the latter effect, the drug is contraindicated in patients with increased intracranial pressure unless methods are used to minimize the pressure increase. These methods may include intraventricular drainage, hyperventilation or administration of osmotic diuretics, or use of a drug such as thiopental, which has been shown to lessen the pressure change with ketamine.

The major deterrent to the use of ketamine is the frequent occurrence of emergence delirium and hallucinations in the postoperative period. Emergence from ketamine anesthesia is rather slow and, during this period, patients may experience unpleasant dreams, hallucinations or distorted images and may evidence confusion, excitement or irrational behavior. This bizarre behavioral pattern seems to be more common in adults than children. There is some evidence that suggests that this adverse reaction can be minimized by the use of tranquilizers, droperidol or diazepam. One should keep in mind also that respiratory obstruction and nausea and emesis also may occur; as a result, precautions for such complications must be taken.

CHAPTER EIGHTEEN

Muscle Relaxants

Current anesthetic practice recognizes that the state of anesthesia includes several elements, such as analgesia, hypnosis and muscle relaxation. The first two of these elements have long been produced by the inhalation anesthetic agents, narcotics and barbiturates. The introduction of the muscle relaxants into anesthetic practice facilitated the production of the third element and accentuated the effort of anesthetists to be more precise in developing the various components of the anesthetic state. Unfortunately, however, this opportunity to be more precise in the management of anesthesia has been ignored by those who elect to use the relaxants inappropriately. Thus, there is no reliable evidence to indicate that muscle relaxants in common use today contribute anything to analgesia or hypnosis; they provide muscle relaxation only and should be used during anesthesia with only that function in mind.

The relative safety of muscle relaxants, the ease of their administration and their ability to block muscular responses associated, for example, with pain and anesthesia that is too light, tempt many anesthetists to use relaxants inappropriately as substitutes for necessary concentrations or doses or agents that are more efficient in providing analgesia and hypnosis. Inappropriate use is manifest in the unfortunately prevalent practice of administering relaxants, instead of analgesics or hypnotics, when the patient moves in response to pain. Relaxants are often used inappropriately when the circulation fails (e.g., in the presence of hypotension) because concentrations or doses of analgesic or hypnotic drugs are poorly adjusted to the patient's physical state. It is, of course, true that relaxants given inappropriately in these circumstances provide the surgeon with optimal conditions in a patient who does not move; unfortunately, however, ample evidence indicates that such misuse of relaxants often means that a patient is paralyzed but not anesthetized—a state that may be satisfactory for the anesthetist and the surgeon but wholly unsatisfactory for the patient. Some anesthetists claim that it does not matter if the patient recalls events during an operation as long as he does not recall pain. Perhaps this is so; but, in our opinion, if the patient moves, grimaces or otherwise gives evidence of response to a potentially painful stimulus, additional pain relief, rather than additional paralysis, should be provided. We submit that neither our senses nor our instruments are yet sufficiently sophisticated to tell us whether or not, during an operation, the patient can or cannot experience or recall pain. The evidence is that some patients can recall not only events but pain.

It is possible, of course, that relaxants can contribute to the total anesthetic state by relaxing muscles and therefore diminishing the input of stimuli from the periphery to the brain. The diminished input of stimuli due to relaxation of the muscles results in a lesser requirement of other agents in producing the desired anesthetic state. As a result, an appropriate state of analgesia and hypnosis can be established or reestablished with concentrations and doses of anesthetic drugs smaller than would be required in the absence of muscle relaxation.

We firmly believe that relaxants should be used only to provide skeletal muscle relaxation, which thereby diminishes the concentration and dose of analgesic or hypnotic drugs, or both, necessary to produce the desired total anesthetic state. Relaxants used to cover up deficiencies in total anesthetic management as in the prevention or treatment of laryngospasm, movement in response to pain and hypotension due to relative overdose of analgesic or hypnotic drugs (for a particular patient) represent an inefficient and inappropriate use of these valuable adjuncts to anesthesia. Use of relaxants is inefficient and inappropriate in the circumstances mentioned only when they are used to cover input of stimuli other than those coming from tense muscles. For example, if a poor-risk patient is given a relaxant to keep him on the operating table for a surgical procedure not requiring muscle relaxation, this is inappropriate use. If, on the other hand, the concentration of an anesthetic agent can be decreased by relaxation of muscles in a surgical procedure in which muscle tension may be stimulated or a hindrance to surgery, use of relaxants is appropriate.

RELAXANTS IN COMMON USE

d-Tubocurarine, gallamine, pancuronium and succinylcholine are the relaxant drugs that are commonly used. Pancuronium has been introduced quite recently; the evidence indicates that it is now a useful and popular relaxant. Traditionally, the relaxants have been separated into two basic classes: *d*-tubocurarine, gallamine, and pancuronium exemplify the class known as antidepolarizers, nondepolarizers or desensitization drugs, while succinylcholine and the infrequently used decamethonium exemplify the other class, known as depolarizers. It is important and useful to know the basic actions and interactions of these drugs in order to administer them safely, efficiently and appropriately. Although all the particulars of action at the neuromuscular junction are not known, there is sufficient reliable information to permit one to formulate a defensible rationale of the administration of these drugs, to recognize contraindications to the use of the drugs in combination and to treat overdose or residual effects.

The critical element in the action of either antidepolarizing or depolarizing drugs seems to be the impact of the drugs on the transmission of and the response to acetylcholine (Fig. 18-1). As a result, one can anticipate some effect of relaxant drugs in any system in which acetylcholine is the chemical

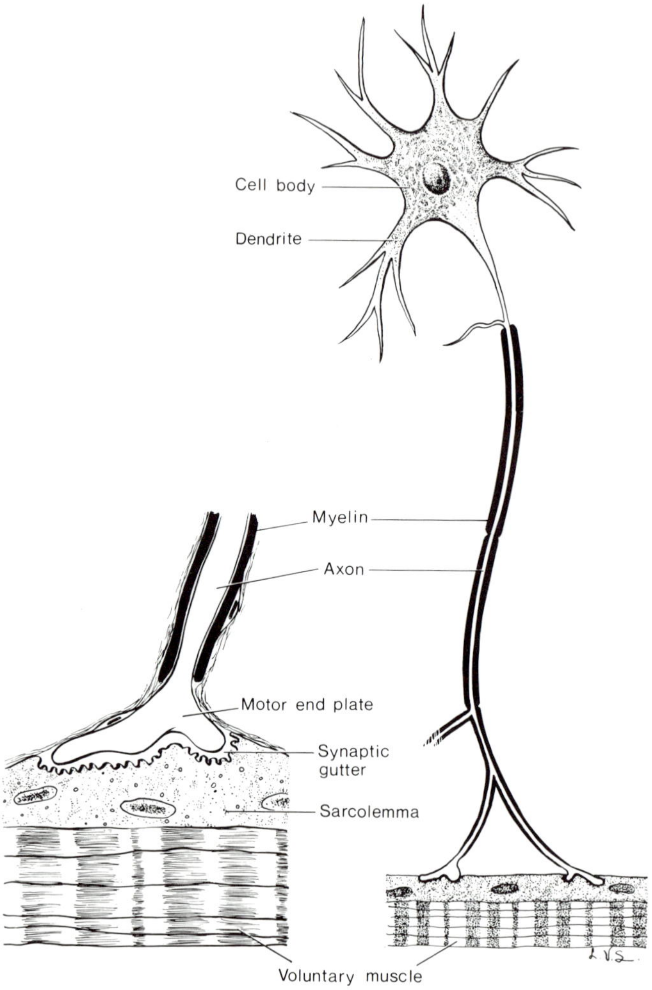

Fig. 18-1.—Schema of neuromuscular junction. Located in motor end plate is acetylcholine, the normal activating substance, in numerous small vesicles. The principal ions involved (K and Na) in changes in potential are located within motor end plate (K) and on outside of nerve structure (Na) in the resting state. Receptors responding to acetylcholine and to muscle relaxants are located in synaptic gutter and to some extent in sarcolemma.

mediator. This means that it is possible that relaxants might block ganglionic action and might even have an impact on cerebral function. The evidence is, however, that in doses used clinically and with the exception of relatively large doses of *d*-tubocurarine, there is no demonstrable clinical effect on ganglia and no demonstrable cerebral effect.

Depolarizing Relaxants

Succinylcholine and decamethonium derive their designation as depolarizing relaxants from the evidence that they function in much the same manner as does acetylcholine. Good evidence supports the concept that relaxant and acetylcholine compete for receptor sites on the postjunctional membrane. Succinylcholine, as does acetylcholine, depolarizes the postjunctional membrane and causes the common fasciculation of skeletal muscles. Subsequently, repolarization occurs but muscle relaxation persists, presumably due to the inability of acetylcholine to gain access to the receptor sites.[1] The relatively short-term action of succinylcholine may be due to the relative weakness (in relation to *d*-tubocurarine) of its bonding action at the receptor site. If the receptor sites are flooded with succinylcholine or if disturbances in blood flow allow succinylcholine to remain in contact with the postjunctional membrane for longer than usual, more receptor sites are occupied by succinylcholine and are therefore unavailable to acetylcholine. As a result, muscle relaxation is prolonged and the situation at the postjunctional membrane is similar to that existing with *d*-tubocurarine, an antidepolarizer. In this circumstance, the postjunctional membrane is insensitive to acetylcholine and the block is a desensitization block. This state has been dubbed "Phase 2 block." Many anesthetists believe that denial of access to acetylcholine, desensitization or Phase 2 block exists to some degree whenever succinylcholine is administered and that the clinical evidence of a Phase 2 block appears only when sufficient receptors are occupied to make the desensitization type block apparent.

Antidepolarizing or Desensitizing Relaxants

d-Tubocurarine, gallamine and pancuronium derive their designation as antidepolarizers, nondepolarizers or desensitization relaxants because they block the access of acetylcholine to receptor sites in the postjunctional membrane without inducing depolarization of that membrane. The popular theory is that these drugs compete with acetylcholine for the receptor sites. Acetycholine will displace the relaxants only when it is present in larger amounts or concentrations (as occurs after the administration of neostigmine). The termination of the action of a relaxant is due to the ultimate displacement of the relaxant from receptor sites by acetylcholine, in proportion not to the concentration of acetylcholine present but rather to the total quanta of acetylcholine to which the receptors are exposed. Occupation of the receptor sites by relaxant, whether it be due to the strong bonding of *d*-tubocurarine and similar drugs or to the overwhelming of receptor sites by succinylcholine, results, as we have said, in prevention of action of acetylcholine and desensitization of the postjunctional membrane.

Feldman has challenged the traditional concept of action of the relaxants at the neuromuscular junction.[2] He postulated that, although succinylcholine and decamethonium do depolarize the postjunctional membrane, the subsequent persistence of relaxation is a function of a relatively short-term bonding at the receptor site. The end result, of course, is a temporary interference with normal action of acetylcholine. According to Feldman, if the receptor sites are flooded with or exposed to succinylcholine (e.g., in cases of circulatory impairment), then succinylcholine—despite its weak bonding property at the receptor site—may bond more firmly and with more receptor sites. By so doing, access to receptor sites by acetylcholine is prevented and

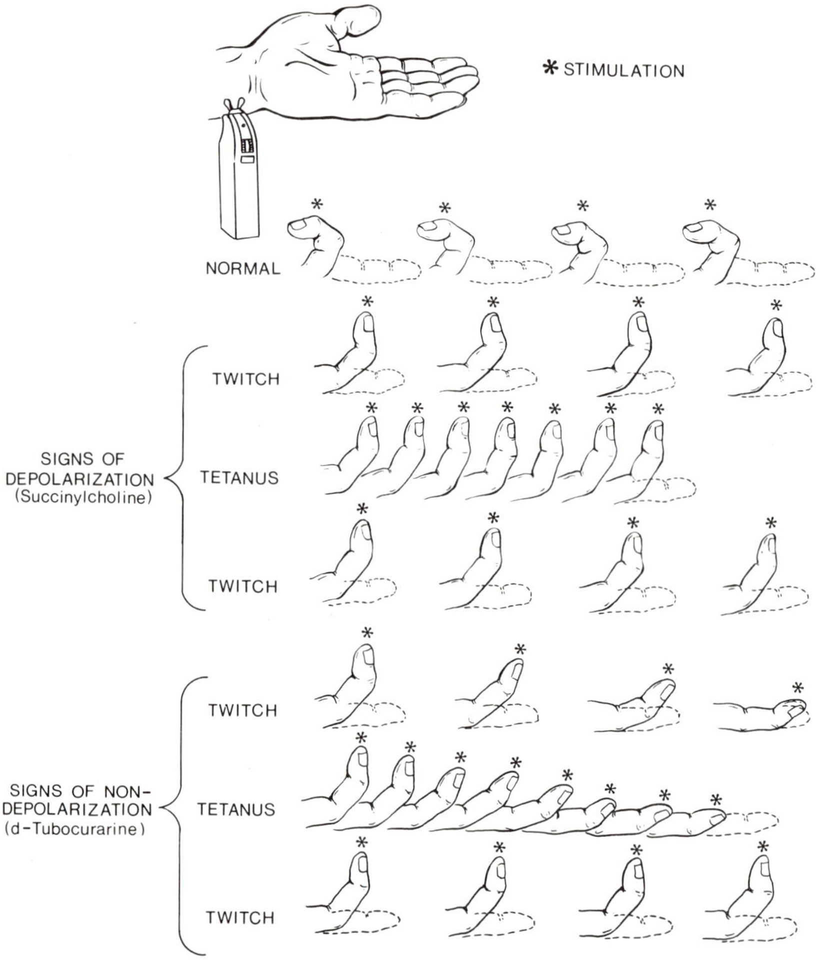

Fig. 18-2.—Changes in finger movement in response to either twitch or tetanic stimulus. Diminution of finger movement with both twitch and tetanic stimuli but no "fade" (successive reduction in extent of finger movement) with a depolarizing drug (e. g., succinylcholine); however, in presence of nondepolarizer (e. g., *d*-tubocurarine) there is not only decrease in extent of finger movement but also "fade" in extent of movement with both twitch and tetanic stimuli. Finally, there is augmentation (facilitation) of extent of finger movement with first twitch stimulus after tetany (*lowest line*). [After Wylie, W. D., and Churchill-Davidson, H. C.: *A Practice of Anaesthesia* (3rd ed.; London: Lloyd-Luke, 1972).]

a block similar to that produced by *d*-tubocurarine is in effect. This hypothesis relative to the desensitizing drugs is attractive also in that it explains the ultimate displacement of drugs such as *d*-tubocurarine from receptor sites on the basis of bonding strength. The bond ultimately becomes weakened, even with a drug such as *d*-tubocurarine, and acetylcholine succeeds in displacing the relaxant.

Recent unpublished evidence indicates that some of the different actions of gallamine (e.g., increased resistance to antagonism with neostigmine) may be attributable to the fact that its major site of action is at the motor nerve terminal rather than the postjunctional membrane. If so, and although it responds to current tests in the same manner as desensitizing drugs, gallamine may represent a different class of relaxant. However, increasing evidence supports the hypothesis that *d*-tubocurarine, as well as gallamine, may act, at least in part, at the motor nerve ending also. Relaxation may be a function of a block of the output of acetylcholine with occupation of receptor sites at the postjunctional membrane. As a result, action of at least two of the antidepolarizing drugs may be presynaptic as well as postsynaptic.[3,4]

Differentiation of the type of block present at the postjunctional membrane is done not only by sophisticated neurophysiologic methods but by a relatively simple clinical test. This test involves application of galvanic current to relatively exposed motor nerves such as the ulnar nerve at the elbow, the radial and ulnar nerves at the wrist or the facial nerve just anterior to the ear. In the presence of nondesensitization block due to succinylcholine, application of a repetitive stimulus will result only in a diminished muscular response with no decrease in successive twitch heights. Application of a tetanic stimulus will result in a diminished muscle response but no fade of the tetanic contraction and no facilitation of the twitch response to a subsequent single stimulus. On the other hand, if the block is of the desensitization type such as occurs with *d*-tubocurarine, there will be a gradual decrease in the height of the twitch response with successive single stimuli. There will also be a decrease (fade) in the muscle response to a tetanic stimulus and a facilitation (increase in height) of the twitch to a single stimulus applied after the tetanic stimulus (Fig. 18-2).[5] Recently, a somewhat more refined and precise use of electrical stimuli was recommended.[6] Evidence indicates that if trains of four stimuli of the same frequency are applied, the ratio of the height of the fourth twitch to the height of the first twitch is a more sensitive indicator of the presence of relaxant effect than the application of either repetitive single stimuli and tetanic stimulus. Unfortunately, current apparatus and technics necessary for successful application of this measure of muscle response do not lend themselves to the rigors and the costs of everyday clinical assessment. Similarly, the electromyograph can be more precise in the definition of neuromuscular block. Its drawbacks, however, are cost and the precision with which it must be used, and it is therefore not currently adaptable to use in the operating room.[7]

APPROPRIATE APPLICATION OF RELAXANTS

By taking into account the basic actions of the relaxants and by remembering that there are initial fundamental differences and that these differences are to some extent time- and dose-dependent, it is possible to use them rationally, safely and efficiently. Accordingly, it makes sense to limit the use of short-acting relaxants such as succinylcholine to situations in which short action is desired. If longer action is needed, *d*-tubocurarine and similar drugs are more appropriate. Succinylcholine also may be used in the form of a continuous infusion over a long period of time. If used in this manner, the anesthetist must remember that the major action will change to that of the desensitizing drugs; as a result, there is little to be gained from attempting to adapt a basically short-acting relaxant to requirements of long duration.

A question often arises as to the appropriateness of using the different types of relaxant in the same patient during the same procedure. Because the postjunctional membrane is desensitized to the action of acetylcholine by *d*-tubocurarine, gallamine and pancuronium, succinylcholine will be less effective in presence of those drugs. Therefore one might expect that larger doses of succinylcholine might be needed if *d*-tubocurarine or a similar drug is present in the body. Fortunately, however, this is clinically insignificant when small amounts of *d*-tubocurarine or a similar drug are used to prevent the twitching associated with administration of succinylcholine.[8] Also, if additional abdominal relaxation is needed for the short period of peritoneal closure, for example, there seems to be little need for significantly larger amounts of succinylcholine if *d*-tubocurarine or a similar drug has been used during most of the operation. Some anesthetists believe that the administration of succinylcholine to a patient who has received *d*-tubocurarine or a similar drug makes the augmentation of the desensitization block more likely. We have seen no convincing evidence of this and, as a result, have no compunction about either using *d*-tubocurarine or similar drugs before succinylcholine or using succinylcholine in patients to whom *d*-tubocurarine or similar drugs have been given—assuming, of course, that common sense is used with respect to dosage and timing. Common sense and proper timing mean that succinylcholine may be used for intubation followed by *d*-tubocurarine or similar relaxants, provided that time is allowed for muscle function to return following administration of succinylcholine before the other type of relaxant is given. Also, if succinylcholine is given while *d*-tubocurarine or a similar drug is still present in the body, one must assess the degree of block from the desensitizing drug before adding succinylcholine. If there is a substantial block attributable to the desensitizing drug, one will need to consider whether the additional necessary relaxation might be more efficiently produced by a small dose of a desensitizing drug rather than by a larger dose of a depolarizing drug. Use of a larger dose of a depolarizing drug in the presence of a slightly ineffective desensitizer might result in protracted relaxation that would be difficult to assess and treat.

THE ACTION OF RELAXANTS

All relaxants are capable of producing muscle relaxation that is limited, for practical purposes, to the skeletal muscles. This, of course, includes the muscles of respiration and one must be prepared always to support respiration. There is an order of impact of relaxants on the muscles: the muscles of the eye and face seem to be most susceptible and the diaphragm most resistant. This difference in response may be due to the physical advantage the muscle may have with respect to origin and insertion and efficiency of pull. The eye muscles, for example, have a poor physical advantage, as do the muscles of the head and neck. The resistance of the diaphragm may be attributable to the relative inaccessibility of the receptors in the circumstance of a less abundant circulation.[2] Clinical effect, determined either by observation or by electrical stimulation, is apparent only when approximately 80% of the receptors are occupied.[9] This evidence makes it clear that there is always a distinct possibility of unrecognized, but effective, residual relaxant effect.

Testing for Relaxant Effect

It is mandatory, therefore, to test for residual effect when any significant amount of relaxant has been used or a relaxant has been knowingly or inadvertently used in susceptible patients (e.g., patients with myasthenia gravis or low or abnormal concentrations of pseudocholinesterase). This can be done either by clinical assessment of the ability of the patient to raise his head and keep it raised for at least 30 seconds or to grasp one's hand vigorously or by testing with an electrical stimulus. It is important to remember that sufficient acetylcholine can be mobilized to displace relaxant at the postjunctional membrane on either one occasion or a short-term basis. This means that a patient may be able to raise his head once for more than 30 seconds or he may be able to grasp one's hand firmly for a few seconds or he may be able to take a few deep breaths. The hazard of residual relaxant, however, is in the patient's inability to sustain muscular effort so that, for example, he can take repetitive deep breaths, can cough effectively and can move about in bed. With the exception of cardiac malfunction associated with hyperkalemia and succinylcholine, abnormalities and deficiencies of cholinesterase and inattention to ventilation, the common hazard in the use of relaxants arises from unrecognized residual effects in the postanesthetic period. Except for the patient's ability to raise and keep his head elevated for 30 seconds or more, the most reliable test for residual relaxant effect is by the electrical stimulator. Such stimulators are readily available on the market (e.g., Blockade Monitor and Churchill-Davidson stimulator).

The best site for making a reliable estimate of the degree and type of neuromuscular block is the ulnar nerve at the elbow or, perhaps, the radial nerve or ulnar nerve at the wrist. There is clinical evidence that using the facial nerve anterior to the ear is distinctly less reliable in assessing the degree of block. Ideally, one should have a reference response at the site and to the degree of electrical stimulus to be used prior to administration of relaxant. Intermittent use of electrical stimuli, provided a base line has been established prior to relaxation, is useful in determining the extent and nature of a neuromuscular block during anesthesia. This objective monitoring helps to prevent one from giving an overdose of relaxant, which may occur with pressure from surgeons for more relaxation. To minimize any overdose, it is usually wise to avoid complete loss of respiratory (diaphragmatic) effort. Rarely, it is necessary to produce a complete block in order to provide satisfactory surgical conditions. If this seems necessary, one should first consider factors such as the depth of anesthesia, the position of the patient, the presence of hypercarbia and the size of the incision. Proper attention to these details often significantly reduces the need for relaxant.

Miscellaneous Influences on Action of Relaxants

pH.—With the exception of gallamine, which acts in exactly the opposite manner, relaxant action is enhanced by a high P_{CO_2} and a low pH and is diminished by a low P_{CO_2} and a high pH. However, it has been shown that a persistently high P_{CO_2} ultimately results in no significant change in response for any class of relaxant.[7] As a result, except when one is using gallamine, it is wise to avoid hypoventilation when attempting to stimulate the patient to breathe again spontaneously.

HYPOTHERMIA.— At temperatures as low as 30° C, hypothermia diminishes the action of *d*-tubocurarine. More intense hypothermia exaggerates the action of *d*-tubocurarine. The action of succinylcholine is minimally affected by cold but, if anything, the reverse action is apparent.

PLACENTAL BARRIER.—Relaxants pass through the placenta. Their diffusibility is dependent upon the chemical structure. The long thin structure of succinylcholine, for example, allows it to pass relatively easily whereas the chunky configuration of *d*-tubocurarine makes it difficult for this relaxant to pass. Pancuronium and gallamine pass easily. Fortunately, the distribution of relaxant administered intravenously diminishes the development of high plasma concentrations, and for practical purposes there is little impact on the fetus.

Detoxification and Elimination

Desensitization relaxants such as *d*-tubocurarine and pancuronium are detoxified in the liver. Gallamine is eliminated in large part by the urine. It is therefore unwise to use gallamine in patients with absent kidneys (prior to transplant) or in patients with poorly functioning kidneys. Decamethonium also is eliminated unchanged in urine. Succinylcholine is destroyed by pseudocholinesterase. This destruction may be limited in patients with low values of esterase (e.g., in debilitated patients and patients with severe liver disease). There also may be abnormal types of pseudocholinesterase. This deficiency is genetically linked and it is wise to inquire into any known sensitivity to succinylcholine. If the sensitivity is encountered unwittingly, one should then test for the presence of an abnormal type of pseudocholinesterase or for low concentrations. If the test reveals genetically related abnormalities it is then wise to make an inquiry into relatives of the patient to alert them to their peculiar sensitivity.

SUCCINYLCHOLINE SENSITIVITY.—Kalow and Genest have concluded that in succinylcholine-sensitive patients the serum cholinesterase is atypical in its properties and probably qualitatively different in structure from the serum cholinesterase present in most people. It seems likely that the low activity of the enzyme in such people is due largely to the decreased, catalytic activity of an abnormal enzyme rather than to a gross decrease in enzyme protein synthesis. They developed a simple test for differentiating enzymes.[10] The percentage inhibition obtained is called the dibucaine number (DN); this is about 20 for the atypical enzyme and about 80 for the usual type of enzyme. Although there are variations, essentially two allelic genes account for the enzyme. One, E_1^u, determines formation of the usual enzyme, whereas E_1^a determines formation of the atypical enzyme. Homozygotes $E_1^u E_1^u$ and $E_1^a E_1^a$ form only the corresponding enzymes whereas the heterozygotes $E_1^u E_1^a$ are thought to synthesize both enzymes.

A more rapid screening method for typical serum cholinesterase suitable for identification of drug sensitive patients and for genetic population studies is available.[11] This has led to the development of a commercially available diagnostic kit that makes use of paper strips.

DETERMINATION OF DOSE

There is a tendency to estimate the dose of a relaxant on a mg/kg basis. Since many factors influence the requirement of relaxant—for example, the anesthetic agent to be used, the level of anesthesia, the site and nature of the operation, the preferences and ability of the surgeon, the stature of the patient, the position of the patient and the presence or absence of hyperventilation—we submit that it is inappropriate to administer the relaxants on the basis of weight. It is necessary, of course, to have some sort of base-line dose; this is discussed in the sections on individual relaxants. In general, if reasonably profound relaxation is needed, as for abdominal surgery, we are inclined to give large doses initially. We base this on the assumption that a better gradient is established between plasma and tissue; this makes for better saturation of receptor sites. Repeated small increments of relaxant (*d*-tubocurarine) tend to increase length of action.[12,13] This latter effect may increase the opportunity for undetected latent effect in the postanesthetic period. We also believe, without objective evidence to support our assumption, that the initial large dose establishes a solid and relatively long-term block thus diminishing the need for subsequent doses and, as a result, a lower total amount of relaxant for a given procedure. We are inclined to believe that the "dribbling in" of doses results in an ultimate larger total amount and more likelihood of residual effect. Obviously, if there is any suspicion of conditions such as myasthenia gravis, general debility, or a low concentration or abnormal type of pseudocholinesterase, we avoid large initial dose. We are disinclined to use test doses routinely, reserving use of a test dose only for those situations in which an abnormal response is suspected. Of the common inhalation agents, ether, isoflurane (Forane) and enflurane (Ēthrane) seem to contribute significant degrees of neuromuscular block so that less muscle relaxant is required. Halothane contributes substantially less to neuromuscular block and more relaxant is required for an equivalent effect. Nitrous oxide contributes essentially nothing to the block and, as a result, relaxants must provide essentially all the relaxation needed.

ANTAGONISM

The approach to reversal of neuromuscular block is based on the following premise. Blocking the breakdown of acetylcholine by acetylcholinesterase will cause the concentration of acetylcholine to increase to such an extent that by mass action acetylcholine can override the occupation of the receptor sites by relaxant and restore muscle tone. As a result, one gives neostigmine (in combination with atropine to negate the muscarinic effect) and observes the restoration of muscle tone. It is convenient to mix neostigmine and atropine in the same syringe, the ratio being 2.5 mg of neostigmine to 1.0 mg of atropine. Usually, an initial dose of 2.0 ml of this combination is given intravenously and restoration of muscle action observed. Repetitive doses are given until satisfactory muscle response is obtained. Except in circumstances of unusual sensitivity to relaxants or overdose, 2.5 mg of neostigmine is sufficient. One may use up to 5.0 mg of neostigmine, but a larger dose may induce additional relaxation rather than antagonism due to the excess acetylcholine produced. If the relaxation is due to succinylcholine or decamethonium through their initial type of action, neostigmine will enhance the block because the actions of the relaxants and acetylcholine are the same. If the relaxation is due to desensitizers such as *d*-tubocurarine or if it is due in large part to the later (desensitizing) action of succinylcholine, reversal of relaxation will take place. Antagonism can be accomplished on a temporary basis by edrophonium (Tensilon). Its action is essentially the same as for neostigmine, but its action is very short. As a result, edrophonium is used primarily to make an assessment of whether neuromuscular block due to relaxants is present and also to differentiate (without inducing a prolonged undesirable effect) depolarizing and desensitization types of block, especially in circumstances in which a substantial element of Phase 2 block may be expected.

Recently, there has been renewed interest in the use of pyridostigmine (Mestinon) as an antagonist of the desensitizing relaxant.[14] It is reported to be superior to edrophonium as an antagonist and equal to neostigmine in efficacy. It does not possess the same degree of muscarinic effects of neostigmine such as heart slowing and production of mucus. As a result, less atropine is needed.

ACTIONS OF SPECIFIC DRUGS

d-Tubocurarine

This relaxant, although the first reliable preparation (as the active ingredient of Intocostrin extract), remains the favorite long-acting relaxant. It is likely that it may be displaced in favor by pancuronium, primarily because of the greater potency and the lack of some of the disadvantages now to be listed.

Hypotension has been associated with use of *d*-tubocurarine. Presumably, hypotension is the result of either a ganglionic blocking action or relaxation of capacitance vessels due to histamine output. There has been some suspicion that the preservative used in preparations of *d*-tubocurarine accounted for the hypotension, but evidence indicates that such is not the case.[15] However, hypotension associated with administration of *d*-tubocurarine usually occurs only when large doses are given to patients with borderline cardiac compensation or hypovolemia. If one encounters hypotension, one should be alerted to the likelihood that some existing but covert circulatory deficiency is made overt by the relaxant. With the aid of more precise continuous measurement of blood pressure, it is now apparent that *d*-tubocurarine causes a rather profound but brief decrease in blood pressure with doses often used for relaxation. Pancuronium does not seem to produce a significant decrease in blood pressure.[16,17]

Histamine output from muscles is a phenomenon peculiar to *d*-tubocurarine. There is no evidence to support the popular notion that histamine output accounts for the hypotension seen. In fact, if the hypotension is dose-related, it is unlikely that histamine is a significant cause. Output of histamine also has been suspected of provoking bronchospasm. We doubt, however, whether there is any clinically significant incidence of bronchospasm following administration of *d*-tubocurarine. Chest stiffness and wheezing coincident with administration of *d*-tubocurarine usually can be assigned to other factors such as an improperly placed endotracheal tube, anesthesia that is too light with straining on an endotracheal tube, reaction to narcotics such as meperidine and preexisting asthma or bronchiectasis. As a result, if bronchospasm is suspected one must look for likely precipitating factors other than *d*-tubocurarine.

A convenient initial dose of *d*-tubocurarine in the "average" 70 kg adult in good condition in whom one is using halothane as the anesthetic agent for an abdominal surgical procedure is from 15 to 30 mg. As has been indicated, this dose should be adjusted if necessary by taking into account the numerous other factors influencing the need for relaxant such as use of another agent and the physical condition of the patient. For example, in the presence of isoflurane (Forane) and ether less relaxant is required. We know of no absolute contraindications to *d*-tubocurarine.

Gallamine (Flaxedil)

Gallamine has proved useful as a substitute for *d*-tubocurarine, primarily because it has a vagolytic action with a consequent increase in pulse rate. Also, it does not cause an output of histamine. It is considered useful in conjunction with halothane because it counteracts the tendency of halothane to produce bradycardia. It seems not to produce hypotension.

Gallamine is eliminated largely through the kidney and, as a result, it should be avoided if kidney function is significantly depressed or absent. The dose of gallamine is equivalent on a volume basis to *d*-tubocurarine (20 mg/ml of gallamine equal to 3 mg/ml of *d*-tubocurarine). A larger dose of neostigmine will be required for antagonism.

Pancuronium

A recently introduced substitute for *d*-tubocurarine is pancuronium. The demonstrated advantages are its lack of histamine output, lack of hypotensive effect and lack of ganglionic blocking.[18] It has a rather rapid onset of action. It interacts with the anesthetic agents and other drugs such as meperidine and thiopental, as does *d*-tubocurarine. The duration of action is approximately the same as that of *d*-tubocurarine. It is, however, five times as potent as *d*-tubocurarine. As a consequence, the equivalent dose for the sample case described for *d*-tubocurarine would be 3.0 to 6 mg. It has less cumulative action than *d*-tubocurarine so that larger sequential doses are required.

Succinylcholine

As the major representative of the class of drugs known as depolarizers or nondesensitizing drugs (except under the circumstances outlined earlier), succinylcholine produces its effect promptly and has a short action. There is evidence that in small children repeated doses provoke profound cardiac irregularities and bradycardia. This is evident chiefly with intravenous administration, and can be avoided usually by subcutaneous or intramuscular injection. Except in the special circumstances outlined later, there is no evidence that hyperkalemia by itself increases the chances of cardiac arrhythmias with administration of succinylcholine. There is debatable evidence that succinylcholine produces a significant increase in the serum potassium concentration in the absence of any other factor. If so, this increase seems to be impeded by the prior administration of any of the desensitizing relaxants. However, the evidence is convincing that in patients with trauma (i.e., until catabolism recedes), burned patients, patients with denervated muscles as in paraplegia or hemiplegia and patients with muscular dystrophy and multiple sclerosis, there is not only an increased serum potassium level but also a pronounced increase with administration of succinylcholine. A substantial degree of hyperkalemia can be eliminated by the prior administration of a desensitizing relaxant.[19-22]

As a consequence of the depolarizing or acetylcholine-like effect of succinylcholine, intragastric pressure may increase. This, together with relaxation of the upper esophageal sphincter, enhances substantially the opportunity for regurgitation of stomach contents. This same action of succinylcholine increases intraocular pressure by contraction of the extraocular muscles. Both of these actions can be effectively eliminated by prior administration of a desensitizing relaxant. As a result, succinylcholine need not be contraindicated in circumstances of a full stomach or in a patient with glaucoma. Myoglobinemia has been reported after intravenous administration of succinylcholine, presumably due to the depolarizing effect.[23] This is much more prevalent in children, which emphasizes a suspected difference in the response of children to this relaxant. Again, however, the output of myoglobinemia can be prevented by the prior administration of a desensitizing relaxant or by giving the drug intramuscularly.

In the average adult, the usual dose needed for relaxation to facilitate tracheal intubation is 60 mg.

Decamethonium

Decamethonium, the other representative of the class of depolarizing drugs, is used relatively infrequently, probably because it has few, if any, advantages over succinylcholine. It has a somewhat longer action than succinylcholine. Perhaps its greatest disadvantage is its inconstancy of action.

SUMMARY

We believe that this outline of the role of muscle relaxants will suffice to encourage and make possible the rational and safe use of these exceedingly useful adjuncts to inhalation anesthesia. The relaxants enjoy a remarkable reputation as safe and useful drugs. They will continue to enjoy this reputation only if they are used intelligently in their proper relationship to the anesthetic state by those who appreciate the role of these drugs in anesthetic practice and are aware of the hazards of indiscriminate and inappropriate use.

REFERENCES

1. Thesleff, S.: Effect of acetylcholine, decamethonium and succinylcholine on neuromuscular transmission in the rat, Acta Physiol. Scand. 34:386, 1955.
2. Feldman, S. A., and Tyrrell, M. F.: A new theory of the termination of action of muscle relaxants, Proc. R. Soc. Med. 63:692, 1970.
3. Sokoll, M.D., Dretchen, K. L., Gergis, S. D., and Long, J. P.: *d*-Tubocurarine effects on nerve terminal and neuromuscular conduction, Anesthesiology 36:592, 1972.
4. Galindo, A.: The role of prejunctional effects in myoneural transmission, Anesthesiology: 36:598, 1972.
5. Miller, R. D., Larson, C. P., Jr., and Way, W. L.: Comparative antagonism of *d*-tubocurarine, gallamine and pancuronium neuromuscular blockades by neostigmine methylsulfate, Clin. Pharmacol. Ther. 13:147, 1972.
6. Hassan, H. A., Utting, J. E., and Gray, T. C.: Quantitative assessment of residual antidepolarizing block (Part I), Br. J. Anaes. 43:473, 1971.
7. De Jong, R. H.: Controlled relaxation, J.A.M.A. 197:393, 1966.
8. Miller, R. D., and Way, W. L.: The interaction between succinylcholine and subparalyzing doses of *d*-tubocurarine and gallamine in man, Anesthesiology 35:567-571 (Dec), 1971.
9. Waud, B. E., and Waud, D. R.: The relation between tetanic fade and receptor occlusion in the presence of competitive neuromuscular block, Anesthesiology 35:456, 1971.
10. Kalow, W., and Genest, K.: A method for the detection of atypical forms of human serum cholinesterase as indicated by dibucaine numbers, Can. J. Biochem. 35:339, 1957.
11. Morrow, A. C., and Motovsky, A. G.: Rapid screening method for the common atypical pseudocholinesterase variant, J. Lab. & Clin. Med. 71:350, 1968.
12. Cohen, E. N., Hood, N., and Canner, P.: Blood pH and plasma levels of *d*-tubocurarine, Anesthesiology 26:727, 1965.
13. Gibaldi, M., Levy, G., and Hayton, W.: Kinetics of the elimination and neuromuscular blocking effect of *d*-tubocurarine in man, Anesthesiology 36:213, 1972.
14. Katz, R. L.: Pyridostigmin (Mestinon) as an antagonist of *d*-tubocurarine, Anesthesiology 28:528, 1967.
15. Stoelting, R. K.: Blood pressure responses to *d*-tubocurarine and its preservatives in anesthetized patients, Anesthesiology 35:315, 1971.
16. Miller, R.: Personal communication.
17. Stoelting, R. K.: The hemodynamic effects of pancuronium and *d*-tubocurarine in anesthetized patients, Anesthesiology 36:612, 1972.

18. Katz, R. L.: Clinical neuromuscular pharmacology of pancuronium, Anesthesiology 34:550, 1971.
19. Mazze, R. I., Escue, H. M., and Houston, J. B.: Hyperkalemia and cardiovascular collapse following administration of succinylcholine to the traumatized patient, Anesthesiology 31:540, 1969.
20. Birch, A. A., Mitchell, G. D., Playford, G. A., and Lang, C. A.: Changes in serum potassium response to succinylcholine following trauma, J.A.M.A. 210:490, 1969.
21. Cooperman, L. H.: Succinylcholine induced hyperkalemia in neuromuscular disease, J.A.M.A. 213:1867, 1970.
22. Schaner, P. J., Brown, R. L., Kirksey, T. D., Gunther, R. C., Ritchey, C. R., and Gronert, G. A.: Succinylcholine induced hyperkalemia in burned patients, Anesth. & Analg. (Cleve.) 48:764, 1969.
23. Ryan, J. F., Kagen, K. J., and Hyman, A. I.: Myoglobinemia after a single dose of succinylcholine, New Eng. J. Med. 285:822, 1971.

PART 5

Respiration and Circulation as Related to Anesthesia

CHAPTER NINETEEN

Respiration

WITH FEW EXCEPTIONS, anesthetic drugs depress respiration. Additional factors such as preexisting pulmonary disease, body position, location of operation, function of anesthetic apparatus and rate and pattern of breathing all may influence the adequacy of ventilation. Consequently, the ability to assess the adequacy of respiration and institute appropriate therapy are important hallmarks of a competent anesthetist.

REGULATION OF RESPIRATION

We believe that the competent anesthetist should have a working knowledge of the regulation of normal respiration in order to assess and treat more effectively the abnormalities encountered in patients as a result of their disease and the impact of anesthesia and surgery. Knowledge of the mechanisms involved in the control of breathing has grown considerably in recent years, and several detailed reviews of this subject are available.[1-3] In this chapter we present a brief description of our current understanding of the mechanisms involved in the regulation of respiration. No attempt will be made to include complex details, not only because it may not be possible but also because, as research in this field continues, currently held ideas may prove to be in error. Moreover, complex details are irrelevant to information appropriate to competent management of anesthesia.

Normal respiration is regulated or influenced by both *neural* and *chemical* stimuli. In 1939, Pitts, Magoun, and Ranson suggested a unified mechanism to explain the neural control of rhythmical respiration. They proposed the existence of a continuously active medullary inspiratory center, which, when unopposed, produced a state of prolonged inspiratory spasm, or apneusis. Periodic inhibition of this tonic activity by the pontine pneumotaxic center and vagal afferent impulses from pulmonary stretch receptors resulted in rhythmic inspiration and expiration. The chemical control of respiration was considered by physiologists to originate from 1) direct stimulation by CO_2 of medullary respiratory neurons, and 2) carotid and aortic body chemoreceptor activity, determined by the P_{O_2}, P_{CO_2}, and pH of perfusing arterial blood. Since their inception, these schemata have been generally accepted as constituting the normal regulatory mechanism for respiration. However, more recent observations, many in serious conflict with this design, have necessitated thorough reevaluation of respiratory regulation.

Neural Control

Most of the recent information about central neural control of respiration has come from the recording of respiratory rate, depth and pattern during certain experimental procedures: progressive ablation of the central nervous system, electrical stimulation of neural areas, with or without subsequent destruction, and intracellular and extracellular microelectrode recordings of neuronal discharges. None of these research technics is technically ideal and the results therefrom are not entirely compatible. The cat has been the predominant experimental animal, but sufficient studies of other animals exist to allow one to conclude that the organization of neural control is probably similar among most mammals.

Located in the reticular substance of the medulla, near its dorsal surface, are cells forming the inspiratory center (IC) (Fig. 19-1). Stimulation of these cells initiates a forceful inspiration; CO_2 breathing increases their discharge frequency, and ablation of this area terminates respiration. Lying slightly more dorsal and cephalad to the inspiratory center are cells comprising the expiratory center (EC) (see Fig. 19-1). Although less discrete in area than the

Fig. 19-1.—Central respiratory mechanisms in medulla and pons of cat. Ventral surface is shown on left and dorsal surface on right. Chemosensitive area (*CSA*) is stimulated by changes in hydrogen ions in cerebrospinal fluid or extracellular fluid of the brain. Medullary chemoreceptors are anatomically distinct from the inspiratory (*IC*) and expiratory centers (*EC*), which are buried within reticular formation near dorsal surface. Location of pneumotaxic center (*PNC*) in pons is also shown. (Scales bordering drawing represent stereotaxic coordinates in millimeters.) (From Severinghaus, J. W. and Larson, C. P.[16])

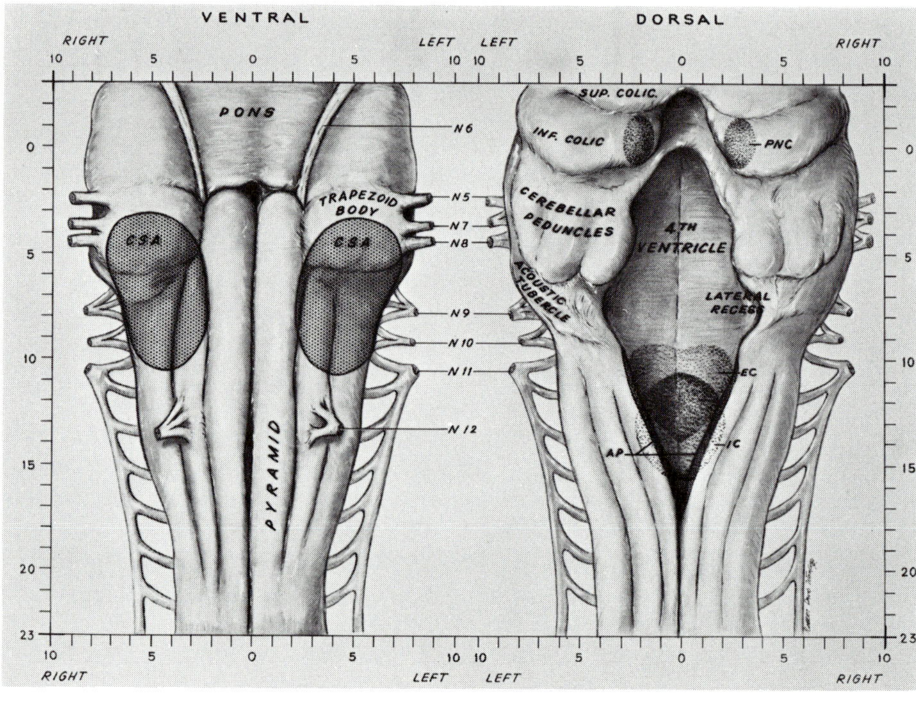

inspiratory center, its function is equally specific. Electrical stimulation of these cells elicits active expiratory spasm.

Transection of the brain stem in the region of the midpons produces apneustic respiration in the cat. This form of breathing is characterized by two alternating phases: a strong inspiratory spasm and a brief expiratory apnea. The usual interpretation of this observation is that the midpontine apneustic center functions to augment, but not supplant, the basic medullary inspiratory drive. To retain a more normal rate and pattern of respiration in the presence of apneustic amplification requires modulation of the inspiratory spasm. Two mechanisms have been postulated, one located in the pons and the other in the lung. The pontine mechanism is called the pneumotaxic center (PNC) (see Fig. 19-1). Electrical stimulation of this area increases respiratory rate and shortens expiratory time, thereby encouraging a more rhythmic respiration. The second mechanism originates from receptors in the airways of lungs and is mediated centrally via vagal nerves and nuclei. These receptors respond to changes in lung volume by inhibiting inspiratory activity, thereby hastening expiration (Hering-Breuer inflation or stretch receptor reflex) or by augmenting inspiratory activity (deflation reflex). The role of the inflation and deflation reflexes in the regulation of respiration is unclear. Recently Phillipson and associates showed that abolition of the Hering-Breuer reflex in conscious dogs has no effect on tidal volume or respiratory frequency.[4] Both the inflation and deflation reflexes from the lungs are thought to be considerably weaker and play a less significant role in respiratory regulation in adult man than in newborn infants or other mammalian species. Under special circumstances in man, such as the sudden development of a spontaneous pneumothorax, lung reflexes may have more profound stimulatory influences on respiration (e.g., increased respiratory frequency and decreased Pa_{CO_2}).[5]

Other neural areas may influence respiration. Certainly, man can exert voluntary control over respiration, probably via cortical pathways. Acts of sneezing, coughing and swallowing also alter respiration through unknown reflex pathways. The state of wakefulness itself may act as an important stimulus to respiration. In the waking state, many forms of sensory stimulation originate from peripheral receptors; for example, cold, pain and limb movement are perceived and evaluated centrally and may alter the rate or pattern of breathing.

All of the impulses from the higher centers and brain stem probably aggregate in a respiratory motor-neuron pool in the spinal cord, where they may be integrated or modified before traveling via phrenic and intercostal nerves to the muscles of respiration.

Chemical Control

Two groups of receptors (Fig. 19-2) participate in the chemical control of breathing.

PERIPHERAL RECEPTORS.—Located in the aortic arch and at the bifurcation of the common carotid arteries are receptors called carotid bodies,

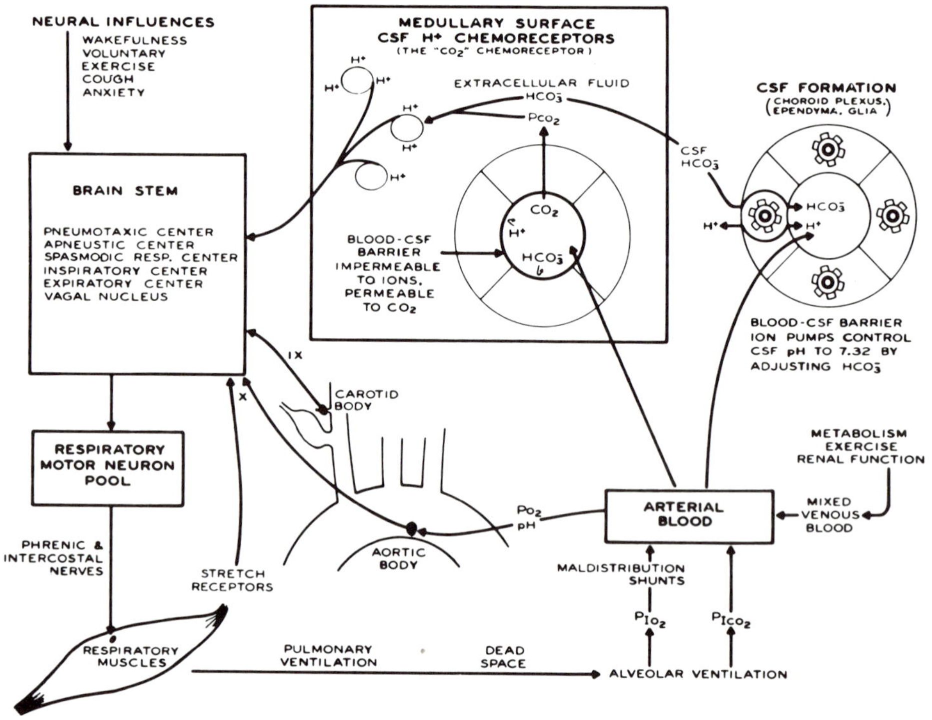

Fig. 19-2.—Schema of neural and chemical control of respiration. See text for details. (From Severinghaus, J. W., and Larson, C. P.[16])

which are capable of modifying respiration in response to changes in composition of perfusing arterial blood. These receptors are active at birth and remain so throughout life. Their impulses are carried to the central nervous system by the glossopharyngeal (nerve of Hering) and vagus nerves.

The physiologic stimuli to which these chemoreceptor cells respond include the following:

1. Decrease in arterial O_2 tension. The relation of chemoreceptive activity to progressive arterial hypoxemia is best described by a sigmoid curve with the maximal rate of discharge occurring at Pa_{O_2} values of 25 to 40 mm Hg. It has recently been shown that, at the Pa_{O_2} of the sea-level environment, chemoreceptors possess tonic activity and contribute a small part toward maintaining man's ventilatory drive.

2. Decrease in arterial pH. Ventilatory response to added hydrogen ions appears to interact synergistically with the hypoxic stimulus; that is, the response to hypoxia and acidosis greatly exceeds that which would be expected from the arithmetic summation of the effects of either stimulus acting alone. An increase in Pa_{CO_2}, which stimulates ventilation, probably results from the acidifying property of CO_2 rather than from the specific action of CO_2 on peripheral chemoreceptors.

3. Decrease in blood flow. The receptor cells have a high oxygen consumption so that any decrease in blood flow (e.g., hypotension and local vasoconstriction) excites chemoreflexes.

4. Change in temperature of the blood perfusing the receptors; warm blood excites the receptors and cold blood has the reverse effect.

The respiratory response to peripheral chemoreceptor stimulation is hyperpnea and tachypnea, and this results in an increase in the minute volume of ventilation. The ventilatory responses to stimulation from aortic and carotid chemoreceptors are qualitatively similar but quantitatively different.

Recent studies indicate that, if aortic bodies do exist in man, they are physiologically inactive. Loss of carotid body function as evidenced by a loss of ventilatory and circulatory responses to hypoxia is a common occurrence following operation at the carotid artery bifurcation for extracranial occlusive cerebrovascular disease.[6] No compensatory respiratory or circulatory responses from the aortic bodies were observed in these patients.

Loss of carotid body responsiveness has been observed recently in two other groups of patients; namely, natives living at high altitudes and children with cyanotic congenital heart disease. Both types of patients show blunted or absent ventilatory responses to hypoxia.

The discovery of carotid and aortic chemoreceptors has generated much interest in exploring the entire arterial and venous system for other active chemoreceptors. Since no consistent relationship has been found between the level of ventilation and the systemic Pa_{CO_2} during exercise, attempts have been made to locate CO_2-sensitive venous receptors to explain the hyperpnea of muscular exercise. The search has been particularly intense about the pulmonary artery, but current evidence is overwhelmingly against the existence of such chemoreceptors.

CENTRAL CHEMORECEPTORS.—Since the respiratory response to inhaled CO_2 could not be accounted for by peripheral chemoreceptors, the brain has been examined for the existence of central chemoreceptors. A chemosensitive area (CSA) has been located on the ventrolateral surface of the medulla (see Fig. 19-1). Perfusing these receptors with mock cerebrospinal fluid (CSF) having a low pH or applying pledgets containing acid, nicotine, or acetylcholine to the receptor area stimulates ventilation. The application of local anesthetics or CSF that is cold (<20° C) has the opposite effect. When apnea is induced with cold or procaine, neither inhalation of CO_2 nor stimulation of the carotid nerve will restore ventilation.

The P_{CO_2} of CSF is determined chiefly by the brain P_{CO_2} because CSF has no blood flow or metabolic activity as a source of CO_2. Being highly diffusible, CO_2 quickly equilibrates between brain and CSF. The brain P_{CO_2}, in turn, is regulated by the Pa_{CO_2}, cerebral blood flow, and brain tissue metabolism, so these factors indirectly influence the CSF P_{CO_2}. However, CSF, unlike blood, has no anions that are readily available to buffer incoming CO_2, and any increase in Pa_{CO_2} increases CSF $H+$ concentration and results in a maximal shift in CSF pH. The resulting ventilatory response is one of hyperpnea and tachypnea in an effort to decrease the arterial and hence the brain P_{CO_2}. The superficial nature of the medullary chemoreceptors, responsive primarily to CSF, and the lack of blood flow to CSF explain the 6- to 10-minute delay in respiration, reaching a new steady state when CO_2 is inhaled.

Recent clinical studies in man either ascending to altitude or made acutely acidotic by ingestion of ammonium chloride indicate that the CSF pH remains relatively constant, despite marked changes in arterial pH. This constancy can only be explained by active transport of ions, presumably HCO_3^-, across the blood-brain barrier. In metabolic acidosis this mechanism works as follows: Acute acidosis stimulates carotid and aortic chemoreceptors, thereby increasing ventilation and decreasing arterial and CSF P_{CO_2}. CSF pH shifts in the alkaline direction, diminishing ventilation and the full peripheral chemoreceptor effect. Within 24 hours, CSF pH is gradually restored to normal by active transport of HCO_3^- out of CSF and breathing increases. If the metabolic acidosis in blood is rapidly corrected, ventilation does not immediately return to normal because any decrease in ventilation results in an increase in arterial, brain and CSF P_{CO_2} and an acid shift in CSF pH. Once CSF pH is restored to normal by active transport of HCO_3^- into CSF, breathing will also return to normal.

EFFECTS OF ANESTHETICS ON RESPIRATION

Evaluation of the Effects of Drugs on Respiration

Evaluation is both clinical and physiologic.

Clinical evaluation.—Clinical evaluation of the adequacy of breathing as applied to the drug depressed, unconscious traumatized or anesthetized patient involves observation of the chest wall and abdomen, auscultation of breath sounds and observation of the movements of the reservoir bag.

Observation of the movements of the chest wall and abdomen.—Normally, the chest wall should rise and the thoracic cage increase in girth during inspiration, the opposite changes occurring during expiration. As outlined in Chapter 7, the magnitude of the respiratory excursions is determined in part by the level of unconsciousness or anesthesia. As this level becomes deeper, the upper thoracic cage ceases to move outward or upward during inspiration and, in fact, may collapse inward at end-inspiration. The inward movement of the upper chest during inspiration probably results from loss of intercostal muscle activity and hence becomes a passive movement in response to the negative intrapleural pressure generated by diaphragmatic action. The lower thoracic cage continues to expand, although expansion is less vigorous as anesthesia is deepened. The characteristic appearance of inward movement of the upper thorax and enlargement of the lower thorax has been likened to a "rocking boat" and is important to observe because it signals the onset of deep surgical anesthesia. The airway obstruction that occurs commonly in this setting mimics this pattern; its characteristic features are described later in this section. Partial muscle paralysis from relaxants or neurologic deficiency may also mimic this pattern.

Auscultation and comparison of the quality and intensity of breath sounds in symmetrical areas of lung.—Breath sounds should be similar in comparable areas of lung. With increasing depth of anesthesia, breathing

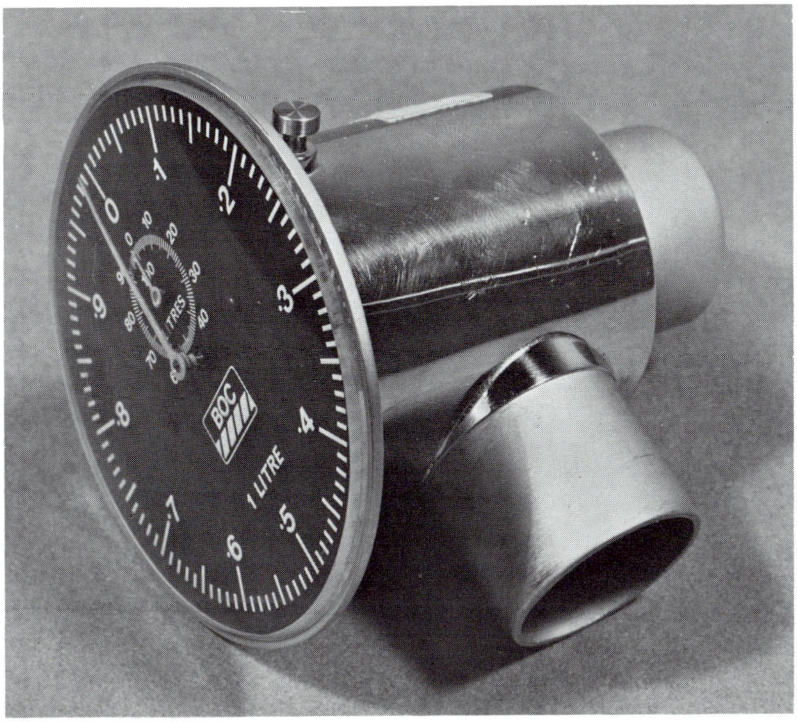

Fig. 19-3.—Wright respirometer for measuring tidal volume and minute ventilation. Device has off-on switch and manual zero reset button. A larger model is available for permanent mounting to an anesthetic machine.

becomes shallower, breath sounds more distant and comparisons more difficult. One can depend on the usual chest piece or esophageal stethoscope for monitoring for evaluation of the presence or absence of breath sounds and their location; however, they fail to measure the volume of air moved. In other words, these monitors can tell whether air is being moved and in what areas of the lung but they cannot tell how much air is being moved. As a result, it is important to correlate the sounds with observation of chest movements and with movements of the rebreathing bag.

Observation of excursions of the reservoir bag.—The anesthetist commonly watches the excursions of the reservoir bag and, with experience, learns to discern adequacy of ventilation and levels of anesthesia by familiarity with the patterns and extent of movement of the bag (Chapter 7). These same patterns can be used by the experienced observer in evaluating respiratory adequacy by using a simple bag and mask applied to the patient's face.

PHYSIOLOGIC EVALUATION.—Reliance on clinical observation for determining the adequacy of ventilation during anesthesia has two major drawbacks. First, while gross changes in the pattern or depth of ventilation are evident, smaller more subtle changes are not. Second, these forms of evaluations lack quantitation. Clinicians have learned that physiologic measurements are more meaningful, reliable and precise in confirming or denying

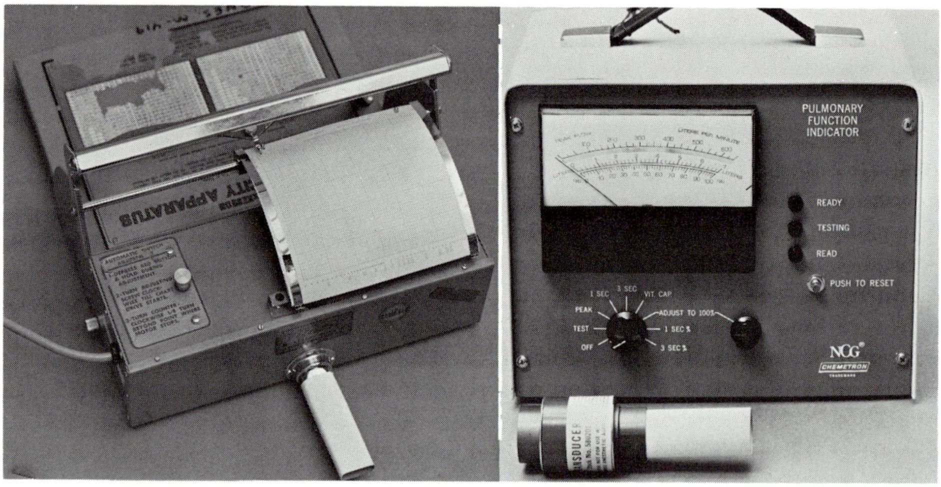

Fig. 19-4.—Devices for measurement of vital capacity, maximal expiratory flow rate and forced expiratory volume (FEV). **Left**, McKesson Vitalor: patient breathes into disposable mouthpiece and flow tracings are recorded on paper that can be removed and placed in patient's chart; average normal values for men and women based on height are inscribed at top of machine. **Right**, electronic spirometer: 1- and 3-sec FEV's can be measured; disposable mouthpiece and transducer in front of machine.

the clinical observations. The physiologic studies most commonly used to evaluate drug action on respiration include spirometry, blood-gas determinations, measurements of ventilatory response to inhaled CO_2 (CO_2 response test) and tests of mechanics of breathing.

Spirometry.—Several devices have been developed for measuring inspired or expired gas volumes, the simplest of which is the Wright respirometer (Fig. 19-3). This device measures tidal volume or vital capacity and its usefulness in operating room and intensive or respiratory care units makes it an essential item in the armamentarium of the anesthetist. More sophisticated mechanical or electronic devices (Fig. 19-4) are available for measuring forced expiratory volume (FEV_1) or maximum inspiratory or expiratory flow rates in addition to measurements of volume. These devices provide rapid, accurate and reproducible values but can be used only when patients are alert and cooperative. Hence the use of the more sophisticated devices is confined to preoperative screening of lung function and to obtaining postoperative values for comparison when the patient has recovered sufficiently from the operation to be pain-free and cooperative.

Significance of changes in spirometric measurements.—Measured decreases in tidal volume or minute ventilation suggest depression of ventilation and increases suggest stimulation. However, one must be cautious when drawing conclusions about the adequacy of ventilation from measurements of tidal or minute ventilation. Decreases in minute ventilation below normal almost invariably reflect a state of ventilatory inadequacy, but the reverse is not necessarily true. Ventilation may be inadequate even though the measured values are normal (5 liters in a 70 kg adult) or above normal. The reasons for this are two. The first is that tidal and hence minute ventilation has two components: that which serves functional alveoli (i.e., alveoli that are ventilated and perfused), and is called "effective" or "alveolar ventilation," and that which serves nonfunctional units, such as unperfused alveoli and conducting airways, neither of which participate in gas exchange. The second of the two components has traditionally been called dead space, but we prefer the term "wasted ventilation" because it denotes the nonfunctional nature of this gas volume. Unless its volume is measured, the fraction of the tidal or minute ventilation that is wasted ventilation is unknown. Normally, the wasted fraction is 40% or less of the tidal volume, but it may become as high as 70 to 80% of tidal volume in certain disease states.

Any events that enlarge the airway size or increase the number of alveoli that are either unperfused or inadequately perfused will increase wasted ventilation. Wasted ventilation is commonly increased to 50 to 60% of tidal ventilation during anesthesia. The possible explanations for this are several. Some anesthetic drugs, such as atropine or scopolamine, increase the size of the conducting airways and thereby the volume of the container for nonfunctional gas. More importantly, events occurring during anesthesia may alter the distribution of the pulmonary circulation and increase the number of alveoli that receive an inadequate supply of blood or no blood at all. Because the pulmonary circulation is a low-pressure system, small changes in pressure within the pulmonary circulation (i.e., 2 or 3 torr) may influence the distribution of blood flow within the lungs. Decreases in cardiac output, increases in intra-alveolar or intrapleural pressure by positive pressure ventilation, or changes in body position (all common events during anesthesia) may shift pulmonary capillary blood flow to the most dependent portions of the lungs and leave the remainder of the lungs inadequately perfused. A portion or all of the ventilation going to these alveoli is then wasted. Because these events are dynamic and constantly changing, wasted ventilation will also change. Hence, only by measuring the volume of wasted ventilation can one be certain of the fraction of tidal volume that is participating in gas exchange.

The second reason why spirometry may be an unreliable indicator of ventilatory adequacy is that the measurement does not provide any information about changes in CO_2 production. General anesthesia decreases whole-body metabolism and hence CO_2 production. This is a dose-related effect, averaging 10 to 15% at light levels of surgical anesthesia and 20% or more at deeper levels. As less CO_2 is produced, less ventilation is required to maintain the same CO_2 excretion via the lungs. Consequently, measured decreases in tidal or minute ventilation without consideration of metabolism may overestimate the magnitude of ventilatory insufficiency. Should hypothermia with shivering or hyperthermia occur in the anesthetized patient, metabolism and CO_2 production may outstrip ventilatory responsiveness. In this case, measurements of tidal and minute ventilation may severely underestimate the degree of ventilatory insufficiency.

Anesthesia and Changes in Ventilation

In view of the limitations of spirometry, what have spirometric studies revealed about the effects of inhalation anesthetics on ventilation? The

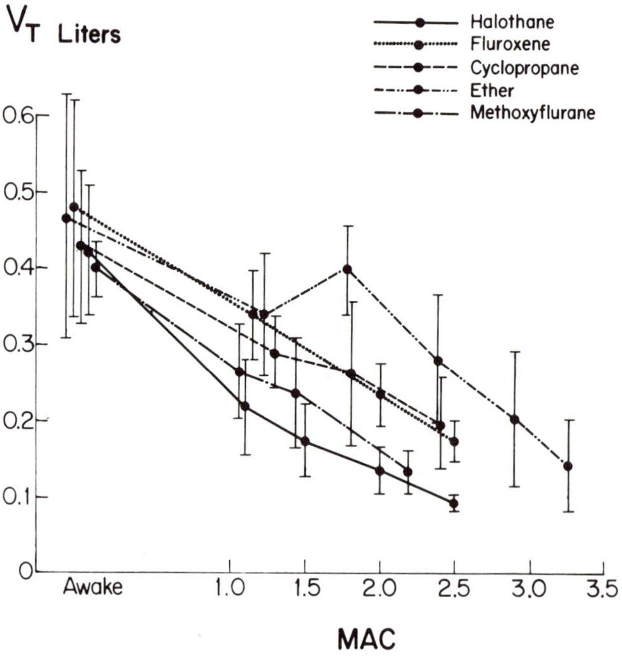

Fig. 19-5.—Effects of depth (dose) of anesthesia on tidal volume in 43 patients anesthetized with one of five agents: halothane, fluroxene, cyclopropane, ether or methoxyflurane. Anesthetic dose expressed in multiples of minimum anesthetic concentration (MAC); tidal volume (V_T) in liters. Decrease in V_T is significantly greater ($P < 0.01$) at all MAC values during halothane than during ether anesthesia. (From Larson, C. P., *et al.*[8])

changes usually observed are those of a decrease in tidal volume and an increase in the frequency of breathing. Recent studies have documented the respiratory effects of the more commonly used inhalation anesthetics in volunteer patients not undergoing surgery and have compared the effects at doses that are multiples of an equipotent concentration (i.e., minimum alveolar anesthetic concentration or MAC).[7, 8] Notwithstanding the evidence that multiples of MAC do not represent continuing (or linear) equipotency for all agents, the observations do give reasonable data on the impact on the various parameters of respiration by the increasing concentrations of agents.

TIDAL VOLUME.—Tidal volume decreases with increasing anesthetic depth with respect to all agents studied, and thus this is a useful clinical sign of relative anesthetic depth. However, the magnitude of this decrease varies among the agents; the decrease is significantly greater for halothane and methoxyflurane than for diethyl ether (Fig. 19-5).

RESPIRATORY FREQUENCY.—Although the respiratory frequency increases with increasing depth in the case of most inhalation anesthetics, the magnitude of the changes with cyclopropane and methoxyflurane is small. This means that with these two agents any change in rate is less useful as a clinical sign of anesthetic depth than it is with halothane, fluroxene, or ether (Fig. 19-6). Except for ether, the increased respiratory rate does not compen-

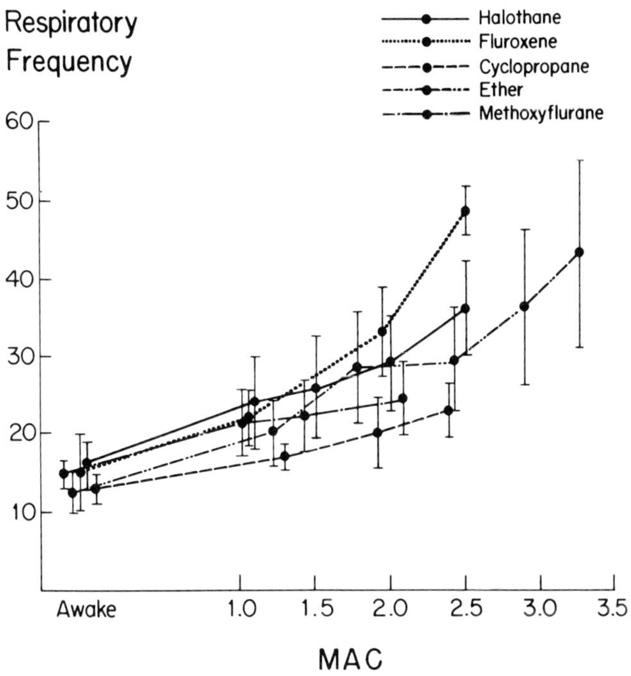

Fig. 19-6.—Effects of depth (dose) of anesthesia on respiratory frequency in 43 patients anesthetized with one of five agents: halothane, fluroxene, cyclopropane, ether or methoxyflurane. Anesthetic dose expressed in multiples of minimum anesthetic concentration (MAC); respiratory frequency in breaths per minute. Changes in frequency are significantly greater during fluroxene anesthesia than during ether, methoxyflurane or cyclopropane anesthesia. (From Larson, C. P., *et al.*[8])

sate fully for the decreased tidal volume and hence the net result is a decrease in minute and alveolar ventilation. Forane, a recently developed inhalation anesthetic, is a potent respiratory depressant; tidal volume decreases with increasing depth and no compensatory increase in respiratory rate occurs.[9]

The tachypnea associated with inhalation anesthesia has been attributed to several mechanisms, as follows: 1) sensitization of the pulmonary inflation and deflation receptors; 2) stimulation of irritant receptors in the airways; 3) stimulation of extrapulmonary sensory receptors such as those that exist in muscle spindles or skin; 4) mobilization of catecholamines that are known to stimulate breathing such as epinephrine; 5) alteration of acid-base balance in the blood or CSF, which thereby stimulates peripheral or central chemoreceptors; and 6) direct central respiratory stimulation. These various mechanisms have been evaluated in dogs anesthetized with ether or halothane.[10] The tachypnea associated with these agents was not abolished by bilateral vagotomy, which would block afferent impulses from lung receptors; by high spinal anesthesia, which would block afferent impulses from extrapulmonary receptors and any neurogenically-induced release of catecholamines; by bilateral carotid body denervation; or by any combination of these maneuvers. Nor was tachypnea necessarily associated with an arterial or CSF acidosis. It was concluded that these anesthetics act on central respiratory mechanisms to increase respiratory frequency.

Because tachypnea occurs so commonly with inhalation anesthesia, anesthetists are naturally inclined to attribute the increase to the pharmacologic effect of the drug on the central nervous system and dismiss other possible mechanisms that also may be active and potentially hazardous to the patient. For example, tachypnea may result not only from the primary action of the anesthetic drugs but also from a preexisting or superimposed hypoxemia, metabolic acidosis or hyperthermia. One must exclude the possibility of these multiple factors before attributing tachypnea to the effect of a drug on the central nervous system.

There is another important precaution. It has been suggested that the efficiency of ventilation might be improved by administering small doses of opiates intravenously in order to lessen the rate of breathing. Opiates decrease breathing frequency in patients anesthetized with halothane but the tidal volume is not increased correspondingly; hence, ventilation and CO_2 elimination are depressed (Munson, E. S., unpublished data). Tachypnea induced by anesthetic drugs should be viewed as a compensatory response to the decreased tidal volume and should not be lessened without simultaneously augmenting tidal volume.

Factors Influencing Blood-Gas Values

The primary function of the lungs is to exchange O_2 and CO_2, the beginning and end products of metabolism. How well the lungs accomplish this function is determined by measurements of blood gases; namely, O_2 (Pa_{O_2}), CO_2 (Pa_{CO_2})and hydrogen ion (pHa).

FACTORS INFLUENCING ARTERIAL O_2 TENSION.—The partial pressure of O_2 in arterial blood (Pa_{O_2}) is determined by the balance between the factors aiding and those impeding the addition of O_2 to blood. These factors are several and must be considered when interpreting a Pa_{O_2} value (Table 19-1).

TABLE 19-1.—FACTORS AFFECTING ARTERIAL OXYGEN TENSION

Inspired oxygen concentration
Concentration of oxygen being delivered
Flow rate of oxygen
Anesthesia circuit
Barometric pressure
Alveolar oxygen tension (PA_{O_2})
Alveolar ventilation
Oxygen consumption
Diffusion anoxia
Ventilation-perfusion abnormalities
Blood temperature, pH, and hemoglobin concentration
Age

Inspired oxygen concentration.—During anesthesia, the inspired O_2 concentration may deviate appreciably from that found in atmospheric air (20.93%). Factors affecting the inspired O_2 concentration include the concentration of O_2 being delivered to the patient from the anesthesia circuit, the flow rate of O_2 delivery to the circuit and the type of anesthesia circuit being used. Inspired O_2 concentrations may intentionally be as low as 30% when 70% nitrous oxide is being administered or as high as 99 or 100% when potent inhalation (halothane, 1.0%) or intravenous (opiates or thiobarbiturates) anesthetics are being used. Moreover, depending upon the anesthetic system used (i.e., open, semi-closed, closed or high-flow vs. low-flow), nitrogen is eliminated or maintained in the system. Any nitrogen present in the lungs will, of course, affect the O_2 concentration in the alveoli. Under special circumstances, such as the first 1 or 2 minutes of induction with nitrous oxide, the experienced anesthetist may choose to decrease the inspired oxygen concentration below 30%. Nitrous oxide, because of its high diffusibility, is rapidly taken up by the blood passing through the lung in the early induction period (3 to 5 minutes). Its rate of uptake is more rapid than that of O_2. As a result, nitrous oxide disappears from the lung faster than O_2 and the concentration of O_2 in the alveoli is greater than that being delivered to the lung. Because of the alveolar hyperoxia, nitrous oxide can be administered safely in concentrations of 80% or more for the first few minutes of induction. Use of O_2 in concentrations less than 30% should be avoided by the inexperienced anesthetist. The commonest cause of failure to deliver an adequate concentration of oxygen to the patient is an incorrect setting of the flowmeters. One must always be alert to this potential error.

Gas flow rates.—At total gas flow rates of 5 liter/min or greater, the inspired O_2 concentration will be essentially identical to the flowmeter concentration, provided the flowmeters are properly calibrated. As total gas flow is decreased below 5 liters/min, the greater is the likelihood that the inspired O_2 concentration will be different from that calculated from the flowmeters. Because under anesthesia, the body consumes from 150 to 200 ml of O_2 per minute, the removal of this amount of O_2 from the anesthetic circuit decreases the O_2 concentration in the circuit. At flows greater than 5 liters/min, removal of 150 to 200 ml of O_2 makes no significant impact on the O_2 concentration in the system. However, as the flow is decreased, the removal of this amount of O_2 does have an impact on the O_2 concentration in the alveolar atmosphere. Furthermore, inaccuracies in the flowmeters are significant at lower flow rates. To take another example, the addition of 100% O_2 at a flow rate of 200 ml/min to a closed anesthetic circuit previously equilibrated with 70% nitrous oxide and 30% oxygen would result in a disparity between metered (100%) and actual (30%) inspired O_2 concentration. In this example, the inflow O_2 just balances that being consumed by the body, none being left to dilute or concentrate nitrous oxide in the anesthetic circuit.

Detailed consideration of the effects of different anesthetic circuits on inspired O_2 concentration are beyond the scope of this chapter, except to indicate that calculated and actual inspired O_2 concentrations inherently tend to be closer when nonrebreathing systems (e.g., Ayre's T-piece or non-

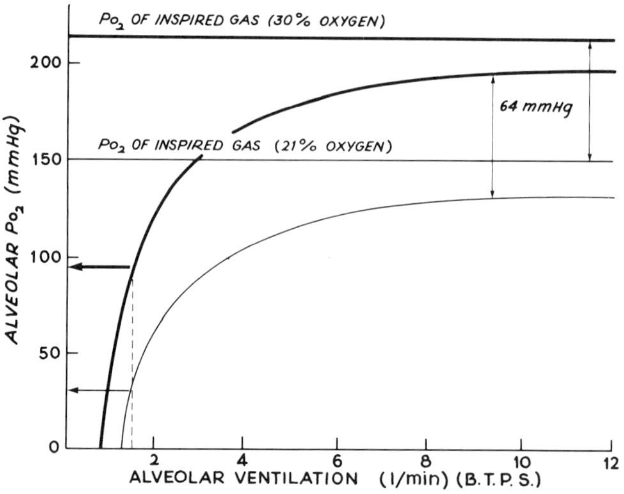

Fig. 19-7.—Effect on alveolar O_2 tension (PA_{O_2}) of increasing the inspired O_2 concentration from 21% (*thin line*) to 30% (*heavy line*) at assumed O_2 consumption (V_{O_2}) of 200 ml/min. In this example, PA_{O_2} decreases to dangerously low value when patient is breathing air at alveolar ventilation of 1 to 5 liter/min; at this point, O_2 enrichment of inspired gas to 30% is sufficient to raise PA_{O_2} almost to within normal range. All points on *heavy line* are 64 torr above corresponding points on *thin line* at same ventilation. (From Nunn, J. F.: *Applied Respiratory Physiology* [New York: Appleton-Century-Crofts, 1969].)

rebreathing valves) are used than when conventional anesthetic circle systems are used. Of course, at total gas flows exceeding 5 liters/min the conventional circle becomes essentially a nonrebreathing system, and calculated and actual O_2 concentrations would be similar. If any question arises about the adequacy of the inspired O_2 concentration, this can and should be checked with an O_2 sensor. Several such devices are available; they are easily calibrated and provide a quick and accurate analysis of inspired O_2 concentrations. In the absence of a sensor, the obvious and vital move is to increase the O_2 concentration. If this fails to correct an obvious O_2 deficiency, air should be substituted for the anesthetic atmosphere until the machine can be checked for malfunction.

Barometric pressure.—Inspired O_2 tension, and hence Pa_{O_2}, will decrease in direct proportion to the decrease in barometric pressure. For example, the barometric pressure in Denver, Colorado (altitude, 5,330 feet) is about 620 torr, which in turn decreases the inspired O_2 tension to about 110 torr.

Alveolar oxygen tension (PA_{O_2}).—Alveolar oxygen tension is determined in part by alveolar ventilation, the exact relationship between the two being best described by a hyperbolic curve (Fig. 19-7). In Figure 19-7 the effect of alveolar ventilation on PA_{O_2} is shown at two inspired O_2 concentrations. As the alveolar ventilation increases, the PA_{O_2} also increases but reaches a plateau before reaching the O_2 tension of inspired gas because of the contribution of inert gas (nitrogen or nitrous oxide) from the wasted-ventilation

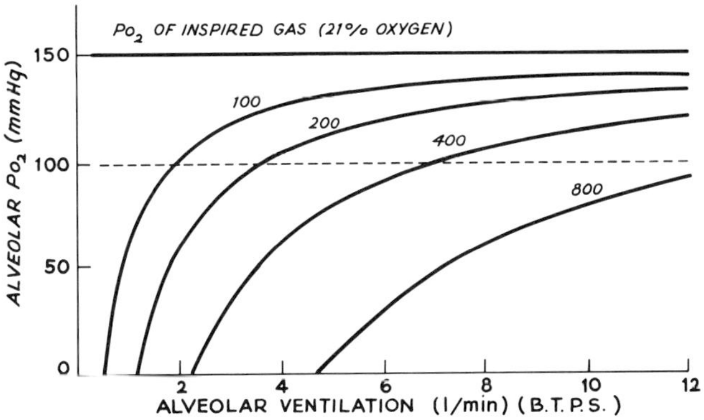

Fig. 19-8.—Relationship between alveolar ventilation ($\dot{V}_A$) and alveolar oxygen tension ($P_{A_{O_2}}$) at four values of oxygen consumption ($\dot{V}_{O_2}$) for a patient breathing 21% O_2 (atmospheric air). Values for $\dot{V}_{O_2}$ are in ml/min. Typical values for $\dot{V}_{O_2}$ in average adult: 200 ml/min at rest; 150 to 175 ml/min during general anesthesia; 100 ml/min during anesthesia and hypothermia (30° C); and 400 ml/min or more with restlessness, struggling, shivering or pyrexia. $\dot{V}_A$ required to attain any particular $P_{A_{O_2}}$ is directly proportional to $\dot{V}_{O_2}$. (From Nunn, J. F.: *Applied Respiratory Physiology* [New York: Appleton-Century-Crofts, 1969].)

compartment. If no inert gas were present (i.e., if pure O_2 were to be inspired), then alveolar and inspired O_2 tensions would be different only by the differences in water vapor and CO_2 tensions between inspired and alveolar gas. In the lower portion of the curve, it is clear that as alveolar ventilation decreases, the $P_{A_{O_2}}$ also decreases. The rate of decline in $P_{A_{O_2}}$ is most rapid at alveolar ventilation values below 3 liter/min. At an alveolar ventilation of 1.5 liter/min, the $P_{A_{O_2}}$ is dangerously low at an inspired O_2 concentration of 21% but is quite adequate if the inspired O_2 concentration is increased to 30%, with no change in alveolar ventilation. If alveolar gas contains only O_2 and the usual tensions of water vapor and carbon dioxide (i.e., inert gases such as nitrogen or nitrous oxide are absent), ventilation can cease for 5 to 10 minutes and the patient still maintain a $P_{A_{O_2}}$ or Pa_{O_2} of greater than 500 torr. As O_2 molecules are absorbed into pulmonary capillary blood from alveoli, alveolar pressure decreases. This decrease in alveolar pressure causes O_2 molecules to move into the alveoli from the airways. This in turn causes O_2 to move from the gas source into the airways. Hence there is a continual flow of O_2 from the O_2 source to the blood stream without any ventilation, provided there is no airway obstruction. This state of affairs has been called diffusion respiration.

In reality, the term diffusion respiration is a misnomer because the effect is one of mass gas movement, not diffusion. Regardless of name, the technic is useful in those circumstances where general anesthesia with or without muscle relaxants is used for endoscopic manipulations in the upper or lower airway. The limiting factor is either dilution with air in the circumstance of endoscopy or the eventual increase in Pa_{CO_2} in "pure" diffusion respiration. It is because Pa_{O_2} can be normal in the absence of ventilation that Pa_{O_2} values cannot be used to evaluate the adequacy of ventilation.

Stated another way, Pa_{O_2} measurements will define the adequacy of oxygenation but not the adequacy of ventilation.

Oxygen consumption.—O_2 consumption also affects PA_{O_2} and hence Pa_{O_2} (Fig. 19-8). As O_2 consumption increases, alveolar ventilation must also increase if a normal PA_{O_2} is to be maintained. Shivering during recovery from anesthesia may double or triple O_2 consumption. If ventilation is not increased by a proportional amount, PA_{CO_2} will decrease and hypoxemia will ensue.

Diffusion anoxia.—A condition peculiar to anesthesia that may affect PA_{O_2} is that of diffusion anoxia. Diffusion anoxia occurs if a patient is allowed to breathe room air immediately upon the conclusion of anesthesia with nitrous oxide. Nitrous oxide, being a relatively insoluble anesthetic, preferentially leaves pulmonary capillary blood in favor of alveolar gas spaces. Nitrogen in the incoming air is only 1/30th as soluble in blood as nitrous oxide and hence also preferentially remains in the alveolar compartment. As the partial pressures of nitrous oxide and nitrogen increase, PA_{O_2} must decrease if alveolar pressure is to remain at 1 atmosphere. The resulting hypoxemia, although brief, may be severe. Diffusion anoxia can be prevented by administering 100% oxygen for a few minutes before the patient is allowed to breathe room air.

Ventilation-perfusion abnormalities.—Ideally, pulmonary ventilation and blood flow should be exactly matched so that mean alveolar and arterial Po_2 values are identical. Practically, this never happens because 1 to 3% of the venous return of healthy man completely bypasses the lungs. The thebesian, bronchial, and pleural veins empty directly into the left ventricle thereby decreasing Pa_{O_2} by 4 to 10 torr below PA_{O_2}. This is termed an alveolar-arterial O_2 tension difference (A-aDo_2). Increases in A-aDo_2 occur commonly during anesthesia and are due either to increases in ventilation-perfusion abnormalities or increases in venous admixture (shunt), or both.[11] For example, acute atelectasis, a common event in surgical patients, causes inadequate or nonventilation of perfused alveoli as evidenced by the development of large A-aDo_2 values. Decreases in cardiac output, which are disproportionally greater than the decreases in body metabolism, also occur during anesthesia. Because of the slowed circulation, more O_2 than usual is extracted at the tissue level and mixed venous O_2 content is below normal. The addition of a fraction of the abnormally desaturated blood to the arterial system by way of normal or abnormal shunts in the lungs causes a large decrease in Pa_{O_2}.

Effects of pH and temperature.—Pa_{O_2} values are affected by blood temperature and pH. The solubility of O_2 in blood is inversely related to temperature, solubility increasing with hypothermia and decreasing with fever. When the temperature of measurement of Po_2 (usually 37° C) is different from the temperature of the patient, the measured Po_2 should be corrected. A useful correction factor to remember is that Pa_{O_2} changes by 6.6% for each degree change in temperature. A sample calculation is as follows:

1) Measured Pa_{O_2} @ 37° C = 70 torr
2) Corrected Pa_{O_2} to 34° C = 70 − (70 × 0.066 × 3° C) = 56 torr

The temperature factor is subtracted from the measured value if the patient's temperature is below that of the measuring instrument and added if the patient's temperature is above that of the measuring instrument.

Both temperature and pH also alter mixed venous PO_2 by their effects on the position of the oxyhemoglobin dissociation curve. This would in turn affect Pa_{O_2} by the effects of venous admixture on Pa_{O_2}. This correction factor is small and not ordinarily applied in clinical practice.

Effect of hemoglobin value.—Changes in hemoglobin concentration can affect Pa_{O_2} by influencing the partition of O_2 between physical solution and chemical combination with hemoglobin. The effect is small and ordinarily no correction is made for it in clinical practice. However, making corrections in Pa_{O_2} is readily facilitated by use of the Severinghaus blood-gas calculator.[12]

Age.—The patient's age influences Pa_{O_2}. Pa_{O_2} decreases with increasing age during air breathing, the relationship being adequately described by the equation,

$$\text{Expected } Pa_{O_2} = 100 - (0.4 \times \text{age}).$$

The progressive decrease in Pa_{O_2} with advancing age is probably the result of deterioration in the ventilation-blood flow relationships that occurs with lung aging.

In summary, anesthetic agents may decrease Pa_{O_2} by decreasing the inspired O_2 concentration or alveolar ventilation, increasing O_2 consumption, altering the normal distribution of ventilation and blood flow in the lungs, or by decreasing cardiac output or body temperature. All anesthetic agents appear to be capable of producing these changes and the anesthetist must be alert to the possibilities of each. These adverse changes are to some extent avoidable. Where this is the case, one must avoid taking the easy way out by merely increasing the inspired O_2 concentration. One should not resort to this maneuver until all reasonable efforts to correct the cause of an abnormally low Pa_{O_2} have been made.

FACTORS INFLUENCING ARTERIAL CO_2 TENSION.—The definitive test for evaluating the effects of anesthetics on ventilation is the determination of arterial CO_2 tension (Pa_{CO_2}). The reason for this is as follows. Most of the metabolically produced CO_2 is excreted via the lungs. In the average adult at rest this amounts to about 200 ml/min, or 5.6% of the total gas volume excreted from the lungs per minute. That is,

$$\begin{aligned}\text{Alveolar ventilation } (\dot{V}_A) &= \frac{CO_2 \text{ output/min}}{\text{alveolar } CO_2 \text{ concentration}} \\ &= \frac{200}{0.056} \\ &= 3570 \text{ ml/min}\end{aligned}$$

The alveolar CO_2 concentration of 5.6% is equivalent to a PA_{CO_2} of about 40 torr (5.6 × [760-47 torr] water vapor). This means that at a constant CO_2 output, any decrease in $\dot{V}_A$ will result in an increase in PA_{CO_2} and hence Pa_{CO_2}. Thus, any increase in Pa_{CO_2} above the normal range of 35 to 45 torr indicates alveolar hypoventilation and a Pa_{CO_2} below this range indicates alveolar hyperventilation.

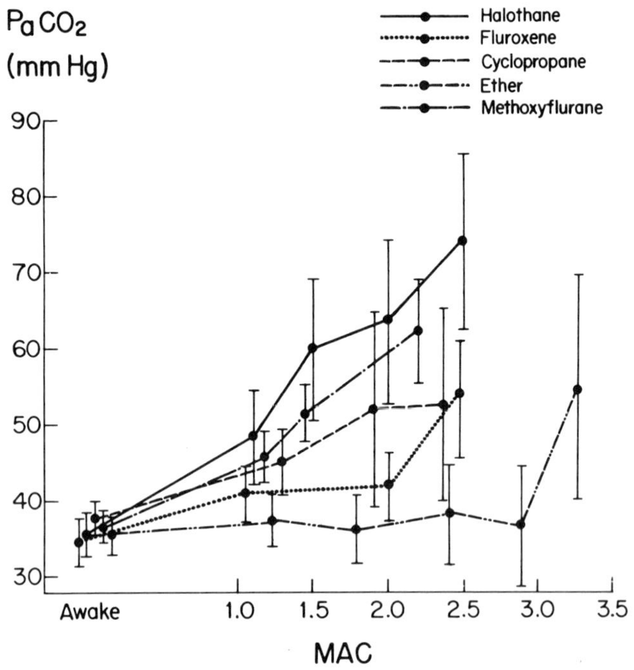

Fig. 19-9.—Effect of anesthetic depth (dose) of arterial CO_2 tension (Pa_{CO_2}) in 43 patients anesthetized with one of five agents: halothane, fluroxene, cyclopropane, ether or methoxyflurane. Anesthetic dose expressed in multiples of minimum anesthetic concentration (MAC). Values for halothane are significantly greater than those for fluroxene or ether at all anesthetic doses. (From Larson, C. P., *et al.*[8])

Anesthetic drugs.—Comparative evaluation of several inhalation anesthetics in volunteer subjects at doses that are multiples of an equipotent concentration (minimal alveolar anesthetic concentration or MAC) shows that anesthetics vary in their effects on Pa_{CO_2}.[8] Halothane and methoxyflurane produce a progressive increase in Pa_{CO_2} with increasing anesthetic depth (Fig. 19-9). At the other extreme is ether, which is unique among the agents studied in that Pa_{CO_2} remains unchanged from the value in the conscious patient until deep levels (2.9 MAC) of anesthesia are attained. Values for Pa_{CO_2} with fluroxene and cyclopropane are intermediate between the other agents. These findings suggest that in the absence of any other impairment to ventilation (e.g., use of muscle relaxants, abnormal body position, and limitation of diaphragmatic excursion), ventilatory support with these agents present is usually unnecessary to maintain a normal Pa_{CO_2}. Such is not the case with halothane or methoxyflurane. With either of these agents, ventilatory support is mandatory in most patients anesthetized with more than 1.5 MAC (1.1% halothane or 0.24% methoxyflurane). In reality, the magnitude of the ventilatory depression may be even greater than indicated from the study conducted on volunteers who did not undergo surgery.

Most other events during anesthesia and surgery also impair ventilation and add to the effects of halothane or methoxyflurane. For example, atropine or scopolamine tend to increase Pa_{CO_2} by enlarging the conducting airways and increasing the wasted ventilation in the lungs. Opiates decrease the respiratory rate and hence alveolar ventilation. The use of muscle relaxants further depresses ventilation by impairing the function of the respiratory muscles. One exception to the principle that anesthesia and surgery impair ventilation is that of surgical stimulation, which has been shown to lower Pa_{CO_2} by an average of 5 torr.[7] However, the stimulatory effect of surgery is usually inadequate to restore Pa_{CO_2} to normal.

The decrease in the required concentration of halothane for an equivalent level of anesthesia by adding nitrous oxide lessens somewhat the ventilatory depression of halothane.[13] The mild ventilatory stimulation provided by nitrous oxide is thought to be a catecholamine response induced by the drug. However, as with surgical stimulation, the effect is inadequate to restore Pa_{CO_2} to normal.

CORRECTION OF Pa_{CO_2} ABNORMALITIES.—Three options are available for management of ventilation of patients anesthetized with an agent such as halothane, which is capable of inducing respiratory depression: 1) to allow spontaneous ventilation to continue, recognizing that some degree of respiratory acidosis may occur; 2) to use assisted ventilation or augmentation of the tidal volume of a patient-initiated inspiration; and 3) to use controlled ventilation in which ventilation is managed entirely by the anesthetist, either manually or mechanically.

In our opinion, the choice is made relatively easily in most circumstances. We find little use for assisted ventilation since it is relatively ineffective as a means for decreasing Pa_{CO_2}.[14,15] Assisted ventilation can only decrease Pa_{CO_2} by 5 to 8 torr before apnea ensues, and such small changes are seldom of any physiologic significance. Controlled ventilation is necessary when ventilation is seriously impaired by muscle relaxants or required by the operative procedure (e.g., thoracotomy and neurosurgical procedures requiring a "slack" brain). Complete respiratory paralysis may occur, of course, with high concentrations of agents but it also occurs with high spinal anesthesia. Decrease in the concentration of the anesthetic, reversal of drug action, and artificial ventilation with oxygen are indicated.

Spinal anesthesia to levels of T2, contrary to rather prevalent opinion, does not impair ventilation. With these high levels, however, patients often complain of being unable to breathe and actually do not breathe voluntarily because the impact of input of peripheral stimuli is blocked. However, when such patients are asked to breathe and when challenged with CO_2, the ventilatory response is not abnormal. Actual paralysis occurs when the concentration of agent in the brain stem is sufficient to block phrenic nerve or medullary chemoreceptor activity.

In circumstances in which controlled ventilation is not essential, we prefer to maintain spontaneous ventilation, even though some increase in Pa_{CO_2} and respiratory acidosis may occur. We believe that in many instances there are fewer hazards to the patient during spontaneous ventilation with halothane than during controlled ventilation, when all respiratory signs of anesthetic depth are lost. The potential danger of anesthetic overdose during controlled ventilation with potent agents is far greater than the risks associated with mild hypercapnia. However, we emphasize that we permit spontaneous ventilation only in circumstances in which the hypoventilation is minimal (Pa_{CO_2}, 55 torr or less). We emphasize also that it is necessary to check by blood gas analysis the level of Pa_{CO_2} whenever there is any doubt about the degree of hypoventilation.

Except for producing a respiratory acidosis, inhalation anesthetics per se have little effect on acid-base balance.[7] We found no appreciable changes in base excess in volunteer subjects exposed to several doses of anesthetics for 5 hours or more (Fig. 19-10).

CO_2 RESPONSE TEST.—Another method for evaluating the effects of anesthetic drugs on ventilation is the measurement of the ventilatory responses to inhaled CO_2. CO_2 is administered in intermittent, graded doses or as a continuously increasing dose (i.e., rebreathing) before and after administration of a drug. Minute ventilation is measured and plotted on the ordinate against Pa_{CO_2} on the abscissa (Fig. 19-11). The increase in ventilation varies from 1.4 to 3.6 liters/min/mm Hg increase in Pa_{CO_2} in healthy awake subjects. During anesthesia, the ability to increase ventilation in response to increased Pa_{CO_2} is diminished. A series of CO_2-response curves that vary with the depth of anesthesia may be obtained. Two kinds of changes may be noted following the administration of an inhalation anesthetic. The first is displacement of the curves to the right of the curve for the awake subject, which indicates an increase in resting (unstimulated) Pa_{CO_2}. This shift or

Fig. 19-10.—Effect of anesthetic depth (dose) on base excess (mEq/liter) in 43 patients anesthetized with one of five agents: halothane, fluroxene, cyclopropane, ether or methoxyflurane. Anesthetic dose expressed in multiples of minimum anesthetic concentration (MAC). No significant differences found among various agents or at varying doses. (From Larson, C. P.: Unpublished observations.)

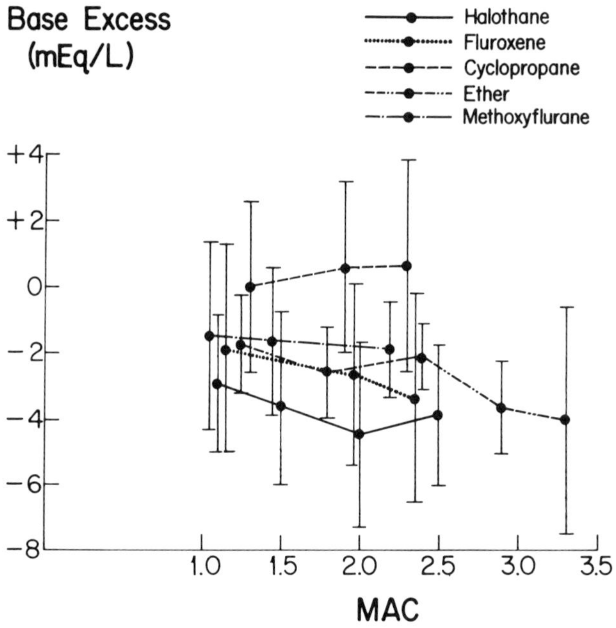

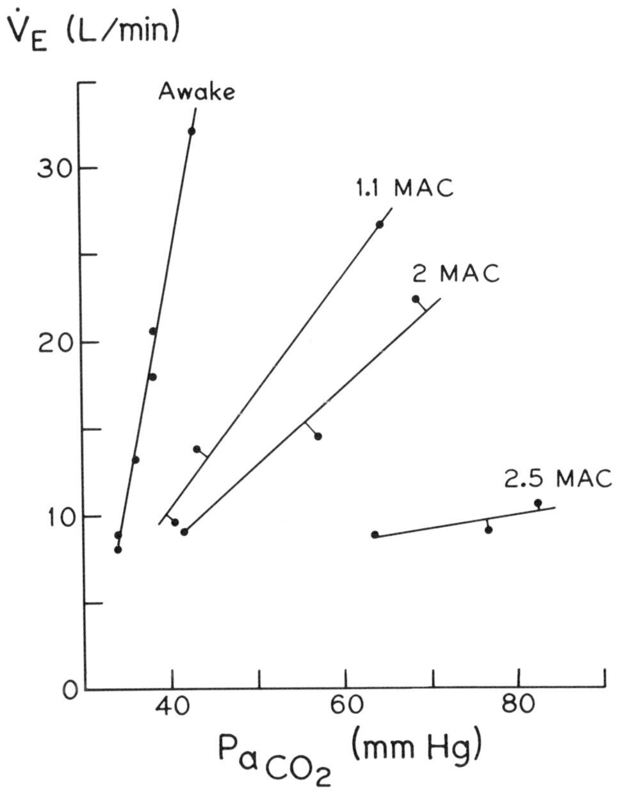

Fig. 19-11.—Family of CO_2 response curves obtained from one patient awake and at three levels of fluroxene anesthesia. Vertical axis, minute ventilation (liter/min) and horizontal axis, Pa_{CO_2} (mm Hg). Note progressive decrease in slope of ventilatory response and displacement to right with increasing anesthetic dose. (From Munson, E. S., *et al.*[7])

displacement of the curve to the right suggests that the level or threshold of CO_2 required to initiate ventilation has increased. In other words, the Pa_{CO_2} at which apnea occurs (apneic threshold) is higher. Recent studies suggest that although the threshold for apnea is higher during anesthesia, the increase does not vary with anesthetic dose.

The second change is a decrease in the slope, which is dose-dependent. In fact, in the example shown (see Fig. 19-11), CO_2 becomes a depressant to ventilation at fluroxene anesthetic doses exceeding 2.5 MAC (8.5% alveolar concentration). Decreases in slope have been interpreted as indicating a change in sensitivity of respiratory control mechanisms in the brain and rightward displacement to indicate an altered CSF H^+ change.[16]

The CO_2 response test is a more sensitive measure of respiratory depression by drugs than isolated Pa_{CO_2} values for three reasons: 1) the degree of changes in slope provides a quantitative measurement of the effect of drugs on ventilation; 2) the test detects subtle degrees of respiratory depression that are not apparent until respiratory function is challenged by CO_2; and 3)

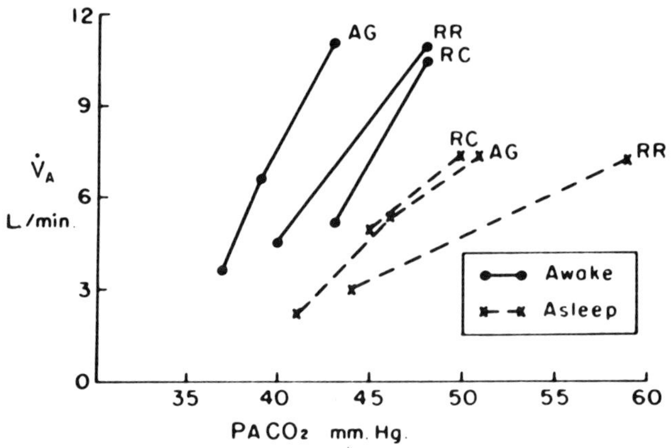

Fig. 19-12.—Effects of normal sleep on ventilatory responses to CO_2 in three healthy adult volunteers. Vertical axis is alveolar ventilation (VA) in liter/min and horizontal axis is alveolar P_{CO_2} in mm Hg. Note downward and rightward displacement during sleep, which reflects both decreased CO_2 production and hence need for less ventilation to maintain normal PA_{CO_2} and slight decrease in responsiveness to CO_2 during sleep. (From Severinghaus, J. W.: Unpublished observations.)

the test can be used to quantify the time course (onset, maximum change, and duration) of the anesthetic effect on respiration. When interpreting CO_2 response tests, however, one must take cognizance of the many factors that may influence the test.[16] Hypoxia, hyperoxia, fever, acidosis, pregnancy, prolonged hyperventilation, norepinephrine and decreases in cardiac output or cerebral blood flow move the curve to the left of control. Increases in wasted ventilation, partial airway obstruction, restriction of the chest wall or lung, or even natural sleep (Fig. 19-12) shift the response curve to the right of the control curve.

All inhalation anesthetics, except perhaps trichloroethylene, appear to decrease the slope of the CO_2 response test; the greater the anesthetic dose, the greater the depression (Fig. 19-13). The magnitude of the effect, however, differs among the various agents. Ability to increase ventilation, when faced with a CO_2 challenge, is significantly greater for patients anesthetized with cyclopropane than for patients anesthetized with other agents.[8] With respect to trichloroethylene, no change was found in CO_2 responsiveness from the awake slope in five patients anesthetized with 1 and 2% trichloroethylene (Fig. 19-14; Talcott, unpublished data). The differences associated with this agent may have been due to an accompanying metabolic acidosis, which would augment ventilation through stimulation of the peripheral chemoreceptors.

EFFECT OF TIME ON CHANGES IN VENTILATION.—The ventilatory depression accompanying halothane anesthesia has been shown to diminish as the duration of anesthesia extends beyond 5 to 6 hours. Fourcade and colleagues found a 20% decrease from maximal in PA_{CO_2} and a leftward shift and increased slope of the CO_2 response test curve after 6 hours of constant-depth halothane anesthesia in volunteers (Fig. 19-15).[17] The explanation for

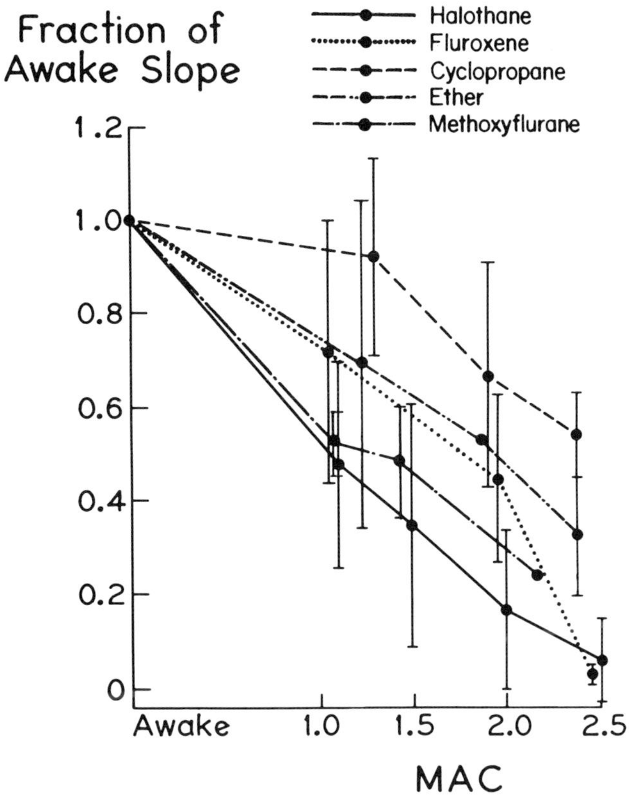

Fig. 19-13.—Effects of anesthetic depth (dose) on ventilatory responsiveness to inhaled CO_2 in 43 patients anesthetized with one of five agents: halothane, fluroxene, cyclopropane, ether or methoxyflurane. Anesthetic dose expressed in multiples of minimum anesthetic concentration (MAC); values on ordinate are expressed as fraction of awake slope. Cyclopropane produced the least depression in CO_2 responsiveness (90% of awake value at 1.5 MAC); halothane had significantly greater effect (< 40% of awake value at 1.5 MAC). (From Larson, C. P., *et al.*[8])

the tendency to recovery from ventilatory depression with time is not known. Several explanations have been suggested, the most plausible being the liberation of a ventilatory stimulant such as norepinephrine or enhancement of existing catecholamine by increased secretion of endogenous corticosteroids. Whether partial recovery from ventilatory depression occurs in anesthetized patients undergoing operation remains to be demonstrated.

Intravenous Anesthetics, Including Narcotics and Other Premedicant Drugs

Intravenous anesthetics vary appreciably in their effects on ventilation. Of the intravenous drugs commonly used, the opiates are generally regarded as having the most profound respiratory effects. Opiates given in the usual therapeutic or premedicant doses produce small but measurable ventilatory changes. Although no changes in resting respiratory rate or volume usually

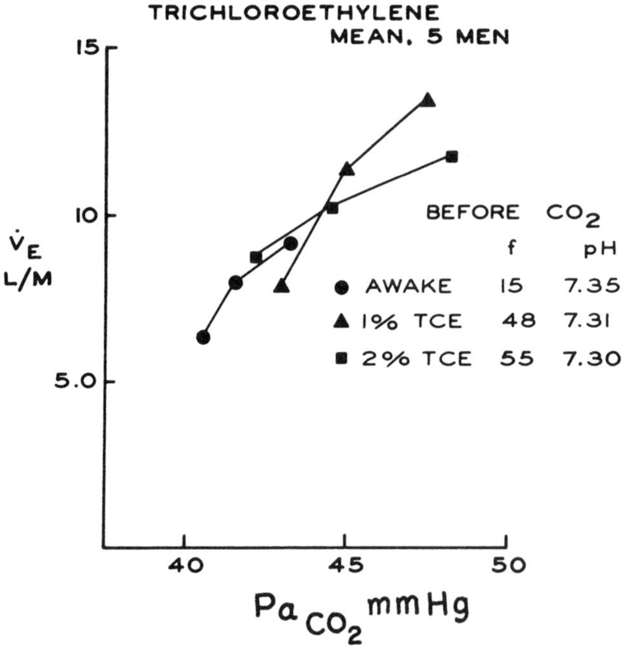

Fig. 19-14.—Mean ventilatory responses to inhaled CO_2 in five healthy patients anesthetized with trichloroethylene. Minute ventilation ($\dot{V}_E$) in liter/min plotted against arterial P_{CO_2} (Pa_{CO_2}). ● represent awake controls; ▲, 1% trichloroethylene; ■, 2% trichloroethylene. No appreciable changes in Pa_{CO_2} or CO_2 response slopes from awake control were observed. Values for respiratory frequency (f) and arterial pH awake and anesthetized but without exogenous CO_2 are shown. (From Severinghaus, J. W., and Larson, C. P.[16])

Fig. 19-15.—Effects of time on the ventilatory responses to inhaled CO_2 during constant-depth halothane anesthesia. Minute ventilation ($\dot{V}_E$) is plotted against Pa_{CO_2}. (From Fourcade, H. E., Larson, C. P., Hickey, R. F., Bahlman, S. H., and Eger, E. I., II: Effects of time on ventilation during halothane and cyclopropane anesthesia, Anesthesiology 36:83, 1972.)

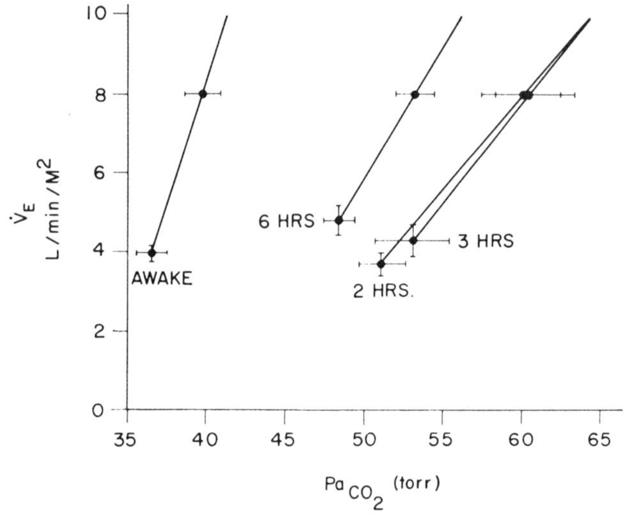

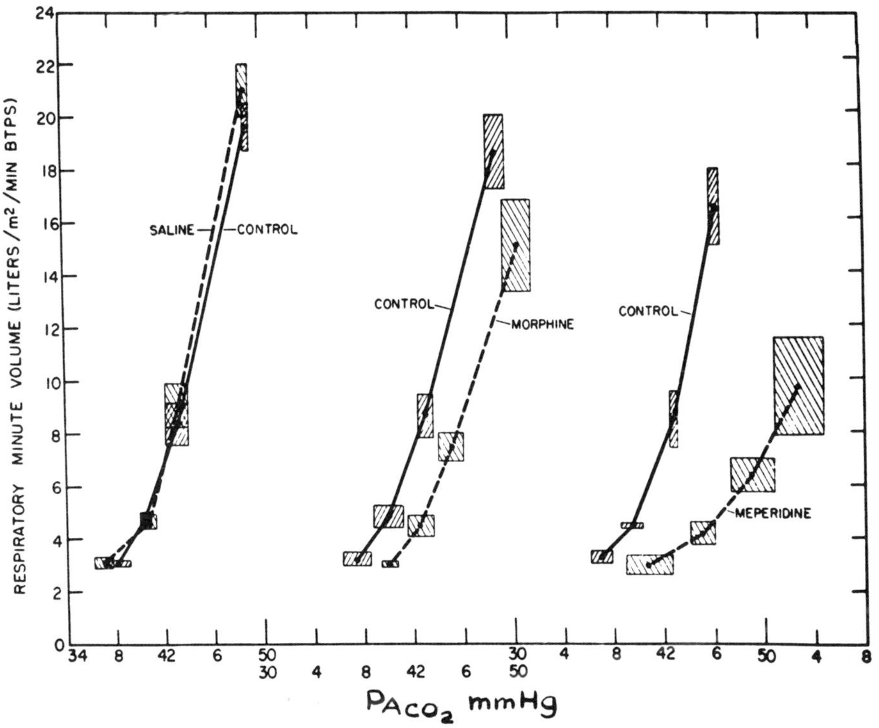

Fig. 19-16.—Mean ventilatory responses to inhaled CO_2 in six healthy patients before and 30 minutes after intramuscular injection of normal saline (2 ml), morphine sulfate (10 mg) or meperidine (150 mg). Shaded areas = 1 S.E.M. At this dose, meperidine depressed CO_2 responsiveness significantly more than did morphine. (From Loeschcke, H. H., Sweel, A., Kough, R. H., and Lambertsen, C. J.: The effect of morphine and of meperidine upon the respiratory response of normal men to low concentrations of inspired carbon dioxide, J. Pharmacol. Exp. Ther. 108:376, 1953.)

occur, Pa_{CO_2} may be increased by 2 or 3 torr and the respiratory responses to inhaled CO_2 are changed. Both morphine and meperidine shift the CO_2 response curve to the right, while meperidine also depresses the curve (Fig. 19-16). Other opiates in premedicant or therapeutic doses appear to produce respiratory changes that are similar to those of meperidine and morphine.

Given in excessive doses, opiates produce a characteristic pattern of breathing. Respiratory frequency becomes slow and tidal volume quite large. If further doses of opiates are administered, apnea will eventually occur. This pattern of breathing is unique to the opiates and can be of great help in establishing the depth of anesthesia during nitrous oxide-opiate anesthesia. Often when the nitrous oxide-narcotic combination is used, the patient will tolerate large doses of narcotic (300 to 500 mg of meperidine, for example) intravenously without apnea until nitrous oxide in nonhypoxic concentrations is added.

Sedatives or tranquilizers are occasionally given in combination with opiates for premedication or tranquilization and analgesia after operation. In some instances, the combination of drugs has a greater depressant effect on

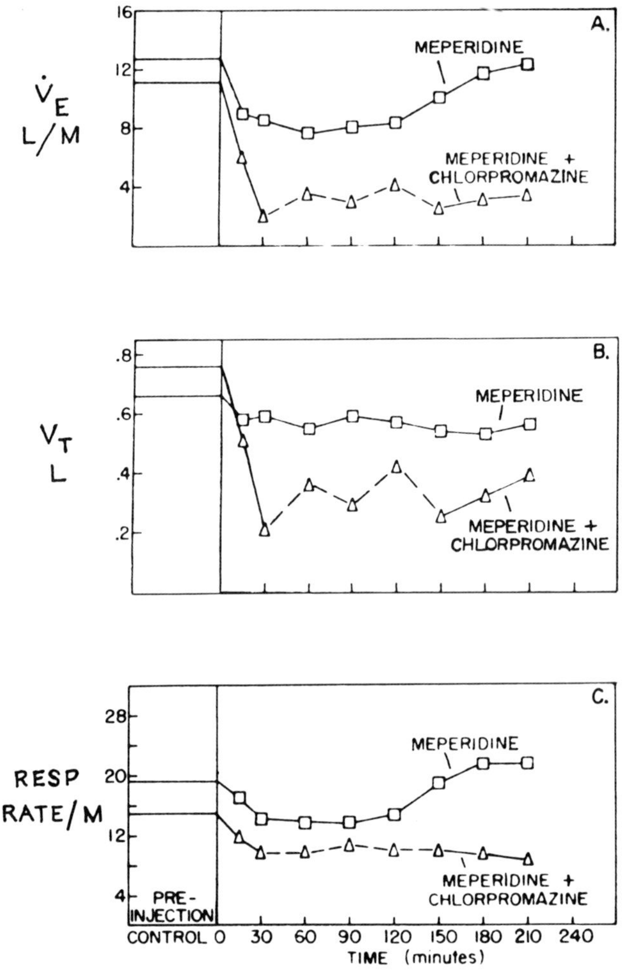

Fig. 19-17.—Effects of meperidine (100 mg/70 kg) alone and meperidine plus chlorpromazine (25 mg/70 kg) on minute ventilation (**A**), tidal volume (**B**) and respiratory rate (**C**) in one patient. Alveolar P_{CO_2} held at 46 torr throughout time period shown. Combination of meperidine and chlorpromazine caused respiratory depression greater both in degree and duration than that produced by meperidine alone. (From Lambertsen, C. J., Wendel, H., and Longenhagen, J. B.: The separate and combined respiratory effects of chlorpromazine and meperidine in normal men controlled at 46 mm Hg alveolar P_{CO_2}, J. Pharmacol. Exp. Ther. 131:381, 1961.)

respiration than the opiate alone (Fig. 19-17), and in other instances the sedative or tranquilizer does not enhance the opiate depression (Fig. 19-18). In general, the short-, intermediate-, and long-acting barbiturates given in sedative doses have little effect on minute ventilation, $P_{A_{CO_2}}$, or ventilatory responses to inhaled CO_2. However, when barbiturates are given in massive doses, as in barbiturate poisoning, respiration may be profoundly depressed or even absent. The ultrashort-acting barbiturates commonly used in clinical anesthesia do depress respiration, and their effects are additive to the other agents being used (Fig. 19-19).

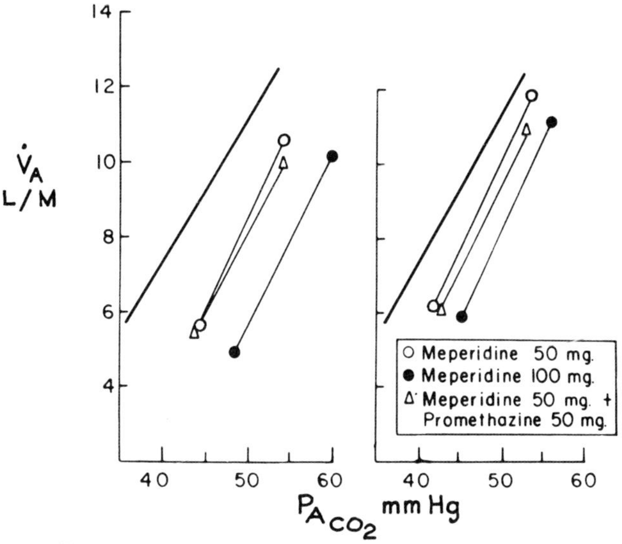

Fig. 19-18.—Effects of two doses of meperidine and meperidine-promethazine combination on mean ventilatory responses to inhaled CO_2 in five patients. $\dot{V}_A$ is calculated alveolar ventilation in liter/min. Meperidine 100 mg produced significantly greater respiratory depression than did meperidine 50 mg alone or combined with promethazine. (From Keats, A. S., Telford, J., and Kurosu, Y.: Potentiation of meperidine by promethazine, Anesthesiology 22:34, 1961.)

Fig. 19-19.—Family of CO_2 response curves obtained following administration of various drug combinations to healthy volunteer. After awake control measurements, anesthetic sequence (experiment 1) was thiopental alone followed by thiopental with nitrous oxide 50% *(solid lines)*. One week later (experiment 2), sequence was control nitrous oxide 50%, morphine 10 mg intramuscularly, morphine-thiopental alone and with nitrous oxide *(broken lines)*. Numbers in parentheses refer to plasma thiopental concentrations in mg/liter. Except for nitrous oxide alone, drug combinations produced varying degrees of respiratory depression. (From Eckenhoff, J. E., and Helrich, M.: Effect of narcotics, thiopental and nitrous oxide upon respiration and respiratory response to hypercapnia, Anesthesiology 19:240, 1958.)

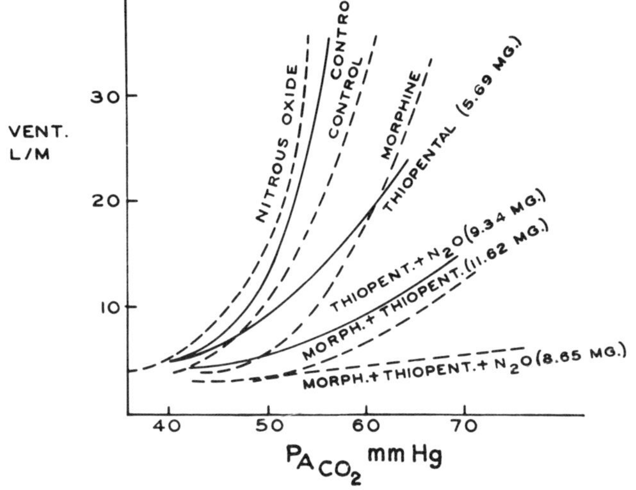

USE OF RESPIRATORY STIMULANTS

Faced with cases of respiratory depression or apnea, physicians are tempted to administer stimulants in the hope that ventilation will return or improve. In general, the use of analeptics or stimulant drugs in these circumstances is to be condemned. Analeptics such as doxapram (Dopram), ethamivan (Emivan) and caffeine are nonspecific antagonists; that is, they do not antagonize depression due to a specific drug. Rather, they stimulate the central nervous system and some increase in ventilation may result. We condemn the routine use of these drugs to stimulate ventilation because the ventilatory responses are unpredictable and evanescent and use of these drugs may evoke other complications, such as convulsions. We prefer to manage drug-induced respiratory depression or apnea with ventilatory support and allow the offending drug, unless this be an opiate, to take its natural course.

Narcotic Antagonists

Respiratory depression or apnea known to be due to opiates requires treatment with narcotic antagonists. These specifically reverse the respiratory depression of opiates. They include nalorphine (Nalline), levallorphan (Lorfan), and naloxone (Narcan). These drugs are N-allyl derivatives of opiates; that is, an allyl group ($-CH_2-CH=CH_2$) is substituted for a methyl group on the basic nitrogen of morphine (nalorphine), levorphan (levallorphan), or oxymorphone (naloxone).

Fig. 19-20.—Effects of morphine and subsequent antagonism by nalorphine on ventilatory responses to inhaled CO_2. Nalorphine produced almost complete recovery of morphine-depressed curve. (From Papadopoulos, C., and Keats, A. S.: Specific and nonspecific antagonism of morphine-induced respiratory depression, Anesthesiology 23:86, 1962.)

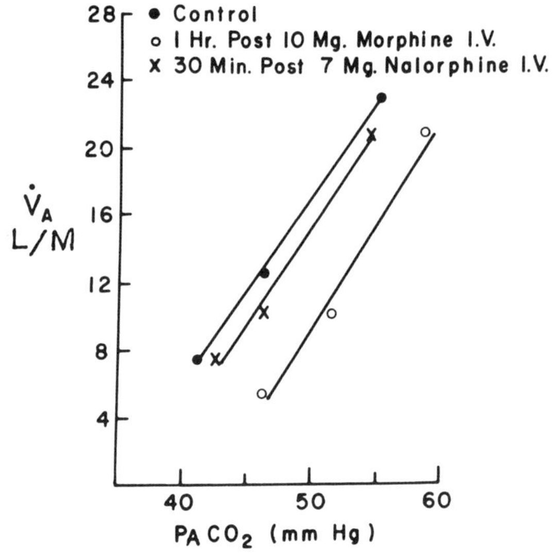

Nalorphine and levallorphan have both antagonist and agonist properties. Administered in doses of 0.15 mg/kg (nalorphine) or 0.02 mg/kg (levallorphan), these drugs will effectively antagonize the respiratory and circulatory depression resulting from an overdose of any of the commonly used opiates (Fig. 19-20). However, given in the absence of prior opiates or when the opiate depression of respiration or circulation is mild, the agonist effects predominate, and depression is augmented rather than reversed.

In contrast, naloxone appears to be a "pure" narcotic antagonist, and is devoid of the agonist actions (i.e., respiratory or circulatory depression, sedation and dysphoria) associated with the other narcotic antagonists. For this reason, naloxone has almost completely replaced nalorphine and levallorphan in clinical practice. Given intravenously in doses of 2.5 to 5 μg/kg (0.2 to 0.4 mg/70 kg), naloxone will reverse the respiratory and circulatory depression from opiate overdose in 1 to 2 minutes.[18] During narcotic-nitrous oxide anesthesia, respiratory depression (from the narcotic) frequently is disproportionately excessive in relation to the desired "anesthetic" effect. In such circumstances, very small doses (0.05 mg) may alleviate the severe respiratory depression without reversing the "anesthetic" effect. Such small doses are useful also in correcting undesired respiratory depression in the immediate postanesthetic period, while useful analgesia is retained. The duration of action varies from 2 to 4 hours, depending on the dose administered, route of administration and the time relationship between administration of the narcotic and of the narcotic antagonist. Because the duration of action of some narcotics may exceed that of naloxone, patients who have responded satisfactorily to naloxone should be kept under continued surveillance for several hours to determine whether repeated doses of naloxone are necessary to maintain reversal. It should be noted that though all of the narcotic antagonists can be administered intramuscularly or subcutaneously, the onset, peak effect, and duration are less predictable than when these drugs are given intravenously.

EFFECTS OF ANTIBIOTICS

The use of certain antibiotics by the intraperitoneal or intrapleural route may result in a sudden, serious impairment of respiration in anesthetized patients or in patients recovering from anesthesia. Several antibiotics have been reported to produce this effect, including neomycin, streptomycin and kanamycin. Respiratory depression seems to be most profound when the antibiotics are used in patients who are also receiving nondepolarizing neuromuscular blocking drugs. Two pharmacologic mechanisms explain the neuromuscular blocking property of these antibiotics: first, antibiotics, like curare, decrease the sensitivity of the postjunctional membrane to acetylcholine; and second, antibiotics inhibit release of acetylcholine from the neural end plate. Favoring the latter mechanism is the finding that calcium alone or, more effectively, in combination with sodium bicarbonate will reverse the neuromuscular block produced by antibiotics. Cholinesterase inhibitors such as neostigmine are only partially effective in reversing the block.

If respiratory depression or apnea occur during or after operation following the use of antibiotics, continuous ventilatory support is mandatory. Since the total duration of respiratory insufficiency may be up to 24 hours, reversal of blockade should be attempted. Calcium gluconate (1 to 2 gm) and sodium bicarbonate (1 to 2 mEq/kg) should be given slowly by intravenous injection. If these drugs prove ineffective, then edrophonium (10 mg) or neostigmine (1 to 3 mg) with atropine may be tried. It is essential to recognize that pharmacologic reversal may not be complete or sustained and that close observation, and possibly ventilatory support, may be necessary.

LUNG MECHANICS DURING ANESTHESIA

The effects of anesthetics on lung mechanics have been studied intensely in recent years. Special interest in this area is the result of a general awareness that anesthesia may alter the mechanical properties of the lungs and also the development of more sophisticated methods for studying changes in lung mechanics.

Airways

Airway obstruction is the most frequent and potentially dangerous respiratory complication of general anesthesia. This problem is discussed in Chapter 6.

Drugs used in anesthesia may have direct or indirect effects on airways. The magnitude of these effects depends primarily upon airway tone at the time the drugs are administered. Bronchial smooth muscle tone is minimal in healthy man, as evidenced by minimal decreases in airway resistance when potent bronchodilators such as isoproterenol, are administered. Inhalation anesthetics like halothane are thought to be bronchodilators but, because airways normally are almost maximally dilated, halothane has little or no effects on airway size or resistance in healthy man.[19] However, halothane appears to be a potent dilator of constricted airways. Thus in dogs, subanesthetic doses of halothane (0.6% or less) prevent bronchoconstriction produced by vagal nerve stimulation or histamine given intravenously.[20] Cyclopropane also has bronchodilating effects, although it is less potent than halothane.

Because of its effects on airways, halothane anesthesia has been advocated as a treatment for status asthmaticus. This, however, must be regarded as radical therapy, and it is rarely, if ever, indicated in clinical practice. The potential risks of hypoxia due to total airway obstruction, hypercapnia and cardiac arrhythmias far exceed the beneficial effects which may occur. Therapeutic efforts are better directed toward the use of more potent bronchodilators such as epinephrine or isoproterenol, the correction of acidosis with sodium bicarbonate, the administration of oxygen with assisted ventilation if hypercapnia is present, and the treatment of any pulmonary infection. On the other hand, halothane seems to be an ideal agent for patients requiring general anesthesia for surgery who have a history of bronchial asthma.

Belladonna alkaloids, such as atropine and scopolamine, relax bronchial smooth muscle indirectly by blocking the constricting effect of acetylcholine. As a result, airway volume (also, wasted ventilation or dead space) increases and airway resistance decreases. Although there is much individual variation, these changes average about 30% of the control values when atropine (0.5 to 1 mg) or scopolamine (0.4 to 0.5 mg) are given. These changes are usually dissipated within 1 hour but may last for 2 or 3 hours.

Lungs

ATELECTASIS.—Atelectasis (pulmonary collapse) is common in patients undergoing general anesthesia and surgery. It occurs with the onset of anesthesia and persists throughout the operative and postoperative periods unless specific measures are taken to prevent its occurrence. It was once thought that the severity of the atelectasis was directly related to the duration of anesthesia, becoming progressively more severe as the anesthesia was prolonged. Recent studies, however, suggest that this is not the case.[21,22]

Atelectasis associated with anesthesia and surgery is generally miliary or diffuse in type; it involves all parts of the lungs, but particularly the dependent portions. It is rarely of sufficient magnitude to be detectable by roentgenographic examination of the chest. Consequently one must rely on physiologic tests to determine its presence. Unfortunately these tests are indirect in that they do not quantitate either the amount or the location of the atelectasis.

Measurement of A-aDo$_2$.—The most commonly used physiologic test is that of measuring the alveolar-arterial oxygen tension difference (A-aDo$_2$). Alveolar collapse is not necessarily associated with a corresponding cessation of pulmonary capillary blood flow to the nonventilated alveoli. Consequently the blood perfusing these collapsed alveoli is inadequately oxygenated. Upon reaching the mixed arterial blood, the desaturated hemoglobin removes oxygen from the normally oxygenated blood, thereby decreasing mean arterial oxygen tension (Pa_{O_2}) below that of mean alveolar oxygen tension (PA_{O_2}). Hence an increase in A-aDo$_2$ is found. The A-aDo$_2$ in awake, healthy man is less than 25 torr, but it is not zero because of blood flowing through normal anatomic right-to-left shunts (i.e., bronchial and thebesian circulations). Larger values for A-aDo$_2$ signify an impairment of oxygen exchange in the lungs, either from abnormal ventilation-blood flow relationships in the lungs or from right-to-left shunts around the lungs. Presumably the greater the A-aDo$_2$ value, the more profound the atelectasis; however, no specific quantitation of this is possible because changes in cardiac output also influence the A-aDo$_2$.

Measurement of FRC.—A second test for detecting the development of atelectasis involves the measurement of functional residual capacity (FRC), which is the volume of gas in the lungs at the end of normal expiration. Several investigators have reported decreases in FRC of about 10% with the onset of anesthesia.[22] More recently, the decrease in FRC has been shown to be due in part to airway closure and gas trapping distal to the collapsed airways.[23] When lung volume decreases to a certain critical volume (closing volume), airways begin to close and gas is trapped behind them. This gas comes into equilibrium with venous blood and is a site of venous admixture or shunt. As yet, there are no studies correlating closing volume or FRC changes with A-aD_{O_2} values. Current evidence suggests that the closing volume varies with age: in childhood it exceeds FRC; in young adulthood it is well below FRC; and with further aging, it increases toward FRC.

Compliance.—A third test of the effects of anesthetics on lung volume is that of compliance. Compliance is an index of the distensibility of the lungs and is determined by measuring the volume change accompanying a known pressure change across the lungs. Measurement of several pressures and volumes permits one to draw a pressure-volume loop, which characterizes the distensibility of the lungs. Decreases in lung volume decrease compliance; increases in lung volume have the reverse effect. The normal compliance of awake man is about 100 ml/cm of H_2O. Anesthesia decreases this value by about 30 to 40%, but this is extremely variable and depends on the inflation history during the several minutes before the measurement is made. Vigorous suctioning of the airway may decrease lung volume and compliance significantly.

Causes of atelectasis.—The cause of atelectasis during anesthesia is unclear and may be multifactorial. Initially, all instances of atelectasis were thought to be caused by airway occlusion from mucus plugs, the distal gas being resorbed. A more recent theory holds that atelectasis is caused by constant small-volume ventilation and failure to take deep breaths or "sighs", as is done in the awake state. Supporters of this theory advocate large tidal-volume ventilation (i.e., greater than 10 ml/kg body weight) or periodic hyperinflation of the lungs to simulate the sigh. Large-volume ventilation is reasonably effective in minimizing the amount of atelectasis that may occur during anesthesia. Although periodic hyperinflation is sometimes effective in increasing FRC and compliance, the benefits are transitory, lasting less than 1 or 2 minutes. Consequently this method is not advocated as a routine form of therapy.

Atelectasis may also occur as a result of active expiratory efforts that are commonly observed in anesthetized patients breathing spontaneously. Other factors such as obesity, chest wall compression or impairment of diaphragmatic excursions may further decrease FRC during anesthesia. In such patients, muscle paralysis and the use of controlled ventilation with large tidal volumes appreciably diminish the tendency for atelectasis.

Continuous positive end-expiratory pressure (PEEP).—If spontaneous breathing is desired, the most effective method of preventing atelectasis is by means of continuous positive airway pressure (CPAP or PEEP). Maintenance of airway pressure at end-expiration of 5 to 10 cm H_2O above atmospheric pressure is an effective means of preventing decreases in FRC and airway closure. Both compliance and A-aD_{O_2} values are also improved.

The principal hazards of CPAP are those of impaired venous return, which results in decreases in cardiac output and blood pressure, and the risk of pneumothorax should the airway pressure become excessive. Provided these risks are recognized, CPAP is a useful technic in the prevention or treatment of atelectasis.

REFERENCES

1. Mitchell, R. A.: Control of respiration, in Frohlich, E. D. (ed.): *Pathophysiology: Altered Regulatory Mechanisms in Disease* (Philadelphia: J. B. Lippincott Company, 1972), pp. 111-126.
2. Leusen, I.: Regulation of cerebrospinal fluid composition with reference to breathing, Physiol. Rev. 52:1, 1972.
3. Sorensen, S. C.: The chemical control of ventilation, Acta Physiol. Scand. [Suppl.] 361, 1971.
4. Phillipson, E. A., Hickey, R. F., Graf, P. D., and Nadel, J. A.: Hering-Brewer inflation reflex and regulation of breathing in conscious dogs, J. Appl. Physiol. 31:746, 1971.
5. Guz, A., Nobel, M. I. M., Eisele, J. H., and Trenchard, D.: The effect of lung deflation on breathing in man, Clin. Sci. 40:451, 1971.
6. Wade, J. G., Larson, C. P., Hickey, R. F., Ehrenfeld, W. K., and Severinghaus, J. W.: Effect of carotid endarterectomy on carotid chemoreceptor and baroreceptor function in man, New Eng. J. Med. 282:823, 1970.
7. Munson, E. S., Larson, C. P., Babad, A. A., Regan, M. J., Buechel, D. R., and Eger, E. I., II: The effects of halothane, fluroxene and cyclopropane on ventilation: A comparative study in man, Anesthesiology 27:716, 1966.
8. Larson, C. P., Eger, E. I., II, Muallem, M., Buechel, D. R., Munson, E. S., and Eisele, J.: The effects of diethyl ether and methoxyflurane on ventilation: II. A comparative study in man, Anesthesiology 30:174, 1969.
9. Fourcade, H. E., Stevens, W. C., Larson, C. P., Cromwell, T. H., Bahlman, S. H., Hickey, R. F., Halsey, M. J., and Eger, E. I.: The ventilatory effects of forane, a new inhaled anesthetic, Anesthesiology 35:26, 1971.
10. Muallem, M., Larson, C. P., and Eger, E. I., II: The effects of diethyl ether on Pa_{CO_2} in dogs with and without vagal, somatic and sympathetic block, Anesthesiology 30:185, 1969.
11. Bergman, N. A.: Components of the alveolar-arterial oxygen tension difference in anesthetized man, Anesthesiology 28:517, 1967.
12. Severinghaus, J. W.: Blood gas calculator, J. Appl. Physiol. 21:1108, 1966.
13. Hornbein, T. F., Martin, W. E., Bonica, J. J., Freund, F. G., and Parmentier, P.: Nitrous oxide effects on the circulatory and ventilatory responses to halothane, Anesthesiology 31:250, 1969.
14. Fink, B. R., Ngai, S. H., and Hanks, E. C.: The central regulation of respiration during halothane anesthesia, Anesthesiology 23:200, 1962.
15. Hickey, R. F., Fourcade, H. E., Eger, E. I., II, Larson, C. P., Bahlman, S. H., Stevens, W. C., Gregory, G. A., and Smith, N. T.: The effects of ether, halothane and forane on apneic thresholds in man, Anesthesiology 35:32, 1971.
16. Severinghaus, J. W., and Larson, C. P.: Respiration in anesthesia, in Fenn, W. and Rahn, H. (eds.): *Handbook of Physiology: Respiration Vol. II,* Amer. Physiol. Soc., Washington, D.C. 1965, pp. 1219-1264.
17. Fourcade, H. E., Larson, C. P., Hickey, R. F., Bahlman, S. H., and Eger, E. I., II: Effects of time on ventilation during halothane and cyclopropane anesthesia, Anesthesiology 36:83, 1972.
18. Foldes, F. F., Duncalf, D., and Kuwabara, S.: The respiratory, circulatory and narcotic antagonistic effects of nalorphine, levallorphan and naloxone in anesthetized subjects, Can. Anaesth. Soc. J. 16:151, 1969.
19. Brakensiek, A. L., and Bergman, N. A.: The effects of halothane and atropine on total respiratory resistance in anesthetized man, Anesthesiology 33:341, 1970.
20. Hickey, R. F., Graf, P. D., Nadel, J. A., and Larson, C. P.: The effects of halothane and cyclopropane on total pulmonary resistance in the dog, Anesthesiology 31:334, 1969.
21. Panday, J., and Nunn, J. F.: Failure to demonstrate a progressive fall of arterial Po_2 during anesthesia, Anaesthesia 23:38, 1968.

22. Don, H. F., Wahba, W. M., Cuadrado, L., and Kelkar, K.: The effects of anesthesia and 100 percent oxygen on the functional residual capacity of the lungs, Anesthesiology 32:521, 1970.
23. Don, H. F., Wahba, W. M., and Craig, D.: Airway closure, gas trapping and the functional residual capacity during anesthesia, Anesthesiology 36:533, 1972.

CHAPTER TWENTY

Circulation

RELATIONSHIP OF CIRCULATORY DISORDERS AND MORBIDITY

DISORDERS OF THE CIRCULATION are common in surgical patients. These disorders may be merely manifestations of the aging process, as is the case with many elderly patients, or they may result from specific disease processes. Such circulatory disorders, regardless of their etiology or nature, augment the problems of management of anesthesia and surgery and increase the likelihood of complications. However, although management may be more difficult, this should not necessarily be interpreted to mean increased risk to the patient. There is little reliable evidence to support the notion that circulatory disorders and anesthetic risk are directly related. Most of the studies relating anesthetic and surgical risk to cardiovascular disease have been retrospective and can be criticized in regard to the criteria used for preoperative and postoperative diagnoses of cardiovascular disease, inconsistent methods of patient evaluation, and lack of satisfactory control groups.[1] In essence, anesthetic risk depends upon management rather than primarily on underlying disease state.

There is, however, reliable evidence that certain circulatory disorders increase the morbidity and mortality rates associated with anesthesia and surgery. Certainly, most congenital cardiac lesions increase the risk of anesthesia and surgery. Likewise, a high mortality is associated with anesthesia and surgery in patients with severe, progressive angina, in patients with a recent history of myocardial infarction (i.e. within the previous 6 months) and in patients with uncontrolled heart failure. Of course, the mortality is high in such patients regardless of surgery and anesthesia. The increase in mortality associated with properly managed anesthesia and surgery is difficult to establish. There is no doubt that these patients offer a challenge to both anesthetist and surgeon to exercise their talents and knowledge to the optimum.

Whenever possible, surgery should be delayed until the cardiac disorder can be brought under control. The question of optimum delay of surgery frequently arises in patients having sustained a proved myocardial infarction. If emergency surgery is required, there can be no delay, but it must be recognized that the mortality associated with anesthesia and operation under these circumstances is high. Of course, these patients would have a high mortality rate even if the emergency operation were not done. Again, it is difficult to establish the contribution of anesthesia and operation to mortality as opposed to the circulatory deficiency itself. For elective surgery, it is recommended that the operation be postponed for at least 6 months after a proved myocardial infarction. One study has shown that in patients who were operated on within 3 months of infarction there was a reinfarction rate of 37%[2]; this rate decreased to 16% in patients operated on between 3 and 6 months of age and, after 6 months, it stabilized at 5%. Other factors, such as the site of operation (thoracic and upper abdominal operations) and postoperative complications (e.g., tachycardia, hypovolemia, hemorrhage, hypotension and hypoxemia) all increase the risk of reinfarction and death. Probably uncontrolled hypertension and cardiac arrhythmias also increase the mortality associated with anesthesia and surgery, and the morbidity and mortality rates in hypertensive patients are lower if antihypertensive medication is continued up to and after anesthesia and operation. It is the practice of most anesthetists, internists and cardiologists to keep patients on their stabilizing dose of antihypertensive (e.g., reserpine and alpha methyldopa) or antiarrhythmic (i.e., digitalis or quinidine) throughout the perioperative period. This is a practice contrary to that of a few years ago, when antihypertensive drugs were discontinued prior to anesthesia and operation under the misapprehension that the hypotension that developed was difficult, if not impossible, to control. Critical observation and experience made it clear that such was not the case.

EVALUATION OF CIRCULATORY CONDITION

If a circulatory disorder is suspected, the anesthetist should seek in his preoperative evaluation a detailed history of circulatory function, with special emphasis on prior chest or arm pains, shortness of breath, palpitations, weakness, dizziness or fainting and headaches. A history of dietary intake, drug habits or evidence of chronic blood loss should be elicited. These symptoms may suggest coronary artery disease or hypertension, the two most common causes of organic heart disease in the elderly. The anesthetist should then examine the patient's circulatory system. This includes taking the blood pressure, checking the rate and fullness of the pulse, observing the fullness of the peripheral and neck veins (and the filling pressure of the heart) and looking for signs of heart failure. Collapsed peripheral veins, for example, may signify serious hypovolemia, a common state in hypertensive patients. The anesthetist also should check the patient's ECG and chest roentgenogram for signs of circulatory derangement. If evidence of a previously unsuspected or undiagnosed circulatory disorder is thus disclosed, elective surgery should be delayed until a full evaluation can be made, usually by an internist or cardiologist.

The preoperative evaluation also alerts the anesthetist to the type and extent of cardiovascular monitoring that should be done in the operative and postoperative periods. Depending upon the circulatory disorder and the location, nature, and extent of the operation, it may be valuable to monitor continuously the ECG, intra-arterial blood pressure and central venous, pulmonary artery or left atrial pressures throughout the operative period and extending into the postoperative period.

ARRHYTHMIAS

Cardiac arrhythmias are common in surgical patients. Occasionally, the anesthetist will detect an arrhythmia at the time of the preoperative visit. Such an arrhythmia may be a normal variant, as with the sinus arrhythmia so often found in children, but often it signifies the presence of a circulatory disorder or organic heart disease, or is an effect of a drug used to treat heart disease. A classification and the characteristic features of the common arrhythmias are shown in Table 20-1; detailed consideration of these arrhythmias, their incidence, etiology and treatment is beyond the scope of this book. Even so, there are certain guidelines that the anesthetist may follow when he detects an arrhythmia in a patient on his preoperative visit. Such a finding should, of course, be followed by a complete cardiovascular evaluation.

Preanesthetic Assessment and Control

Arrhythmias are not necessarily a contraindication to anesthesia and surgery. Certainly, rapid rates should be brought under control by drugs or cardioversion before operation. Before attributing a sinus tachycardia to preoperative anxiety, the anesthetist must be certain that this is not a sign of hypovolemia or excessive use of stimulant drugs. Sinus bradycardia may suggest the need for atropine or scopolamine in the premedication or, if heart block is present, the anesthetist should be prepared to administer a chronotropic agent such as isoproterenol intravenously. It may be advisable to insert a transvenous pacemaker under local anesthesia before major surgery is undertaken in elderly patients with bradyarrhythmias. Stable arrhythmias that do not impair coronary circulation or myocardial performance (i.e., cardiac output) are not likely to be worsened by anesthetic drugs, provided hypotension, hypoxemia, respiratory or metabolic acidosis and sudden exposure to abnormally high concentrations of anesthetic drugs are avoided. Continuous electrocardiographic monitoring is advisable during operation, even though the arrhythmia appears stable preoperatively, because arrhythmias may herald impending trouble.

Intraoperative Assessment and Control

Arrhythmias may occur during operation in patients who otherwise have normal cardiac rhythm. The incidence of arrhythmias during operation depends largely on the technics used to detect them. When continuous electrocardiographic monitoring is used, the incidence varies from 16 to 60%. In general, cardiac arrhythmias are more frequent under the following circumstances: during operation; in patients who have arrhythmias or heart disease before operation; in patients taking digitalis regularly; in patients in whom a tracheal tube is in place; in patients undergoing surgery of the eye or thorax; and in patients in whom the operation lasts for more than 3 hours.[3] Every type of arrhythmia (see Table 20-1) may occur during operation, but the most common types are the slow supraventricular arrhythmias and premature ventricular contractions.

TABLE 20-1.—CLASSIFICATION AND CHARACTERISTIC FEATURES OF ARRHYTHMIAS

TYPE OF ARRHYTHMIA	RATE/MIN	ORIGIN OF IMPULSES	ECG PATTERN	CHARACTERISTIC FEATURES
		Rapid Regular Pulse		
Sinus tachycardia	100 to 150 (adults) >180 (newborns)	SA node	Normal	
Supraventricular tachycardia	140 to 250	Ectopic atrial foci	Abnormal P wave	History of prior attacks paroxysmal tachycardia
		AV node	No P wave or inverted P from retrograde conduction	
		Ectopic atrial foci with block	Multiple P waves/QRS complex	AV block common with digitalis toxicity
Atrial flutter	250 to 350 (atrial) 70 to 160 (ventricular)	Ectopic atrial foci	Saw-tooth P waves Normal QRS	AV block common
Ventricular tachycardia	140 to 250	Ectopic ventricular foci	No P waves Wide QRS complexes	Common with myocardial ischemia
Ventricular flutter	200 to 300	Ectopic ventricular foci	Sine-wave pattern	
		Slow Regular Pulse		
Sinus bradycardia	<60 (adults) <100 (newborns)	SA node	Normal	Abolished by exercise or atropine
Nodal bradycardia	50 to 60	AV node	No P waves	
Heart block	<60	SA or AV node	Long PR interval (>0.2 sec)	1st degree block
			Two or more P waves/QRS complex	2nd degree block
			Independent atrial & ventricular rates	3rd degree block
			Widened QRS with two R waves	Bundle-branch block
		Irregular Pulse		
Sinus arrhythmia	60 to 80	SA node	Normal	Accelerates on inspiration Slows on expiration Abolished by exercise

TYPE OF ARRHYTHMIA	RATE/MIN	ORIGIN OF IMPULSES	ECG PATTERN	CHARACTERISTIC FEATURES
Wandering pacemaker	Variable	Ectopic atrial foci	P wave shape changes	
Premature atrial contractions	Variable	Ectopic atrial foci	Abnormal P wave	
Premature ventricular contractions	Variable	Ectopic ventricular foci	Wide QRS No P wave or retrograde P	Slow conduction time
Atrial fibrillation	Variable	Ectopic atrial foci	Indistinct or absent P	Irregular, irregularity
Ventricular fibrillation	Variable	Ectopic ventricular foci	Indistinct QRS complex	Equivalent to cardiac arrest

During operation, most arrhythmias are caused by imbalances of the autonomic nervous system, either an excess of sympathetic or parasympathetic tone in the heart. Factors such as hypoxia or hypercarbia, which liberate endogenous catecholamines, may precipitate an arrhythmia during anesthesia. Anesthetic drugs vary greatly in their ability to produce arrhythmias, either alone or when combined with exogenous catecholamine administration. Arrhythmia is common with excessive doses of cyclopropane or trichloroethylene, making this a valuable sign of overdosage. Halothane, methoxyflurane, ether, fluroxene, enflurane and isoflurane are less likely to produce arrhythmias, even when administered in excess. These anesthetics, however, may decrease the dose of endogenous or exogenous catecholamine required to precipitate an arrhythmia; they are said to "sensitize" the heart to arrhythmias. Cyclopropane and halogenated hydrocarbons sensitize the myocardium to adrenergic agents such as epinephrine, norepinephrine, metaraminol and dopamine but not ephedrine, phenylephrine or mephentermine.

Stimulation of the parasympathetic nervous system, such as that associated with intubation of the trachea, insertion of a nasogastric tube, traction on intraabdominal or intrathoracic structures, manipulation of the extraocular muscles of the eye or carotid sinus stimulation, occurs commonly during anesthesia and operation. The responses to such stimulation may include bradycardia, other arrhythmias and hypotension. Arrhythmias are more likely if the patient is lightly anesthetized, a state not uncommonly seen with the liberal and inappropriate use of muscle relaxants.

Other causes of arrhythmias include electrolyte imbalance, especially hypokalemia or hyperkalemia, stimulation of the brain during neurosurgical operations and the use of drugs like succinylcholine that have cardiac actions. Arrhythmias due to succinylcholine usually occur after the second or third injection of the drug. Such arrhythmias are usually seen much more often in children and with the intravenous rather than the intramuscular injection of the drug. Several mechanisms have been proposed, including loss of potassium from myocardial cells, postganglionic sympathetic stimulation, ganglionic stimulation and a direct myocardial effect of succinylcholine. The arrhythmic action of succinylcholine is not necessarily prevented by the prior administration of a nondepolarizing muscle relaxant such as *d*-tubocurarine.

Most arrhythmias occurring during operation are short-lived, benign, and do not require treatment. Overanxiety to initiate therapy usually complicates the problem unnecessarily, especially if the therapy involves administration of a cardiac depressant or antiarrhythmic drug. Most such arrhythmias will subside spontaneously within a few minutes of their onset. Persistent arrhythmias, particularly those of ventricular origin, should be regarded as a sign of serious derangement and a search should be made for a possible cause. Correction of inadequacies in ventilation and oxygenation, aberrations in acid-base and electrolyte status, and adjustment of level of anesthesia (increase or decrease) should be made as first steps. Excluding cardiac surgery, it is rarely necessary to resort to the use of antiarrhythmic drugs such as lidocaine or propranolol to control intraoperative arrhythmias.

Monitoring by ECG

Consideration of arrhythmia during anesthesia brings up the question of the need for routine monitoring of the ECG in every anesthetized patient. It is our belief that by means of careful preanesthetic evaluation, knowledge of the factors precipitating arrhythmias and close attention to cardiac function through precordial or esophageal monitoring the anesthetist can detect aberrations in rhythm, and that these arrhythmias can then be further assessed by use of the ECG, especially if they persist. We support routine monitoring by ECG but do not believe that it is mandatory for proper and safe patient management during anesthesia. As we have indicated in Chapter 5, the ECG as used in the operating room is usually capable only of revealing changes in rhythm.

EFFECTS OF ANESTHETICS ON CIRCULATION

With the exception of blood, body tissues have little or no storage capacity for oxygen and consequently are highly dependent upon the circulation for their necessary oxygenation. Hence, circulation must be adequately maintained if highly metabolically active tissues such as brain, heart and kidneys are to remain viable. Unfortunately, there is no easy or reliable means to assess the adequacy of circulation to these various tissues. Measurement of systemic blood pressure does not provide the answer because flow, not pressure, is the critical determinant of tissue oxygenation. We do not even have well-defined upper and lower limits of blood pressure to assure ourselves of adequate tissue oxygenation in most patients. With greater effort, measurements of central venous pressure, left atrial pressure or cardiac output can be made. As with blood pressure, the absolute values for these measurements are less informative than the directions of change. Lacking specific, sensitive indices of circulatory impairment, the anesthetist routinely follows the simpler signs of circulatory homeostasis such as blood pressure, pulse, heart sounds, skin color, temperature and capillary refill time. When indicated, he may monitor the ECG, central venous pressure, urine output, left atrial pressure or pulmonary artery pressure or even cardiac output. Regardless of the measurements, it is the trends rather than the absolute values that are of primary concern to him. The anesthetist also learns to arrive at decisions about the state of the patient's circulation from the net result of measurements and observations rather than from any single measurement or observation.

Inhalation Anesthetics

Anesthetics have varied and sometimes profound effects on circulation. Eger, Stevens and colleagues, for example, have made extensive studies of the effects of inhalation anesthetics on the circulation in young adult, healthy volunteers who were not exposed to surgery.[4, 5] The drugs were administered in multiples of equianalgesic doses, the MAC concept being used to permit comparative evaluation of the various drugs (Table 20-2). These authors found that, at light levels of surgical anesthesia, the inhalation anesthetics can be divided into two groups: those that either have no effects or stimulate the circulation and those that depress the circulation. Cyclopropane, fluroxene and diethyl ether are included in the former category while halothane, methoxyflurane, enflurane and, to a lesser extent, isoflurane make up the latter category.

CYCLOPROPANE.—Cyclopropane produces the least change in circulatory function in healthy man.[4] After 1 hour of moderate cyclopropane anesthesia (1.7 MAC or 17%), cardiac output, heart rate and muscle blood flow were unchanged from normal. Mean arterial blood pressure increased 30%, primarily because of an increase in total peripheral resistance. Only when very high concentrations of cyclopropane were administered (3.6 MAC or 37% cyclopropane) did cardiac output show any decrease from normal (15%); the decreased cardiac output resulted from decreases in both heart rate and stroke volume. After 4 hours of cyclopropane anesthesia, blood pressure and peripheral resistance had returned to values that were close to the awake values. Cardiac output had increased by 10%, much of it probably being directed to muscle, which showed a 50% increase in flow.

FLUROXENE AND DIETHYL ETHER.—Fluroxene and diethyl ether produce similar circulatory changes.[4] At light levels of anesthesia (1.4 MAC), cardiac output, blood pressure, total peripheral resistance and muscle blood flow were essentially unchanged from the awake values for both agents (see Table 20-2). Ether produced a 25% increase in heart rate while fluroxene caused a slight decrease. Cardiac output, blood pressure and heart rate were maintained above awake values, even at deep levels of anesthesia (2.8 to 3.2 MAC). Left ventricular work and stroke work increase above the awake

TABLE 20-2.—CIRCULATORY EFFECTS OF COMMONLY USED INHALATION ANESTHETICS IN HEALTHY VOLUNTEERS; NORMAL Pa_{CO_2}

AGENT	HOURS OF ANESTHESIA	ALVEOLAR CONCENTRATION %	MAC %	CARDIAC OUTPUT(a)	HEART RATE(a)	MEAN ARTERIAL PRESSURE(a)	TOTAL PERIPHERAL RESISTANCE(a)	MUSCLE BLOOD FLOW(a)
Cyclopropane[4](b)	1	17	1.7	No change	No change	30↑	30↑	No change
	4	17	1.7	10↑	No change	10↑	No change	50↑
Fluroxene[4]	1	5.3	1.4	No change	10↓	No change	10↓	No change
(Fluoromar)	5	5.3	1.4	40↑	20↑	15↓	40↓	300↑
Isoflurane[5](c)	1	1.2		No change	20↑	25↓	25↓	100↑
(Forane)	5	1.2		No change	20↑	30↓	25↓	200↑
Halothane[4]	1	1.01	1.2	20↓	No change	25↓	10↓	No change
(Fluothane)	5	1.01	1.2	No change	10↑	25↓	25↓	40↑
Ether[4]	1	3.0	1.4	No change	25↑	No change	No change	No change
	5	3.0	1.4	40↑	55↑	15↓	35↓	180↑
Methoxyflurane[6]	1	0.22	1.4	15↓	10↑	25↓	10↓	
(Penthrane)	3	0.22	1.4	15↓	15↑	25↓	10↓	

(a) Values represent percentage increase or decrease from control.
(b) Superscript numbers are reference numbers (see end of chapter).
(c) Comparable data for enflurane (Ethrane) in man are not available.

values with fluroxene (and also cyclopropane) and to a lesser extent with ether.

HALOTHANE.—Halothane causes the greatest depression of circulation at any level of anesthesia (see Table 20-2).[4] Halothane decreases cardiac output, entirely by decreasing stroke volume. Left ventricular work and stroke work decrease during halothane anesthesia as a result of depression of myocardial contractility. Halothane has been shown to decrease the maximal initial velocity of isotonic shortening (Vmax) and the tension developed isometrically. Halothane also decreases the blood pressure, owing in part to a decrease in cardiac output and in part to a decrease in total peripheral resistance. These changes are dose-dependent; the larger the dose, the more profound the circulatory changes. If profound halothane anesthesia (1.2 MAC) is continued for 5 hours, spontaneous recovery of cardiac output occurs, due to an increase in both stroke volume and heart rate. Spontaneous increases in cardiac output were observed with prolonged cyclopropane, fluroxene and diethyl ether anesthesia as well. It is not known why the depressant effects of halothane were reversed or why the stimulant effects of cyclopropane, fluroxene and ether were augmented by prolonging the anesthesia. The recovery from halothane depression can be prevented by propranolol, suggesting that stimulation of the sympathetics, especially the β receptors in the heart, may be the primary mechanism. The increase in heart rate seen with prolonged anesthesia with all of these agents would explain much of the recovery response seen.

METHOXYFLURANE.—Methoxyflurane produces circulatory changes that are similar to but less profound than those produced by halothane (Table 20-2).[6] At light levels of anesthesia (1.4 MAC), cardiac output is decreased, despite an increase in heart rate. This decrease is due entirely to a decrease in cardiac contractility and hence stroke volume. Both arterial blood pressure and peripheral resistance are also decreased by methoxyflurane. With prolonged methoxyflurane anesthesia, cardiac contractility (Vmax or rate of tension development [dp/dt] ratios) improves but this is not reflected in an increase in cardiac output, probably because of the continued depression of peripheral resistance.

ISOFLURANE.—Isoflurane has circulatory effects that are unique.[5] Isoflurane decreases stroke volume but, because of the concomitant increase in heart rate, cardiac output remains unchanged. Blood pressure is decreased because of the decrease in peripheral resistance. This change is dose-dependent. Much of the decrease in peripheral resistance appears to occur in muscle and skin, in which blood flow is appreciably increased. Except for some increase in muscle blood flow, prolongation of isoflurane anesthesia appears to produce little change in the circulatory variables.

Isoflurane, methoxyflurane and cyclopropane exhibit the least amount of temporally-related cardiovascular stimulation. These drugs have little in common that would explain this observation. It has been speculated that the circulatory stimulant may be a metabolite of the anesthetic.[5] Since neither isoflurane nor cyclopropane undergoes any appreciable biotransformation, there would be no metabolite to stimulate recovery. Acceptance of this theory, however, necessitates an explanation as to why methoxyflurane, a metabolically active anesthetic, also shows little circulatory recovery with time.

ENFLURANE.—Enflurane, an isomer of isoflurane, has not been subjected to critical evaluation in volunteers similar to that reported for the other inhalation anesthetics. Laboratory studies in animals and studies in the clinical setting suggest that the cardiovascular effects of enflurane are similar in kind to those for halothane; namely, depression of myocardial contractility, cardiac output and systemic blood pressure. It is dissimilar from halothane in that enflurane increases total peripheral resistance, probably because of less depression of peripheral sympathetic activity.

NITROUS OXIDE.—As an adjuvant to the more potent inhalation anesthetics, nitrous oxide has been regarded as being impotent and innocuous in its circulatory effects. Several studies would indicate that this is not the case. Nitrous oxide (70%), when added to a stable halothane anesthetic in human volunteers, produces signs of sympathetic stimulation, particularly of the peripheral vasculature.[7] Values for arterial blood pressure, right atrial pressure, systemic vascular resistance, and forearm vascular resistance all increase; the pupils also usually dilate and the plasma norepinephrine concentration may increase. In general, myocardial function remains unaltered by 70% nitrous oxide in volunteers; in patients with cardiovascular disease, however, nitrous oxide may produce cardiovascular depression. Major decreases in arterial pressure, heart rate, cardiac index and stroke volume index have been shown to occur in patients with coronary artery disease or valvular heart disease given 60% nitrous oxide.[8] Circulatory function may remain depressed for some time after discontinuation of nitrous oxide in these patients. Such observations reemphasize the fact that drugs may act differently in different settings; physicians must be alert to the varied backgrounds under which the drugs they give are being administered.

General Considerations of the Circulatory Effects of Inhalation Anesthetics

In general, inhalation anesthetics increase right atrial pressure: halothane and ether increase mean pressure by 2 to 4 torr, and fluroxene and cyclopropane increase mean pressure by 6 to 10 torr. These changes are dose-related; the greater the dose, the higher the value for right atrial pressure. This finding suggests that all of these inhalation anesthetics produce some degree of cardiovascular depression.

The basis for the diverse circulatory effects of different anesthetics is unknown. Controversy still exists regarding the actions of anesthetics on circulatory control mechanisms. Price has concluded that cyclopropane (and presumably other sympathomimetic-like anesthetics) increases sympathetic activity by selectively inhibiting the depressor area.[9] Markee, on the other hand, found the pressor area of the medulla to be the more sensitive to the depressant effects of cyclopropane.[10] This difference in findings remains to be resolved.

The circulatory effects of halothane are probably of both central and peripheral origin. The central effects are disputed, some studies showing depression of medullary vasomotor neurons by halothane and others showing no effects on these neurons. It is generally accepted, however, that halothane acts peripherally by depressing ganglionic transmission and myocardial contractility and dilating vascular smooth muscle. Whether halothane causes vasodilation directly or in part by the release of vasopressin is not known.

Although clinical studies of drug effects in volunteers are basic to our understanding of the circulatory pharmacology of these drugs, one must be cautious when attempting to derive clinical implications from these findings. These kinds of studies do not tell us which anesthetic is safest for the patient with cardiac insufficiency. One might speculate that halothane, because it decreases myocardial work more than it decreases cardiac output or blood pressure, would be the ideal agent for patients with coronary insufficiency. On the other hand, if perfusion pressure to the heart or other organs (e.g., brain and kidneys) is the critical factor, then anesthetics that increase sympathetic activity (e.g., cyclopropane, fluroxene and ether) may be more beneficial. However, we have few reliable indicators as to how good or how poor circulatory function may be. None of the agents studied produce any appreciable alterations in base excess, a finding that suggests that, despite the extreme variability in circulatory function, whole-body perfusion is adequate.

Quite aside from the anesthetic drugs themselves, there are many other factors in the clinical setting that may influence the cardiovascular effects of anesthetics. Some factors, such as hypovolemia, advancing age, catecholamine depletion by drugs or chronic stress and mild hypothermia that commonly occurs during anesthesia and surgery, may augment the cardiovascular depression of anesthetic drugs. In contrast, surgical stimulation or hypercapnia associated with the use of combinations of opiates and inhalation anesthetics may stimulate the sympathetic nervous system and thereby the cardiovascular system. There are few studies that analyze the impact of such factors individually in the clinical setting.

REGIONAL BLOOD FLOW.—*Cerebral Blood Flow.*—Inhalation anesthetics have pronounced effects on regional blood flow as well. *Halothane* increases cerebral blood flow (CBF) and decreases cerebral vascular resistance and cerebral metabolism (CMR_{O_2}), the magnitude of these changes increasing with increasing anesthetic depth.[11] At a 1.2% halothane concentration, CBF increases from 15 to 25% above normal and CMR_{O_2} decreases by about the same amount. The changes in flow and resistance are presumed to be due to direct cerebral vasodilatation by halothane. Even though halothane may be a cerebral vasodilator, there is no evidence that it can cause a loss of cerebral autoregulation or an intracerebral steal of blood from ischemic brain like that produced by CO_2, provided serious hypotension does not occur. If mean arterial pressure is allowed to decrease below 60 to 70 torr, cerebral autoregulation may be lost because of maximal cerebral vasodilation. Whether the increase in CBF produced by halothane is beneficial to patients is not known; however, there is mounting evidence that, under some circumstances, it may be hazardous. Cerebral vasodilatation from any agent causes an increase in cerebrovascular volume and an increase in intracranial pressure. In the healthy patient, increases in intracranial pressure are minimized by the compensatory displacement of cerebrospinal fluid from the intracranial to the spinal subarachnoid compartment. Such compensatory mechanisms may be impaired in patients with intracranial space-occupying lesions. In these patients, intracranial pressure may increase to values of 500 to 800 mm H_2O, the increase being dose-dependent. Inhalation agents thus far identified that increase intracranial pressure include *halothane*, *methoxyflurane* and *trichloroethylene*. For this reason, it is advisable to avoid these drugs or use the lowest doses required in patients with intracranial lesions. Hyperventilation should also be considered in such patients, as it may counteract the anesthetic-induced cerebral vasodilatation.

Cyclopropane and *diethyl ether* have biphasic effects on CBF, decreasing CBF below awake values at low (subanesthetic) concentrations and increasing it well above awake values (i.e., a 60% increase) at high concentrations. Both drugs decrease $CMRo_2$ by 20 to 40%. *Enflurane* is unique among inhalation agents in that, while it has no effects on CBF, it is the most potent depressant of $CMRo_2$; a concentration of 3% decreases $CMRo_2$ by 50%. Unlike all other inhalation agents, *nitrous oxide* (70%) has little or no effect on CBF or $CMRo_2$.

Unfortunately, present knowledge about the effects of anesthetic drugs on flow and metabolism does not allow us to select the ideal agent for administration to patients who are undergoing operative procedures that may cause cerebral ischemia. We have no rational basis for making such a choice. We do not know whether changes in cerebral flow or metabolism offer protection against cerebral ischemia or increase the risks of a neurologic deficit should an ischemic episode occur. For the present, selection of an anesthetic for a patient with a potential or actual neurologic disorder is made, for the most part, on criteria other than its neurocirculatory effects. The only major exception to this is the use of special precautions or the avoidance of drugs that increase intracranial pressure in patients with raised intracranial pressure.

Splanchnic and renal blood flow.—Inhalation anesthetics decrease splanchnic and renal blood flow. Although the effects of anesthetics on visceral blood flow have been studied with only a few agents, the findings are qualitatively similar. Both *halothane*, a sympathetic nervous system depressant, and *cyclopropane*, a sympathetic nervous system stimulant, decreased hepatic blood flow 30% below awake values in lightly anesthetized healthy volunteers (halothane 1.5%; cyclopropane 18%).[12] The decrease with halothane is caused by a decrease in systemic arterial pressure while with cyclopropane it is caused by an increase in regional vascular resistance. However, regardless of the mechanism of the decrease in blood flow, no evidence for splanchnic ischemia could be found. No hazardous or toxic effects from decreases in splanchnic blood flow by anesthetics have been identified.

Inhalation anesthetics depress renal function in man, the magnitude of the depression depending upon the prevailing conditions. Under the usual conditions of surgical anesthesia with halothane, it can be expected that renal blood flow and glomerular filtration rate will be decreased by 50% or more below awake values. Even in young, healthy, well-hydrated volunteers, light halothane anesthesia (1.5%) decreases renal blood flow by 40% and glomerular filtration rate by 20%.[13] These abnormalities in renal function are probably the result of decreases in arterial pressure and cardiac output, although vasopressin release or activation of the renin-angiotensin-aldosterone mechanism cannot be excluded. Studies in patients undergoing renal transplantation have reemphasized the importance, for renal survival, of maintaining renal function at about normal during anesthesia and operation. When called upon to anesthetize patients with borderline renal function, it would seem prudent that the anesthetist use every means required to maintain a urine flow at about normal. These may include vigorous hydration before operation as well as during and after operation, use of light anesthesia to avoid hypotension and the judicious use of osmotic diuretics such as mannitol. Certainly, anesthetic drugs known to be metabolized to inorganic fluoride ions (*methoxyflurane*, a known nephrotoxin, and probably *enflurane*) should be avoided.

Intravenous Anesthetics

THIOPENTAL AND SIMILAR DRUGS.—Like the inhalation anesthetics, the intravenous anesthetics have varied and sometimes profound effects on the circulation. In general, the effects depend primarily on the state of the circulation prior to drug administration, the dose and rate of drug administration and the compensatory circulatory responses that occur. Thiopental, for example, is a myocardial depressant, decreasing myocardial contractility and cardiac output in proportion to the dose administered. In healthy adults, doses of 250 mg or less given intravenously usually have little effect on circulatory function as manifested by changes in blood pressure. Any decrease in stroke volume is usually compensated for by a modest increase in heart rate. However, administration of doses as small as 25 to 50 mg may cause cardiovascular collapse in patients with dehydration, hypovolemia or already impaired myocardial performance. Because the net effects of the rapid-acting barbiturates are so varied, they should always be administered cautiously and slowly. In general, use of repeated small doses rather than single large doses is preferred.

Thiopental may have profound effects on CBF and $CMRO_2$, again depending upon the dose.[11] In large doses (35 mg/kg), thiopental decreases CBF and $CMRO_2$ by 50 to 60% below awake values, without altering the blood flow responses to changes in Pa_{CO_2}. Thiopental does not increase intracranial pressure, provided ventilation and Pa_{CO_2} are maintained at normal. Because of its cerebral circulatory effects, thiopental or other rapidly acting barbiturates may prove to be the ideal anesthetic drugs for patients undergoing operations in which cerebral ischemia may possibly occur. However, because for patients with present or potential cerebral ischemia it is useful to be able to assess the responses as soon as possible after anesthesia and surgery, the use of even short-acting barbiturates may interfere with assessment of responses after operation. Here, as in many other circumstances, one must take into account all the factors involved rather than make decisions based upon the action of an agent on one organ.

MORPHINE AND MEPERIDINE.—The opiates, like the barbiturates, may produce appreciable changes in the circulation but, unlike the barbiturates, the principal site of action is on the peripheral vasculature rather than on the heart. Existing evidence indicates that the opiates have no major depressant effects on the heart, provided hypercarbia and respiratory acidosis are avoided. It is primarily for this reason that the use of large doses of opiates (e.g., morphine 1 to 3 mg/kg) has become a popular anesthetic technic for critically ill patients undergoing cardiac surgical procedures. Studies in such patients have shown that morphine (1 mg/kg) may mildly stimulate the heart, increasing stroke volume and cardiac output and decreasing peripheral vascular resistance.[8] Hypotension usually will not occur unless there is a serious degree of hypovolemia. Because peripheral vasodilatation is the only major circulatory effect of morphine, a declining blood pressure following its administration signals the need for augmented fluid therapy.

The hemodynamic effects of meperidine (Demerol) and other opiates resemble those of morphine with one exception. Meperidine has a molecular configuration resembling atropine and in large doses (10 mg/kg) may cause a profound tachycardia. Should this occur, heart rate can usually be effectively slowed by edrophonium (Tensilon), the dose being 2 to 5 mg intravenously.

Premedicant doses of opiates have no overt effects on the circulation unless there is hypercarbia and respiratory acidosis or a serious degree of hypovolemia. Even so, the normovolemic patients can still become acutely hypotensive by the combination of opiate-induced peripheral vasodilation and sudden shifts in body posture from supine to sitting or standing or by sudden forward acceleration or deceleration. Patients given opiates should be moved about slowly.

Little is known about the effects of opiates on the regional distribution of blood flow. CBF is unaltered by premedicant or mild anesthetic doses of opiates, provided Pa_{CO_2} is not changed. Opiates may cause a mild decrease in cerebral metabolism.

KETAMINE.—Like most anesthetic drugs, ketamine is a myocardial depressant when studied in the isolated dog heart-lung preparation. In intact man, however, it is clearly a circulatory stimulant. At doses of 1 to 2 mg/kg intravenously, ketamine has both central and peripheral effects, the former predominating.[14] Ketamine increases the cardiac index and mean arterial blood pressure by 30%, primarily by increasing heart rate. Both myocardial contractility and oxygen consumption are increased by ketamine. Changes in peripheral vascular resistance are small and quite variable. At these doses, ketamine may increase CBF by as much as 80% above normal and $CMRO_2$ by a smaller amount (16%). The increase in CBF, although transient, will induce potentially hazardous increases in intracranial pressure. Hence, this drug should be used cautiously in patients with intracranial aneurysms or increased intracranial pressure. Because of its general circulatory support, ketamine would appear to be an ideal agent for use in the presence of hypovolemia, hemorrhage, or shock.

DIAZEPAM.—Diazepam (Valium), a drug that is commonly used for sedation and amnesia, has mild, but occasionally unpredictable, circulatory effects. In most patients, the circulation is unchanged, which leads to the use of diazepam in patients undergoing cardioversion, as an amnesic drug for seriously ill patients undergoing cardiac surgery and as a sedative-amnesic drug for patients undergoing regional block anesthesia. However, one must keep in mind that the usual doses of diazepam may provoke significant hypotension in some patients with or without coexisting hypovolemia.

FLUID THERAPY

It is dangerous to generalize about the ideal fluid therapy for the surgical patient because the needs for fluids vary greatly among patients with surgical diseases and during the course of therapy for any specific surgical disease. To describe the fluid needs for every type of patient or every common surgical condition is beyond the scope of this book. Rather, we will consider the major kinds of fluids available and their general indications for usage.

Blood (Whole Blood or Components)

Whole blood is the obvious fluid of choice for administration to patients who are in hemorrhagic shock or are actively bleeding, either before or during operation. Some therapists have recently used, in lieu of whole blood, red cells specifically for replacement of hemoglobin and colloids for fluid replacement. The argument in favor of this practice hinges largely on the advantage of preserving, for use in other patients needing specific therapy, elements in the plasma rather than, in a sense, wasting valuable plasma elements simply for volume replacement.

DETERMINATION OF REPLACEMENT VOLUME.—Much more difficult is knowing how much whole blood or blood components to administer. Before operation, symptoms and signs of shock clearly indicate the need for more blood. However, during anesthesia symptoms are absent and signs also may be absent, diminished or masked. Blood pressure changes seem to be the most reliable. Changes in pulse rate and quality and changes in the quality of heart tones also are useful in the anesthetized patient. Remaining for assessment, but less prominent in the anesthetized patient, are changes such as those of skin color, skin temperature and perspiration. These latter observations may help one to distinguish between hypotension due to blood loss and hypotension due to anesthetic overdose or a reflex action. In the latter circumstances, the skin often remains warm and dry, and the color may be reasonably normal. Estimation of blood loss during operation is usually notoriously in error unless special efforts are made to measure it accurately. This involves keeping a continuous tally of blood lost into the suction apparatus and of the volume of other fluids aspirated into the suction, and also the weighing of sponges, drapes and gowns. Careful, continuous tally of blood loss is especially important in infants and children, in whom a sudden loss of seemingly small amounts of blood during operation can result in profound shock or cardiac arrest. Blood should be replaced in these patients as it is lost, so that one is not suddenly faced with a loss that far exceeds the amount transfused. The administration of whole blood *before* as well as during major aortic vascular surgery has greatly lessened the frequency and severity of the hypotensive episodes that occur with the declamping of major vessels.

Administration of a single unit of whole blood is frequently condemned as bad medical practice because the patient is exposed to the hazards of transfusion (e.g., allergic reaction and hepatitis) in a circumstance in which he could, with less hazard, restore his own loss of red cells. While this may be true outside the operating room, it does not necessarily apply in the operating room. Blood replacement in the operating room generally begins when the estimated blood losses and projected losses exceed 10% of the patient's blood volume. If, after the first unit of blood has been administered, the revised projected losses amount to less than those of the previous estimate (usually because the nature of the operative procedure changes), then this may become an example of a single unit transfusion. As difficult as it is to estimate blood loss in the operating room, it is even more difficult to estimate future losses—yet the latter must be done to avoid placing the patient in jeopardy from hemorrhagic shock. In determining the need for blood, the anesthetist should include an estimate of the losses that may occur in the early postoperative period.

COMPLICATIONS OF TRANSFUSION.—The complications of blood transfusion are of five major types: allergic reactions, nonspecific febrile reactions, hemolytic reactions, disease transmission and circulatory disorders. *Allergic reactions* occur in about 1% of transfusions and, in the anesthetized patient, they will usually be manifest as erythema and urticarial rashes of the skin. Generally, no treatment is necessary other than immediate cessation of infusion of that unit of blood, but antihistamines can be given if the patient should complain later of itching.

Febrile reactions are rare since the advent of plastic disposable blood banking equipment. This is fortunate because their diagnosis is difficult in the anesthetized patient. A sudden fever or convulsive-like movements within 15 to 30 minutes of the start of blood administration suggest this diagnosis. If this is the suspected cause, the transfusion should be stopped and vigorous treatment of the hyperthermia begun; also, blood should be taken for bacterial cultures.

Hemolytic reactions are the most dreaded complication of blood transfusion therapy because of the serious morbidity and high mortality associated with them. They result from incompatibilities of the ABD or Rh systems or from reactions to rare erythrocyte antigens. Most reactions are due to human errors of mislabeling or misreading labels in which the wrong blood is transfused. Anesthetists must be especially cautious to avoid errors in transfusion because hemolytic reactions are especially difficult to diagnose in the anesthetized patient. The opportunity for such reactions is enhanced in circumstances of multiple transfusions, probably because of the interaction of blood in the different units and also because of frequent errors in determining compatibility of blood given in the circumstances requiring multiple transfusion. The anesthetized patient may show signs of tachycardia, tachypnea, fever or hemoglobinuria. The only sign may be that of excessive bleeding during operation caused by intravascular defibrinogenation and thrombocytopenia. If a hemolytic reaction is suspected, the transfusion should be stopped immediately and the remaining blood and a fresh sample of the patient's blood should be sent to the blood bank for study. Laboratory studies of blood urea nitrogen, serum electrolytes, serum bilirubin and blood and urine hemoglobin should be made. High urine output should be produced by the vigorous administration of fluids intravenously, supplemented with mannitol if necessary.

Transmission of hepatitis remains a problem because whole blood accounts for about 90% of all transfusion-associated cases. The attack rate of viral hepatitis from the transfusion of whole blood may vary from 1 to 16 cases per 1000 units administered. Careful screening of blood donors is the most effective means for minimizing this problem.

Of the *circulatory disorders,* the complication of the greatest concern is that of overloading the circulation. Special care must be taken to avoid too rapid replacement of blood in those patients susceptible to heart failure; namely, infants, the elderly and those with cardiac or pulmonary disease. The massive transfusion of blood to any patient offers the hazards of hypothermia, myocardial depression and cardiac arrest. The body core temperature can fall rapidly by several degrees if several units of refrigerated blood are infused quickly. To minimize this problem and if the administration of multiple units is anticipated, whole blood should be warmed to 30 to 35° C immediately before infusion. There are several methods for warming blood, the simplest being to immerse the blood bag or its delivery tubing in a basin of warm water. More sophisticated devices such as a water bath with a thermostat or microwave warmers are available. These devices must be checked periodically as they can cause overheating and hemolysis.

It was thought for many years that the massive transfusion of stored blood containing acid-citrate-dextrose solution would cause citric acid intoxication, citrate-induced hypocalcemia or a generalized acidosis. These fears are, for the most part, unfounded. Citric acid and citrate are freely diffusible substances that are rapidly metabolized in the liver and excreted. Citrate, of course, prevents blood from clotting by binding its calcium, an essential element in the clotting mechanism. It was reasoned that the massive transfusion of blood containing no free calcium might result in a dilutional hypocalcemia that, in turn, might cause a bleeding diathesis or cardiac arrest. Subsequent studies have shown that body stores of calcium are adequate to provide all of the necessary ionized calcium for clotting purposes and to stabilize serum calcium values. Except in exchange transfusions, the empiric administration of calcium with blood is unnecessary. Massive blood transfusion may cause a bleeding diathesis but the cause is usually a dilutional thrombocytopenia rather than a calcium deficiency.

Bank blood is acidotic (pH, 6.5 to 6.9 after 14 to 21 days of storage), and great concern has been expressed about the possibility that the massive transfusion of such blood may cause a serious systemic acidosis. Some authors therefore have advocated the prophylactic administration of sodium bicarbonate (44 mEq for every five units of blood transfused). Others have reported that this is usually unnecessary and may cause a troublesome metabolic alkalosis.[15] We advocate the periodic measurement of acid-base status if there is a special reason for concern.

BLOOD COMPONENTS.—*Packed cells.*—Packed red blood cells are a valuable substitute for whole blood when the primary purpose of giving blood is to increase the erythrocyte count and hence the oxygen carrying capacity of the recipient's blood. Packed cells minimize the chance for circulatory overload and greatly lessen the risk of transfusion reactions from plasma agglutinins. Use of packed cells instead of whole blood should be considered in the preoperative preparation or postoperative care of the anemic patient. Packed cells are seldom used during operation because whole blood is often the more logical replacement for surgical blood loss. Packed cell preparations also are extremely viscous and can only be administered slowly.

Plasma.—Plasma is indicated in two major situations in the surgical patient: 1) to supply sufficient clotting factors, and 2) to increase plasma protein values in cases of decreased production or increased loss of protein. The advantage of plasma over whole blood for treating clotting deficiencies is that plasma will supply the needed clotting factors without increasing the patient's hematocrit. All of the clotting factors are present in fresh or fresh frozen plasma and all factors but V and VIII remain active in plasma frozen to $-20°$ C. To minimize the incidence of hepatitis, plasma is processed from single units of donor blood. Fluid therapy in surgical conditions in which the primary deficit is plasma proteins, such as after major burns or intestinal obstruction with peritonitis, might best be managed with plasma or human serum albumin. Albumin (thermally treated to render it hepatitis-free) is available in a 5% buffered saline or a 25% "salt poor" solution; 25 gm of albumin is the osmotic equivalent of 500 ml of citrated plasma.

Platelet concentrates and fibrinogen.—Platelet concentrates and fibrinogen are rarely used during operation, most surgeons and anesthetists preferring to rely upon fresh whole blood or plasma to treat unexpected bleeding disorders. Low-molecular-weight dextrans are likewise seldom used in the surgical patient. The exceptions to this are when a lessening of cellular aggregation and a decrease in blood viscosity as well as volume expansion are desired. Dextrans are especially useful in patients susceptible to acute thrombophlebitis; for example, in patients undergoing orthopedic surgery of the lower extremities. Low-molecular-weight dextran is usually given as a 10% solution at a rate of 10 to 15 ml/kg/24 hr.

Intravenous Fluids

Every patient being maintained on intravenous fluids has a basic need for water, salt and glucose. The daily water requirement averages 1000 ml/m^2 and the sodium and chloride requirements about 60 mEq/m^2. The daily potassium requirement averages about 35 mEq/m^2. If the patient is febrile and sweating or losing extraordinary amounts of fluid from one or more body compartments, fluid requirements will increase. In addition to the loss of fluid from obvious sites (e.g., urine and nasogastric suction), fluid can also be lost *into* the body.[16] As a result of major trauma (including major surgical trauma), functional extracellular fluid volume may decrease by as much as 30%. The lost fluid is sequestered into third-space compartments, which may include the bowel lumen, the extracellular fluid space surrounding the traumatized area, and perhaps the intracellular space. Because both water and electrolytes are lost, replacement with lactated Ringer's solution, a balanced salt solution, has been advocated; the suggested intraoperative fluid schedule is 4 to 6 ml/kg/hr for mild trauma, 6 to 8 ml/kg/hr in cases of moderate trauma, and 10 to 12 ml/kg/hr in cases of major trauma.

LACTATED RINGER'S SOLUTION.—While we strongly support the need for fluid therapy before and during operation in order to prevent oliguria from stimulation of the ADH mechanism by anesthesia and surgery, we do not support the concept that lactated Ringer's solution is the ideal fluid for operative use. Our reasons for not recommending lactated Ringer's solution, with or without glucose, are several. First, lactated Ringer's solution contains potassium, presumably to prevent dilutional hypokalemia from occurring. However, this small amount of potassium (3 to 5 mEq/liter) is totally inadequate to match daily losses of potassium (50 to 150 mEq/day). As a long-term replacement fluid, the potassium content is totally inadequate and, as a short-term replacement fluid, the potassium content is totally unnecessary. Second, advocates of lactated Ringer's solution emphasize its value as a buffer against acidosis. Lactated Ringer's solution (per liter) contains about 28 mEq lactate, 10 mEq of which are in the form of D-lactic acid to acidify the solution and prevent caramelization of the glucose during sterilization. The D-lactate is not convertible to bicarbonate, leaving only the 18 mEq of L-lactate as the effective buffer. As with potassium, this quantity of buffer is ineffective in treating an acidosis and unnecessary when no acidosis exists. Third, the use of lactated Ringer's solution has deluded physicians into believing that the solution is therapeutic when it is not. This is our greatest concern. For ease and convenience, physicians may use lactated Ringer's solution in place of preparing specific solutions to meet specific patient needs. Finally, because of the many steps involved in its manufacture, the cost-benefit ratio for lactated Ringer's solution is unacceptably high.

RECOMMENDED FLUIDS.—What intravenous fluid do we prefer? For the routine operative procedure in a healthy patient, the type of fluid administered is of little importance. Fluids such as water with 5% glucose or half-normal saline with 5% glucose are quite acceptable. For patients requiring special electrolytes or buffers we prefer half-normal saline containing 5% glucose. We then add to this solution those quantities of cations or anions calculated to meet the patient's specific needs. One can add up to 90 mEq of bicarbonate and still maintain the solution at the osmolality of plasma. This solution will remain in the intravascular compartment for essentially the same time as lactated Ringer's solution and is more effective than lactated Ringer's solution in treating third-space loss. Perhaps most importantly, it forces the physician to adapt fluid therapy to the specific needs of each patient. Preloading with salt solution in the early period of anesthesia will lessen the incidence of hypotension during operation in patients who are hypovolemic or in whom large fluid shifts may be expected. Preloading with blood offers the same benefits in patients undergoing major vascular operations in whom a large blood loss may be anticipated. Preloading, of course, should be done slowly and with awareness of central venous pressure in patients with cardiovascular disease.

For infants and small children, our standard intravenous solution is one-quarter normal (0.2%) saline with 5% glucose. This solution provides the daily salt and water requirements for infants; special ions can be added as needed. A useful formula for fluid replacement in infants is the following: 100 ml/kg/24 hr for the first 10 kg of body weight, 50 ml/kg/24 hr for the second 10 kg, and 25 ml/kg/24 hr for any additional weight.

USE OF VASOPRESSORS

In the last 20 years, the use of vasopressors in clinical medicine has undergone a dramatic reversal. When first introduced into clinical medicine, pressor drugs were used to treat every conceivable type of circulatory instability, the belief being that organ flow was adequate provided systemic blood pressure was maintained. In time, the deleterious effects of pressor drugs became evident. The excessive vasoconstriction produced by pressor drugs sometimes decreased blood flow to some organs to flows below those required to maintain viability. This occurred commonly with the kidneys and resulted in anuria and renal failure. The intense vasoconstriction also decreased blood flow to skeletal muscle to the extent that anaerobic metabolism and lactic acidosis occurred, which in turn lessened the effectiveness of the pressor drug on the heart. Prolonged pressor therapy also increased capillary pressure and filtration, thereby decreasing intravascular volume. The resultant hypovolemia caused a decrease in cardiac output.

Recognition of the hazards of vasopressor therapy precipitated a reactionary movement against their use, again to the detriment of patients. In recent years with a greater understanding of normal circulatory dynamics and the pharmacologic actions of the various pressor drugs, the role of these drugs in patient care is more sharply defined.

Choice of Vasopressor Drug

Pressor drugs can be classified three ways, according to 1) the target organ stimulated, 2) the type of action, and 3) the type of adrenergic receptor stimulated.[17] The target organ may be the heart, the strength of contraction (inotropy) or the rate (chronotropy) being increased, or the peripheral vessels, or both. The type of action of the pressor drug may be a direct one in

TABLE 20-3.—CLASSIFICATION OF PRESSOR DRUGS

DRUG	TARGET ORGAN	TYPE OF ACTION	ADRENERGIC RECEPTORS STIMULATED	MAJOR DISADVANTAGES	USUAL DOSE
Epinephrine	Heart, blood vessels	Direct	β-low doses α-high doses	Arrhythmias	0.1 mg (I/V) 0.2-0.3 mg (I/M)
Norepinephrine	Heart, blood vessels	Direct	α β	Tissue necrosis Cardiomyopathy Hyperkalemia Metabolic acidosis Tachyphylaxis	8-16 mg in 500 ml D/5/W
Metaraminol (Aramine)	Heart, blood vessels	Direct, indirect	α β	Tachyphylaxis	0.05-0.1 mg (I/V) 0.1-0.3 mg (I/M)
Methoxamine (Vasoxyl)	Blood vessels	Direct	α	Myocardial depression	2-5 mg (I/V) 5-10 mg (I/M)
Phenylephrine (Neo-Synephrine)	Blood vessels	Direct	α		0.01 mg (I/V) 10-20 mg in 500 ml D/5/W
Ephedrine	Heart, blood vessels	Direct, indirect	α β	Tachyphylaxis	5-25 mg (I/V) 25-50 mg (I/M)
Mephentermine (Wyamine)	Heart, blood vessels	Direct, indirect	α β		300 mg in 500 ml D/5/W
Angiotensin	Heart, blood vessels	Direct, indirect	α β	Coronary vasoconstriction, decreased renal blood flow	2.5 mg in 500 ml D/5/W
Isoproterenol (Isuprel)	Heart, blood vessels	Direct	β	Arrhythmias Cardiomyopathy	2.5 mg in 500 ml D/5/W
Dopamine	Heart, blood vessels	Direct	α β		

which the drug itself acts as the receptor site. In contrast, the action may be indirect because the drug acts by releasing endogenous catecholamines, which in turn produce the pressor effect. Some pressor drugs have both direct and indirect actions. Finally, pressor drugs differ in their effects on the alpha and beta adrenergic receptors. Stimulation of alpha adrenergic receptors causes peripheral vasoconstriction, mydriasis and myometrial contraction; stimulation of the beta adrenergic receptors causes smooth muscle relaxation, inotropy and chronotropy, hyperglycemia and central nervous system excitation. Some pressor drugs may stimulate both types of receptors, depending on the dose administered.

The individual pressor drugs commonly in use are classified in Table 20-3. In general, we prefer *ephedrine* for routine vasopressor therapy if transient increases in blood pressure and myocardial contractility are needed until circulatory homeostasis is spontaneously or therapeutically re-established. Ephedrine is commonly used for the prevention or correction of transient hypotension from spinal or epidural anesthesia. Likewise, when a pressor drug is needed in obstetric cases, ephedrine is the ideal agent, because of its minimal deleterious effects on the fetus. As an alternative to ephedrine, we prefer *metaraminol*. Although more potent than ephedrine, its sites and mechanisms of action are similar to those of ephedrine. Occasionally, sustained pressor therapy is needed during anesthesia and operation; for example, to maintain a high systemic pressure during temporary interruption of a portion of the cerebral circulation. Under these circumstances, we prefer an infusion of *phenylephrine* because of its minimal effects on the heart and hence no tendency to produce arrhythmias. The antiarrhythmic property of *mephentermine* makes it also a useful drug for this purpose. We urge that, if repetitive or sustained administration of pressor drugs is required to maintain pressure, a physician search diligently for the reason for this. Hypovolemia, for example, often results in hypotension inappropriately treated by pressor drugs. Prolonged pressor therapy, regardless of the drug used, can be only deleterious to the patient.

Isoproterenol is a valuable pressor drug when the desired action is an increase in heart rate. Isoproterenol has a potent chronotropic action, which will usually result in an increase in blood pressure even though it causes vasodilation by its beta action on peripheral blood vessels. Isoproterenol is commonly used to maintain somewhat increased heart rates (and presumably cardiac output) in patients who have undergone cardiac surgery and in patients with heart block.

We mention *methoxamine* only to condemn its use. Although this drug increases blood pressure by peripheral vasoconstriction, it induces a negative chronotropic effect on the heart by stimulation of baroreceptors. Evidence indicates that it enriches flow to nonvital organs, such as muscle, at the expense of vital organs like the heart.

REFERENCES

1. Goldstein, A., and Keats, A. S.: The risk of anesthesia, Anesthesiology 33:130, 1970.
2. Tarhan, S., Moffitt, E. A., Taylor, W. F., and Giuliani, E. R.: Myocardial infarction after general anesthesia, J.A.M.A. 220:1451, 1972.
3. Katz, R. L., and Bigger, J. T.: Cardiac arrhythmias during anesthesia and operation, Anesthesiology 33:193, 1970.
4. Eger, E. I., II, Smith, N. T., Cullen, D. G., Cullen, B. F., and Gregory, G. A.: A comparison of the cardiovascular effects of halothane, fluroxene, ether and cyclopropane in man: a resume, Anesthesiology 34:25, 1971.
5. Stevens, W. C., Cromwell, T. H., Halsey, M. J., Eger, E. I., Shakespeare, T. F., and Bahlman, S. H.: The cardiovascular effects of a new inhalation anesthetic, Forane, in human volunteers at constant arterial carbon dioxide tension, Anesthesiology 35:8, 1971.
6. Libonati, M., Cooperman, L. H., and Price, H. L.: Time-dependent circulatory effects of methoxyflurane in man, Anesthesiology 34:439, 1971.
7. Smith, N. T., Eger, E. I., II, Stoelting, R. K., Whayne, T. F., Cullen, D., and Kadis, L. B.: The cardiovascular and sympathomimetic responses to the addition of nitrous oxide to halothane in man, Anesthesiology 32:410, 1970.
8. Stoelting, R. K., and Gibbs, P. S.: Hemodynamic effects of morphine and morphine-nitrous oxide in valvular heart disease and coronary artery disease, Anesthesiology 38:45, 1973.

9. Price, H. L., Warden, J. C., Cooperman, L. H., and Miller, R. A.: Central sympathetic excitation caused by cyclopropane, Anesthesiology 30:426, 1969.
10. Markee, S., Wang, H. H., and Wang, S. C.: Effects of cyclopropane on the central vasomotor mechanism in the dog, Anesthesiology 27:742, 1966.
11. Smith, A. L., and Wollman, H.: Cerebral blood flow and metabolism: effects of anesthetic drugs and techniques, Anesthesiology 36:378, 1972.
12. Price, H. L., Deutsch, S., Davidson, I. A., Clement, A. J., Behar, M. G., and Epstein, R. M.: Can general anesthetics produce splanchnic visceral hypoxia by reducing regional blood flow? Anesthesiology 27:24, 1966.
13. Deutsch, S., Goldberg, M., Stephen, G. W., and Wu, W.: Effects of halothane anesthesia on renal function in normal man, Anesthesiology 27:793, 1966.
14. Tweed, W. A., Minuck, M., and Mymin, D.: Circulatory responses to ketamine anesthesia, Anesthesiology 37:613, 1972.
15. Miller, R. D., Tong, M. J., and Robbins, T. O.: Effects of massive transfusion of blood on acid-base balance, J.A.M.A. 216:1762, 1971.
16. Shires, T., Williams, J., and Brown, F.: Acute changes in extracellular fluids associated with major surgical procedures, Ann. Surg. 154:803, 1961.
17. Smith, N. T., and Corbascio, A. N.: The use and misuse of pressor agents, Anesthesiology 33:58, 1970.

PART 6

Conduction Anesthesia

CHAPTER TWENTY-ONE

Regional Anesthesia

NERVE TRANSMISSION AND MODE OF ACTION OF LOCAL ANESTHETICS

TO HAVE A BETTER APPRECIATION of the mode of action of local anesthetic drugs and to apply them safely and satisfactorily, it is useful to have some idea of the mechanism of nerve transmission and the manner in which local anesthetic drugs induce a state of analgesia. The nerve fiber consists of a cylinder constructed of a membrane of lipid and protein containing a semi-fluid cytoplasm (axoplasm). In the resting state there is a difference of potential between the interior and exterior of the cylinder, the membrane being the boundary. The inside of the cylinder is negatively charged and the exterior positively charged (Fig. 21-1). An asymmetric distribution of ions on either side of the membrane accounts for the difference in charge, which is the result of an active mechanism (sodium pump) that extracts sodium ions. The concentration of potassium ions inside the cylinder exceeds that of the outside by 20 to 50 times, whereas sodium ions are 3 to 15 times as numerous on the outside. The resting membrane potential arising out of these differences is approximately 60 to 90 millivolts. At initiation of transmission of a nerve impulse, the potential across the membrane decreases by about 15 mv to a value of approximately 45 mv. At this point, ionic exchange becomes active; there is a loss of permeability of the membrane, potassium ions pass out of the cylinder and sodium ions enter. This activity induces an action potential of approximately 100 mv, which results from a shift in polarity and the development of a positive internal charge and a negative external charge. The process is called depolarization, although it is more properly a reversal of polarization (Fig. 21-2). This local process of exchange of ions is reversible; potassium and sodium ions return promptly to their pre-existing relationships internally and externally. However, the "depolarization" initiated by the stimulus provokes similar ionic exchange and changes in permeability along the course of the nerve in a sequential manner. The transmission along the nerve is assisted by the locally induced amplification of the signal in much the same manner as do booster stations along a telephone transmission line.

Nerve fibers are classified into three main groups. *A* fibers are myelinated somatic fibers (diameter, 1-20 μ). *B* fibers are preganglionic myelinated fibers in the autonomic nervous system (diameter, 1-3 μ). *C* fibers are non-

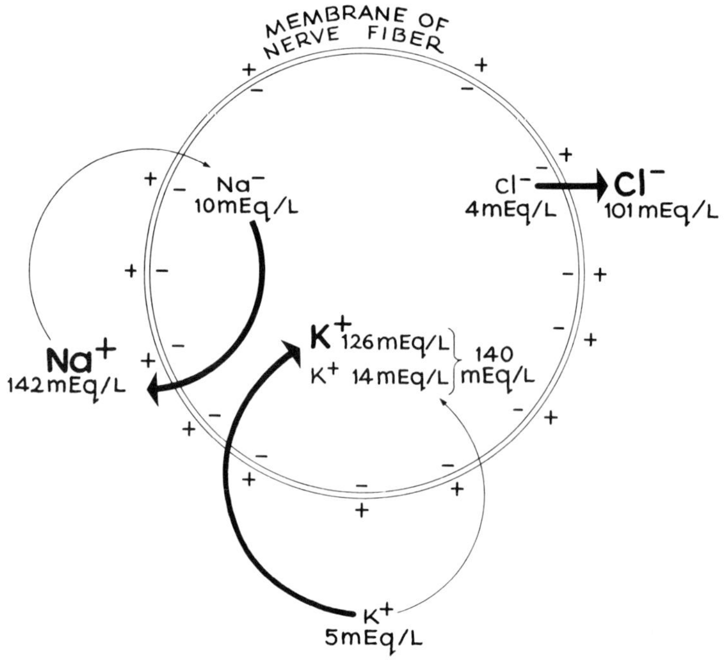

Fig. 21-1.—Diagrammatic representation of ionic state and exchanges during resting state and state permitting nerve transmission.

Fig. 21-2.—Diagrammatic representation of potential changes associated with nerve transmission.

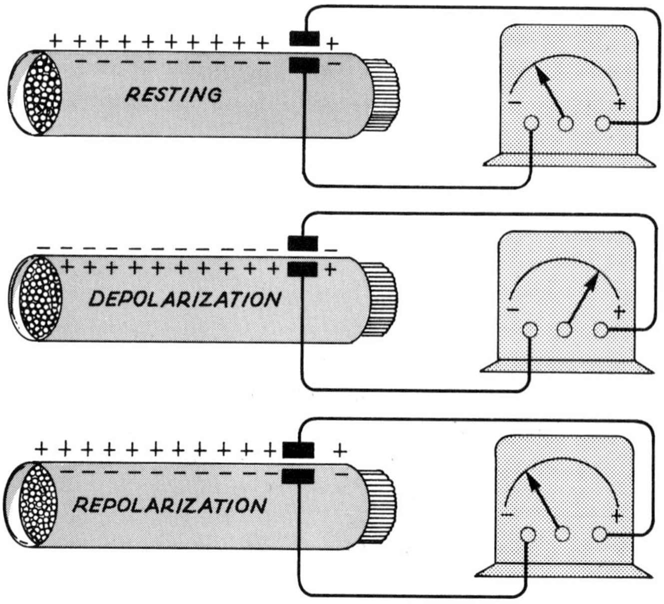

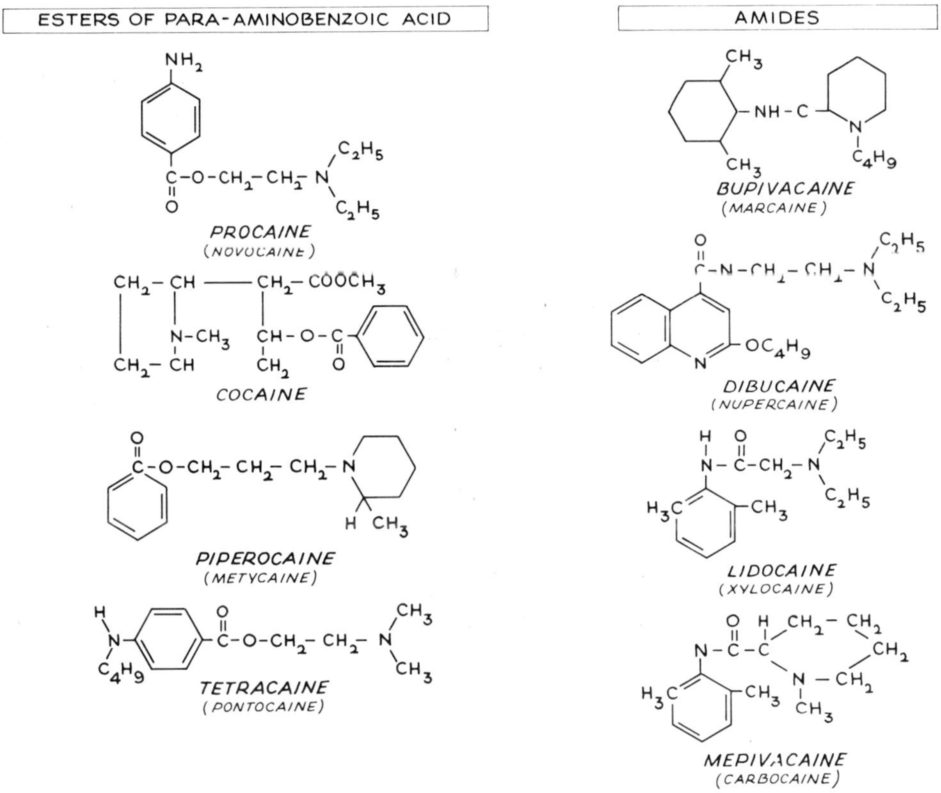

Fig. 21-3.—Basic classes and chemical structures of commonly used local anesthetics.

myelinated and may be either somatic or autonomic in distribution (diameter, 1 μ or less). Pain impulses probably travel in the smaller nonmyelinated *C* fibers or in the smaller *A* fibers. Because block of transmission by local anesthetic drugs depends to a large extent upon the number of molecules of drug that gain access to the membrane, the small nonmyelinated *C* fibers and the smaller *A* fibers are more susceptible to effective concentrations of drug and a differential effect can be produced. Thus, pain, which is transmitted by *C* fibers, can be blocked with lower concentrations and lower amounts of drug than can motor function, which is transmitted through the myelinated and larger *A* fibers. Similarly, touch and proprioception may be retained because these senses are transmitted through *A* fibers. In myelinated nerves, ionic transmission occurs only at the nodes of Ranvier, which are constrictions in the myelin covering of the cylinder occurring at approximately 1-mm intervals. Local anesthetic drugs are effective only at the nodes in myelinated fibers, probably because access to the membrane is easier there. Presumably, the local anesthetic drug acts by preventing the loss in permeability of the membrane and thereby preventing the exchange of ions, the development of the action potential and the transmission of the impulse along the nerve.

TYPES OF LOCAL ANESTHETIC DRUGS

To be effective, a local anesthetic must have hydrophilic properties; that is, it must be soluble in the extracellular fluid surrounding the nerve so that it can get to the nerve. It must also have lipophilic properties, so that when it reaches the nerve it can penetrate the lipid structure surrounding the nerve. Chemically, the local anesthetic drugs in common use are either hydroxy compounds or amines. Derivatives in the hydroxy groups are satisfactory mostly for topical application only. This group is represented by phenol. They are usually irritating to tissue and are labeled with the suffix *-ol*.

Amines constitute the more significant group of local anesthetics. The chemical configuration most consistently associated with local anesthetic activity comprises an aliphatic chain of two or more carbon atoms. One end of the chain has a hydrocarbon nucleus, usually of the aromatic or alicyclic type; the other end has a nitrogen atom, usually in the form of a secondary or tertiary amino group. The chain is sometimes referred to as the pivot, and separates a hydrophilic nitrogen atom from a lipophilic hydrocarbon residue. The majority of local anesthetic drugs are esters of aromatic acids and amino alcohols. Dibucaine (Nupercaine) and lidocaine (Xylocaine) are exceptions; in these, the amide linkage unites the hydrocarbon to the pivot chain. Nitrogen containing local anesthetics of the types mentioned usually are named with suffix *-caine*.

The esters and amides used for local anesthesia can be classified according to the type of acid used to form the ester or amide (Fig. 21-3).

Benzoates

Of the benzoates, cocaine is the most widely used. Attempts to diminish the toxicity induced presumably by the ecgonine portion of the benzoate structure resulted in the piperidine series, of which piperocaine (Metycaine) and cyclaine (Hexylcaine) are the best-known representatives.

Aminobenzoates

The aminobenzoate configuration includes most of the local anesthetics in common use. Within this group, the para-aminobenzoates are the most satisfactory and widely used. The soluble para-aminobenzoates are the most effective. Tetracaine is the most common drug in this series, procaine having been supplanted by the amides.

Amides

The amide configuration is a feature of common drugs such as dibucaine. (Nupercaine) and lidocaine (Xylocaine). More recent introductions are mepivacaine (Carbocaine), prilocaine (Citanest) and bupivacaine (Marcaine). Prilocaine, although an efficient local anesthetic, causes significant methemoglobinemia.

Effectiveness of Local Anesthetics

Salts of local anesthetics are crystalline substances, the majority of which dissolve in water to form acid solutions. The pH of these aqueous solutions varies from 4.0 to 7.0, depending on the base and the acid used to form the salt. Hydrochloric acid is the acid most commonly used and, as a result, the common salt is the hydrochloride. The basic form of the local anesthetic is released from the acid when the drug is injected into tissue. The basic form enters the nerve to produce the stabilization of the membrane that is associated with the action of local anesthetic drugs. Tissue fluids have considerable buffering capacity, and the pH of the salt becomes adjusted upward to the hydrogen ion concentration of the tissue into which it is injected; similarly, the pH of an alkaline solution is adjusted downward. Attempts have been made to increase the effectiveness of local anesthetic solutions by adjusting the pH as far as possible to the alkaline side without precipitation; the buffering action of the tissue, however, negated this attempt. Recently, an attempt has been made to enhance the effectiveness of local anesthetics by decreasing the pH by carbonation, and some success in decreasing the time of onset and the spread of analgesia in epidural anesthesia has been reported.[1,2] Local anesthetics are usually ineffective when injected into inflamed tissue. It is believed that the ineffectiveness may be due either to increased absorption and removal from the site because of hyperemia or to acidity of the inflamed tissue, which interferes with release of the base.

A minimal or "threshold" concentration of the local anesthetic drug must surround the fiber to cause block. The threshold value differs for each drug, but conduction is on an "all or none" basis. Exceeding the threshold concentration does not increase the intensity of the block of whatever fiber is exposed to that concentration. The attainment of the threshold concentration is influenced by the presence of myelin and the size of the fiber. Exceeding the threshold concentration may, however, increase the duration of action. Decrease to the minimum critical concentration is slowed because more time is required by the extracellular fluid to remove the amount of drug present. This effect probably accounts for the practical observation that the amount of drug used for a spinal anesthetic is more important in determining the duration of action than the height of the spinal. Similarly, the achievement of the threshold value is time-dependent and is related to the amount of drug used, its passage by means of extracellular fluid, the distance between the injected deposit of drug and the affected nerve and the ability of the drug to penetrate myelin and membrane. However, once the critical threshold has been achieved, the block is complete. This may account for the fact that, once spinal anesthesia has been obtained, lowering the head will not appreciably extend the level of the block. Correlation between penetration and development of anesthesia is not uniform. Procaine and lidocaine, for example, have equal penetration but different onsets of block and duration of action.

Detoxification

The ester and amide types of local anesthetics are partially or completely detoxified by the tissues of the body. A drug that is not detoxified is eliminated unchanged in the urine. The primary organ for detoxification is the liver. The chemical reactions involved are hydrolysis and then conjugation. Detoxification is accelerated by enzymes in the liver, blood and other tissues. Procaine hydrolysis, for example, is catalyzed by procaine esterase, which is presumed to be identical with pseudocholinesterase. As a result, if there is a low concentration of pseudocholinesterase, there may be delay in the hydrolysis of a drug such as procaine. This may lead to what may be looked upon as a "sensitivity" of an individual to a local anesthetic drug. Impairment of hydrolysis due to a low enzyme concentration may lead to a relatively more rapid accumulation of drug to that level which provokes a toxic reaction. In other words, the amount of drug needed to develop the critical blood level is less than that ordinarily required and, as a result, the patient is "sensitive." Detoxification or hydrolysis and conjugation of the local anesthetics proceed at different rates, according to the susceptibility of the particular drug to breakdown. For example, procaine is readily detoxified, lidocaine is detoxified at a somewhat slower rate, tetracaine is catabolized at one fifth of the rate of procaine, and cocaine and dibucaine are catabolized very slowly.

REACTIONS TO DRUGS

Allergic Reactions

There seems to be a popular, but erroneous, impression that reactions to procaine and similar drugs are due to a sensitivity of the patient and that most reactions are allergic. If a reaction is allergic, it is characterized by the sudden onset of wheals, edema, hypotension and other phenomena associated with this type of reaction from any cause. If a patient gives a history that includes symptoms and signs of this order, it is advisable to avoid the use of the offending drug or one with a similar chemical structure; but if a patient gives a history of, or is observed to have, a reaction of the type to be outlined later, it is not necessary to avoid repetition of the drug. The incidence of true allergic reactions to procaine or similar drugs is extremely low.

The patient may be "sensitive" in another sense; this is the "sensitivity" associated with a slow breakdown of a local anesthetic. Use of local analgesic drugs is not contraindicated in these patients, but must be administered with extreme caution.

THE TYPICAL REACTION.—The usual reaction to procaine or similar drugs is due to absorption of a sufficient amount of the drug into the blood stream to cause symptoms and signs of varying severity in direct proportion to the blood concentration and the rapidity of its attainment. This is a fundamental principle that will facilitate prophylaxis, recognition and treatment of these reactions.

In the application of local anesthetic drugs—especially those with high levels of toxicity—a useful procedure is to place the local anesthetic solution at a distance from the patient. The time taken in walking from one side of the room to another, for example, gives opportunity for the development of early signs of reaction.

Absorption of local anesthetics is increased in areas in which circulation is abundant. Examples of such areas are the upper respiratory passages, the urethra and the caudal canal (which contains a large venous plexus). A good general rule for prophylaxis is to avoid, whenever possible, use of large amounts of these drugs in areas in which absorption into the blood stream will be rapid.

The reactions to procaine are duplicated by the other drugs listed for use in regional, infiltration and topical analgesia. Development of a reaction is directly proportional in time to the rapidity with which the toxic blood concentration is reached.

An immediate reaction is due to accidental intravenous injection of the analgesic solution or to absorption of a large quantity in a very short time. The reaction appears within a few seconds of the injection or topical application of the drug and is characterized by abrupt and complete deterioration of circulation and respiration.

Most reactions occur 5 to 10 minutes after injection or topical application. If a reaction has not developed within 30 minutes of injection or topical application, it is not likely to develop. The symptoms and signs appear with varying degrees of rapidity and severity, depending on the rate of absorption and the quantity absorbed.

Early signs.—The patient becomes somnolent; the somnolence gradually develops into coma. A few patients have enough insight to realize that all is not right and, in the earliest phases of the reaction, they describe themselves as being uncomfortable and somewhat apprehensive. Another small group of patients will become euphoric and elated, most frequently after the application of cocaine. It is always good practice to maintain verbal contact with the patient during induction of regional, infiltration or topical analgesia. By so doing, one can ascertain the patient's mental state and detect premonitory signs of a reaction. If a patient who has been complaining about the insertion of needles or the topical application of a drug abruptly becomes less voluble and apparently more cooperative, one should not breathe a sigh of relief but rather become apprehensive about the state of the patient.

Later signs.—When somnolence or a delay in response develops, one should palpate the pulse. It may be of good quality and at approximately the same rate as before the injection, or it may be of poor quality and somewhat slower than normal. Bradycardia rather than tachycardia is the usual finding. If the pulse is of poor quality, one should check the blood pressure; this will be lower than normal if the reaction is progressing, but hypotension may become extreme. Associated with the hypotension will be pallor, perspiration, clamminess of the skin and syncope. Accompanying the development of hypotension are respiratory irregularities characterized by shallow breathing, sighing, periods of apnea and occasional dyspnea. Twitching about the face and in the fingers may appear and may ultimately develop into a generalized convulsion. Respiratory and circulatory failure succeed the convulsions if the latter are not controlled.

The foregoing symptoms and signs comprise the complete reaction. Minor degrees of this major reaction may occur, depending on the blood concentration of the drug.

TREATMENT OF REACTIONS.—If only the mental changes develop, no therapy is required. The injection or topical application of the drug should, of course, be discontinued. One should, however, be alert to progression of symptoms and signs and have material ready for treatment if the reaction becomes more severe.

Hypotension must be treated with a vasopressor drug. Any of the common vasopressors may be used such as metaraminol and ephedrine. We prefer ephedrine in small increments (15 mg) because it is often effective and there is less likelihood of overshoot. Administration is preferably intravenous to ensure prompt and effective response; the drug should be administered in repeated doses (as needed) until the blood pressure is satisfactory. If hypotension is severe, massive total doses of vasopressor drugs may be needed to restore and stabilize blood pressure. It is extremely important to raise the pressure because persisting low tensions may cause enough tissue hypoxia to produce permanent damage. The administration of oxygen helps to minimize the danger of anoxia during the period of hypotension and respiratory irregularities. A mask and bag are satisfactory, particularly if assistance to pulmonary ventilation is required. Endotracheal intubation is useful in maintaining an airway in the presence of severe and prolonged reactions.

Respiratory irregularities are treated with oxygen and artificial respiration if needed.

Twitchings and convulsions are controlled by the intravenous administration of a soluble barbiturate. The dose of barbiturate must be sufficient to diminish the convulsion. This amount may stop respiration also, but artificial respiration can be done easily and it is essential that the convulsions be stopped. Administration of the barbiturate may be repeated until there is no indication that convulsions will recur after use of the barbiturate has been discontinued. Severe convulsions may be controlled with as little as 0.15 gm of thiopental sodium or thiamylal sodium. Succinylcholine also may be used, but this may be less pleasant for the conscious patient than a barbiturate.

It is important to realize that all of the means for resuscitation must be immediately at hand whenever one contemplates using regional, infiltration, or topical analgesia. Prompt and courageous therapy can prevent fatal termination of the reaction in a large majority of patients, whereas minimal delays in instituting therapy and in using it properly will unnecessarily increase the incidence of fatal outcome.

Minimal equipment that should be instantly available whenever one intends to use analgesia of the types under discussion includes oxygen, a mask and rebreathing bag, a pharyngeal or nasopharyngeal airway, a vaso-

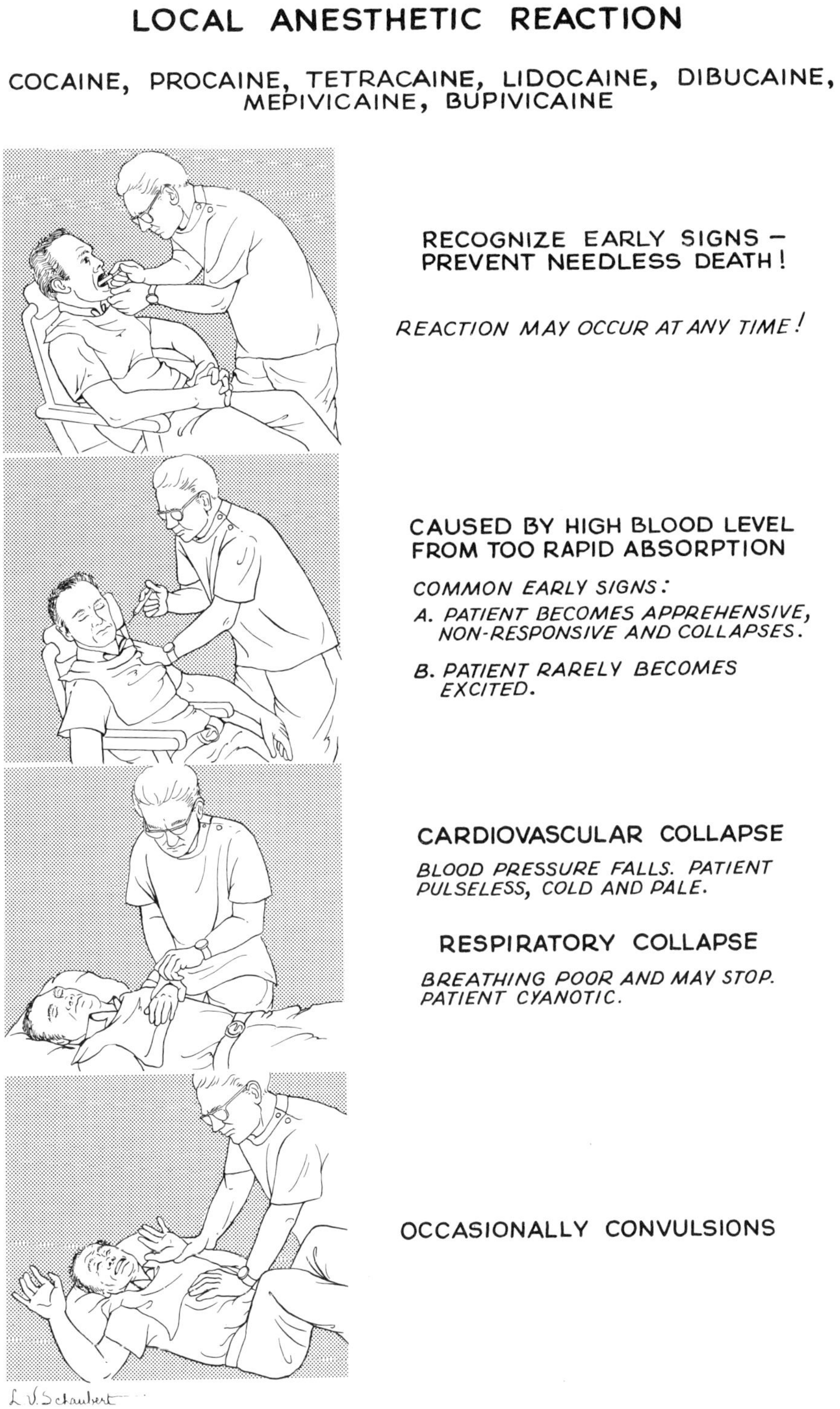

Fig. 21-4.—A, signs of local anesthetic reaction. *(Continued.)*

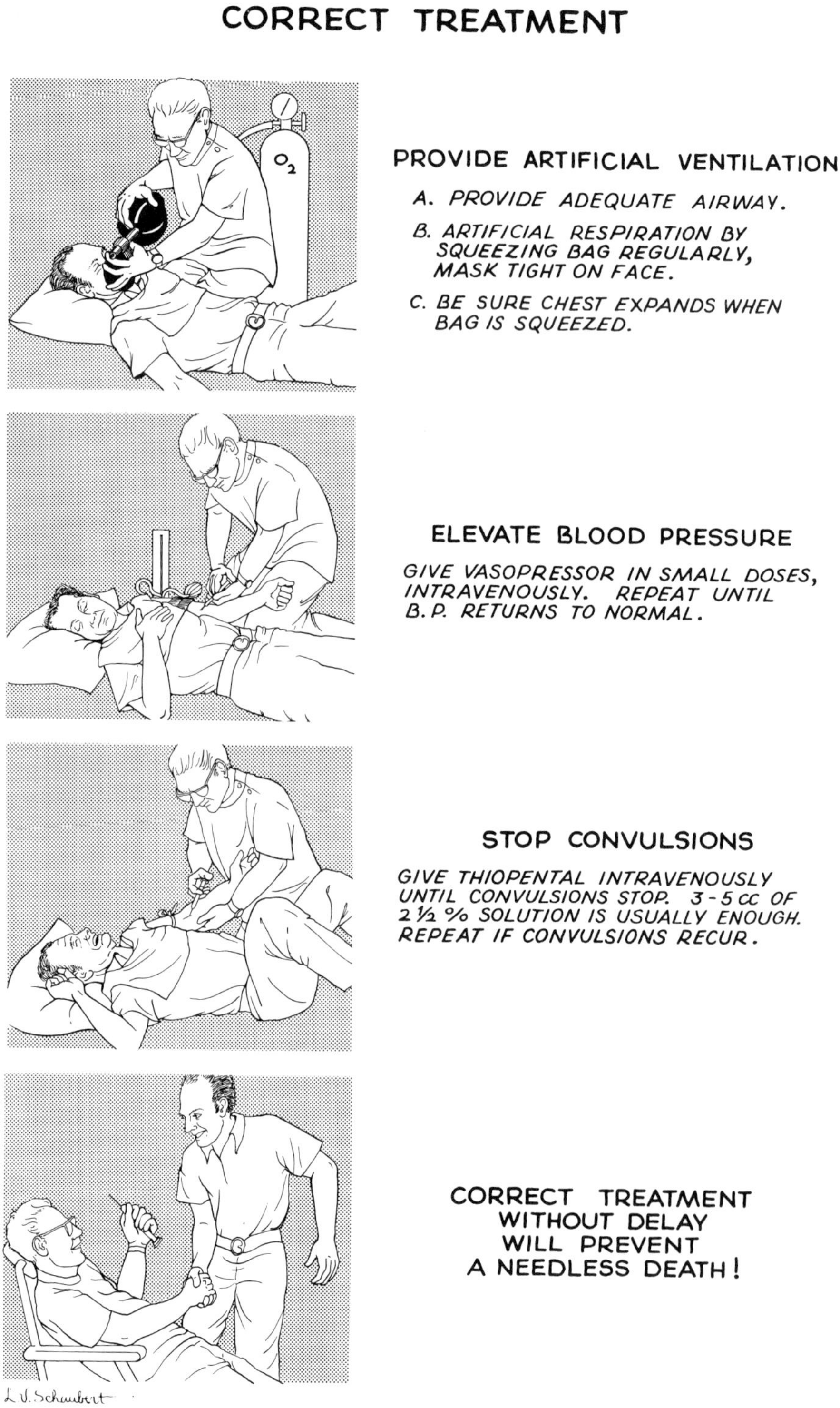

Fig. 21-4 (cont.).—B, correct treatment of local anesthetic reaction. *(Continued.)*

INCORRECT TREATMENT

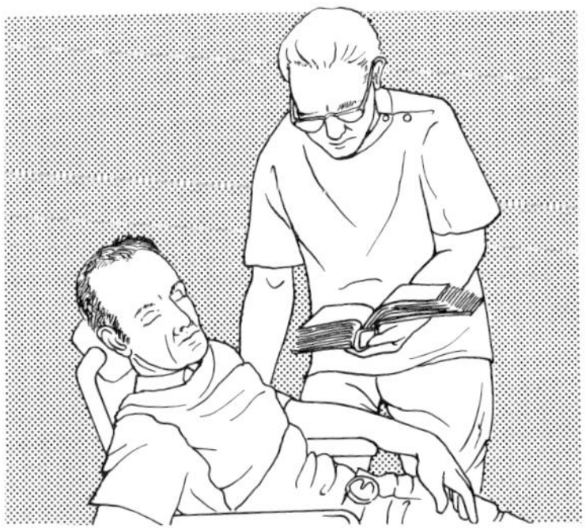

FAILURE TO DO YOUR HOMEWORK BEFOREHAND!

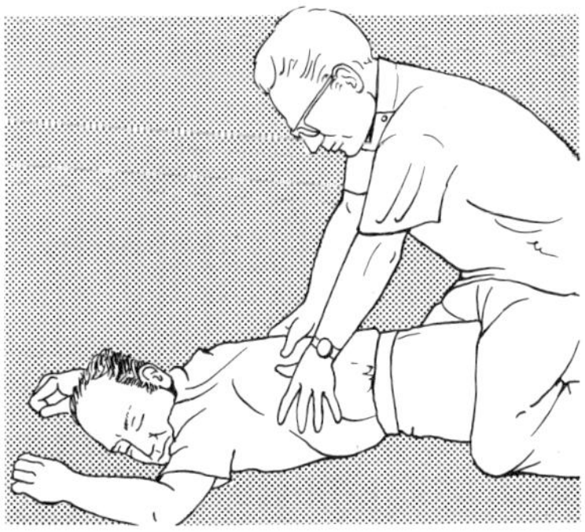

LACK OF VENTILATION BAG AND MASK.

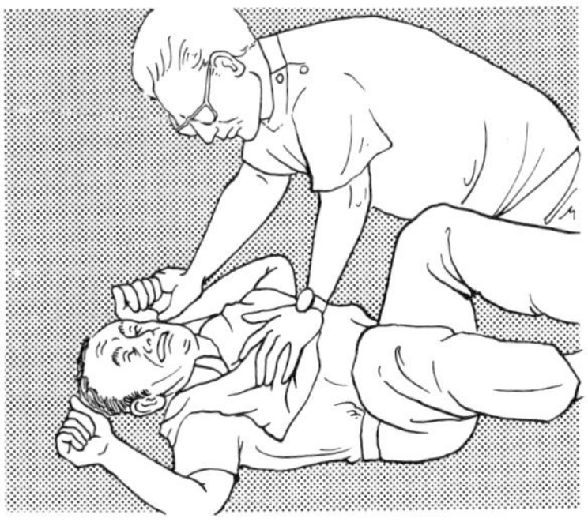

FATAL DAMAGE TO BRAIN FROM ASPHYXIA IF CONVULSIONS ARE NOT CONTROLLED.

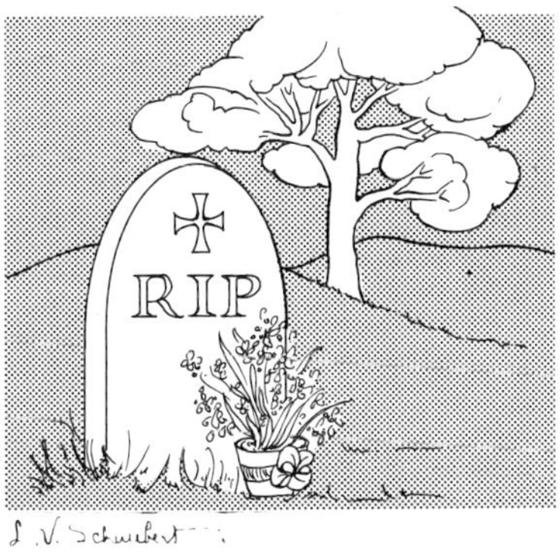

DELAY AND BUNGLED TREATMENT ARE ALL THAT'S NEEDED.

Fig. 21-4 (cont.).—C, incorrect treatment of local anesthetic reaction.

pressor drug and a soluble barbiturate. Whenever regional, infiltration or, particularly, topical analgesia with cocaine or tetracaine is used frequently, it is advisable to have the soluble barbiturate in solution in a syringe ready for instant injection. The equipment mentioned may not be used for years; but if it is used only once and a life is saved because it was there for immediate use, it will justify its relatively minimal cost. Such equipment should be available in every physician's office (Fig. 21-4).

Toxicity Versus the Chances of a Reaction

The foregoing material on reactions to local anesthetics has been oriented to the standard pharmacologic concept of toxicity. In other words, a ratio or index exists between the amount of drug absorbed and the development of toxic reactions. This basic information is, of course, essential to the safe use of these drugs, but use of this standard of "toxicity" tends to make anesthetists and other physicians using local anesthetic drugs to be wary of the more "toxic" drugs and sometimes careless with those drugs with a lower "toxicity." We introduce at this point consideration of another approach to the application of local anesthetic drugs that will not only help in diminishing undesirable reactions in patients but also increase the number of drugs that can be used successfully and more efficiently. This concept evolves from the practice of attempting to determine, for each patient and for each drug used, chances of a reaction. In essence, it does not matter how toxic a drug is if it is used properly. One is interested primarily in providing satisfactory anesthesia in the patient while minimizing chances of a reaction. To decrease the chances of a reaction and, at the same time, to make it possible and safe to apply the available drugs efficiently (for example, cocaine instead of lidocaine for topical use) two basic principles should be kept in mind:

(1) A toxic reaction is usually a function of a critical blood level, and
(2) attainment of this critical blood level is dependent on the following factors: a.) the time taken to apply the drug; b.) the concentration of drug (i.e., the dose or number of molecules of drug); c.) the site of application (relates to speed of absorption); d.) the patient's esterase value; and e.) blood flow related to distribution and redistribution.

If one keeps these factors in mind, one can use drugs such as tetracaine and cocaine safely, effectively and efficiently with the patient's chances of having a toxic reaction being no greater than they would be if drugs with lower toxicity, such as lidocaine, were used. One can then avoid a less satisfactory and less efficient, but rather common, practice of attempting to achieve with the less toxic anesthetic certain effects, such as good topical anesthesia, simply because the anesthetist is inappropriately impressed with the pharmacologic toxicity rather than with the chances of a reaction.

USE OF EPINEPHRINE IN ANESTHETIC SOLUTIONS

The foregoing discussion raises the question of the advisability of combining epinephrine with anesthetic solutions. It is recognized that epinephrine permits the use of lower concentrations and lengthens action, presumably by delaying absorption. All of these factors tend to prevent accumulation of sufficient quantities in the blood stream to cause reactions. The use of epinephrine in concentrations of 1:100,000 or 1:200,000 is effective and probably beneficial. Higher concentrations (e.g., 1:50,000) do not significantly intensify or prolong action of local anesthetics but do add significantly to the likelihood of tissue ischemia and reactions to epinephrine itself. The ischemia of higher concentrations may be sufficient to precipitate gangrene. Secondary vasodilation also may occur, with consequent hemorrhage in the postoperative period. Epinephrine reactions should be differentiated from procaine or similar drug reactions when the drugs are used together. In the dentist's chair, many patients confuse an epinephrine reaction with a local anesthetic reaction. Reactions to epinephrine are characterized by tachycardia, palpitation, apprehension, shivering and hypertension. It is therefore probably unwise to use epinephrine in appreciable quantities in patients with hypertension.

Treatment of a reaction to epinephrine is symptomatic. Oxygen inhalation supports the heart through a period of overactivity, and sedatives allay apprehension. The reactions are seldom fatal and do not last long. Phentolamine (Regitine) may be used to control severe hypertension. Phenothiazine drugs, such as chlorpromazine, may be useful also.

It is possible to prolong the action of the anesthetic solution and induce vasoconstriction through the use of levo-nordefrin (Cobefrin) with it. This drug does not have the cardiac and circulatory effects that epinephrine does and is a satisfactory substitute. It is used in concentrations of 1:5,000 to 1:40,000. It is strange that this excellent vasoconstrictor is not more widely used.

INTRAVENOUS USE OF PROCAINE

Infrequently, local anesthetics are used intravenously as a basis for nitrous oxide inhalation anesthesia. The presumed advantages are production of good analgesia, a decreased frequency of cardiac arrhythmias, profound depression of the cough reflex, prompt awakening and limited depression of respiration. However, the doses required to achieve these advantages and significant support for nitrous oxide approximate those levels of drug concentrations at which reactions may occur, and critical attention must be paid to administration.

Some local anesthetics, particularly lidocaine, when given intravenously are useful in controlling arrhythmias (see Chapter 20).

PRINCIPLES OF REGIONAL, INFILTRATION AND TOPICAL ANALGESIA

Regional analgesia (conduction anesthesia) results from the blocking of nerves at sites distant from the proposed operative site. Infiltration analgesia is analgesia accomplished by blocking nerves at the site of the proposed operation. Topical analgesia results from the blocking of nerve endings by application of an agent on the surface of mucous membranes.

These types of analgesia are useful when it seems advisable to anesthetize regions of the body and thus limit the impact of anesthesia on overall physiologic mechanisms. Complete relaxation can be achieved by proper use of these technics, and bleeding during surgery is probably minimized.

Factors Influencing the Use of Regional, Infiltration, and Topical Technics

A patient must be cooperative and able to distinguish between sensations of touch, pressure, traction and pain. Some patients are incapable of differentiating these sensations and often interpret them as distressful; they are not good subjects for regional or infiltration analgesia. As a general rule, any patient who does not want local analgesia is a poor candidate for such anesthesia. If regional or local technics are used in spite of the patient's dislike of them, analgesia is often unsatisfactory. Suitable preparation of the patient for analgesia for these technics is essential. The patient must understand the procedure and be informed as to what to expect (and what not to expect). Sedative and/or analgesic drugs given prior to or during anesthesia often add to success of the technics. Excessive drug use, however, may result in an uncooperative or severely depressed patient. Narcotics and scopolamine given intravenously are extremely beneficial during analgesia produced by these methods. The narcotic enhances the analgesia and helps to minimize any discomforts of position, pressure or traction—discomforts that are often present, particularly during long procedures, despite completely satisfactory analgesia at the site of operation. Scopolamine is helpful in dissipating some of the apprehension that is present in some patients and contributes to amnesia. The combination of fentanyl and droperidol (Innovar) also is effective. On occasions, it is useful to produce light hypnosis with barbiturates.

These technics are, however, often inconvenient to the surgeon, and they frequently are discomfiting to the patient and add little to the patient's safety. Their use is confined most practically to the following situations: when the patient's cooperation is needed; when the patient prefers to be "awake"; when establishment and maintenance of the airway by artificial means is difficult and unwieldy; when nausea and emesis are likely to endanger the patient or the results of surgery after operation; when proposed surgery is minor; and when the patient is moribund. These technics should not be forced on patients except in rare instances in which safety of the patient otherwise would be imperiled. Forcible application of these technics can result only in unsatisfactory completion of the surgery, and may directly or indirectly cause death. We have no intention of decrying the use of these technics, because they have a valuable and useful function in anesthesia; but there is a general tendency to overrate their safety features, to the ultimate detriment of the patient and inconvenience of the surgeon. The incidence of postanesthetic pulmonary complications is not reduced by use of these technics. Induction of analgesia is often time-consuming and the length of action is limited.

We have deliberately overemphasized the disadvantages of conduction

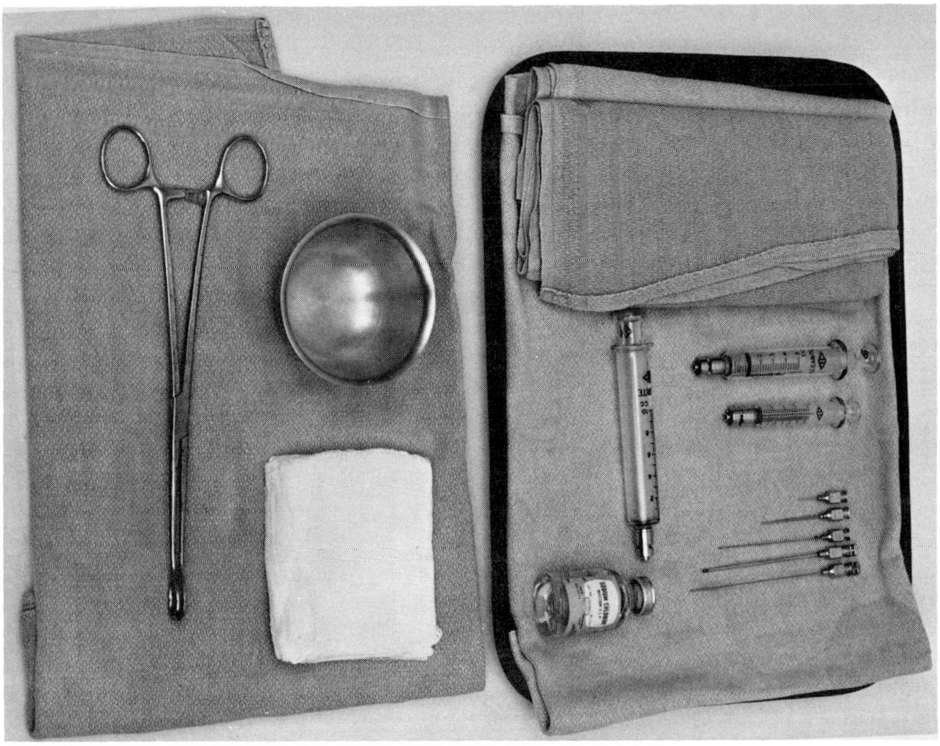

Fig. 21-5.—Simple tray with minimal equipment necessary for performing most regional and infiltration blocks.

anesthesia because of the common but erroneous belief that use of "local anesthesia" somehow magically eliminates all the problems associated with inhalation anesthesia and automatically enhances safety to the patient. The evidence does not support this concept. We do want to make it clear, however, that conduction anesthesia, among its various benefits, can be satisfactory, safe and effective; it can limit the impact of the anesthetic on respiration and circulation, it enables the patient to cooperate and to remain "awake" if he so desires and it minimizes postanesthetic discomfort. It is an important and useful part of the total anesthetic armamentarium and should be included as a possible solution to individual anesthetic problems.

Requirements

Certain fundamental requirements for consistently successful regional, infiltration and topical analgesia cannot be ignored. The anesthetist must have a complete working knowledge of the pertinent surgical anatomy. He must understand the elemental principles of block technic. He must be familiar with the properties of the agents used and be trained to recognize and treat untoward reactions to these drugs. His patient must be properly prepared and cooperative, and the surgeon must be aware of the necessity for gentleness in the surgical manipulations.

A description of the anatomic features that must be known for successful performance of the blocks we outline cannot be included in this book; for these details the reader is referred to the texts of Labat,[3] Lundy,[4] Pitkin,[5] Adriani,[6] Bonica,[7] Moore,[8] and De Jong.[9] It cannot be emphasized too strongly that blind poking with a needle and dependence on diffusion of unnecessarily large quantities of analgesic solution often result in incomplete analgesia, an increased likelihood of reactions and, possibly, permanent damage. There is no substitute for a direct approach based on a knowledge of anatomy. Checking of needle placement and diffusion of anesthetic solution by radiographic methods is useful, but a knowledge of anatomy still is necessary for suitable interpretation.

Block Analgesia

There are three bases of good technics of block analgesia: (1) good equipment, which is kept in good condition; (2) adeptness and finesse in handling the equipment and (3) awareness of aseptic principles.

EQUIPMENT.—A number of sets of block syringes and needles are available, probably the best of these being the syringes and needles devised by Labat.[3] Equipment made after Labat's original specifications is difficult to obtain, but equipment of this type as modified by Lundy[4] is available. It is possible, however, to perform satisfactory injections with standard B-D needles and Luer-Lok syringes (Fig. 21-5). Disposable needles and syringes can be used, but the syringes often stick and the connections between needle and syringe often leak. Disposable syringes do not have the locking devices that prevent exasperating experiences of leaks, a syringe that detaches itself from the needle and sprays solution widely, or the tip of a syringe that breaks off in the hub of a needle properly placed with some difficulty and with discomfort to the patient.

Two syringes are useful: one is a 5-ml and the other, a 10-ml syringe. They should work freely and be well marked. They should have been cleaned with soap, water, alcohol and ether, and thoroughly dried before autoclaving or gas sterilization. Barrel and plunger may be autoclaved together if both are perfectly clean and dry before sterilization.

The needles should be no. 22 gauge in caliber; the most useful lengths are 1.5 to 2.0 cm, 5.0 to 6.0 cm, 8.0 to 9.0 cm and 12.0 cm. Their bevels should be sharp and moderately long. The needles should be made of the best steel and quite flexible. They should be sterilized by autoclaving after thorough cleaning and drying. Disposable needles are sterile in their packages.

Adeptness and finesse in handling the equipment not only facilitate successful introduction of the needles and injection of solutions but also diminish the discomfort to the patient and minimize wear and tear on the equipment. Rough handling of needles will result in unnecessary breakage, damage to their points and needless trauma to the tissues. Much can be told about position of the needle in tissue by transmission through the needle to the fingers of variations in factors such as pressure, tension and resistance, and these can be felt only if the needle is advanced or retracted steadily and gently.

TECHNIC FOR PLACEMENT OF NEEDLES.—Wheals for the introduction of the block needles are best made by attaching the no. 25 gauge hypodermic needle to a syringe and introducing the needle tangential to the skin surface with local anesthetic flowing and with the bevel down. This procedure permits infiltration of analgesic solution into dermis as soon as the point of the needle pierces skin. Wheals should be raised in the uppermost layers of the dermis so that a pigskin-like elevation is made. Deeper infiltration for this purpose is needless and usually unsatisfactory.

After the wheal has been raised, the needle is introduced without the attached syringe. This facilitates handling of the needle; moreover, if the needle is kept in the subcutaneous layers, the patient feels no pain as the needle is advanced. The needle should be grasped at the hub by the thumb and first two fingers and advanced steadily and firmly. Jerky movements should be avoided. If the needle is to be placed deeply, changes in direction of the needle should be made by retracting the needle until it is free of underlying tissue before readvancing it; merely bending the needle at the hub end will not change its direction if the point or main body of the needle is firmly engaged in a mass of tissue. If the needle encounters bone, the point should be brought against it gently to avoid damaging the point and hurting the patient by irritating the periosteum. The needle point should not be repeatedly pricked against a bone. Nor should one ever advance a needle to such a depth that the whole shaft is buried in tissue; most needles break at the junction of shaft and hub, and the retrieving of needles buried in soft tissue is a difficult and embarrassing task. This is particularly true of short fine needles, such as hypodermic needles. A needle should never be placed in a nerve; all injections, except when destruction of nerve tissue for therapeutic purposes is intended, should be perineural. If paresthesias are induced, it is advisable to retract the needle slightly until the paresthesias cease. Intraneural injection causes postinjection neuritis; this can sometimes be relieved by repeated injections of procaine in the affected area.

Once the needle is in position, injection into subcutaneous tissue, as for a field block or infiltration of a line of incision, can be done as the needle is withdrawn. It is seldom necessary to aspirate under these circumstances. In infiltration analgesia, it is important to include the superficial layers of the skin as well as the subcutaneous tissue—inadequate intradermal infiltration is a common cause of unsuccessful infiltration analgesia. If the needle is placed deeply, as for a regional block, aspiration should be done in two planes; that is, suction should be applied with the needle in its original position, and then the needle should be rotated at least 90° and suction again applied. This is essential because the needle may be in a vessel with the bevel against the vessel wall in such a position that aspiration causes the wall to occlude the needle and prevent aspiration of blood into the syringe. If the needle is rotated so that the bevel is away from the vessel wall, it is frequently possible to demonstrate blood in the syringe. Repeated aspiration is good practice because intravenous injection of procaine or similar drugs may cause severe reactions. It is important also to fix the needle as injections are being made, so that there is little tendency for the needle to change position.

ASEPSIS.—There is little need to mention asepsis except to emphasize its importance in regional or infiltration anesthesia. The equipment must be sterile, the anesthetist's hands clean and sterile-gloved, and the skin area properly prepared. With respect to the last, it is a good rule to use whatever preparation of the field for block or infiltration the surgeon deems suitable for preparation of the operative site. Many serious and fatal infections that could have been avoided have followed regional and infiltration procedures.

As a general rule, needles should not be introduced in or near a site of infection; not only will analgesia be unsatisfactory because of the low pH of the tissues but also infection may be disseminated.

A distressing and sometimes fatal accident may accompany regional or infiltration analgesia if proper precautions are not taken to identify the solution injected. If commercially prepared solutions are used, the labels should be checked immediately before use.

Topical Analgesia

Topical analgesia is used most often for surgery about the upper respiratory passages and for ophthalmic surgery. It also may be used in urologic practice, as for instillation in the urethra; in such a circumstance, however, topical analgesia may be hazardous because of the rapid absorption of drug.

Analgesia results because certain drugs have the property of anesthetizing small nerve endings that are close to the surface. This type of analgesia is suitable for use only on mucosal surfaces.

A knowledge of anatomy is invaluable for the proper application of topical analgesic methods because it is often possible, particularly in surgery of the upper air passages, to apply the drug precisely to essential ganglia. The drug is usually applied by means of cotton swabs on applicator sticks or by means of an atomizer.

Because the mucosal surfaces are rich in capillaries and absorption into the systemic circulation is relatively rapid and because the drugs employed for topical analgesia are often quite toxic, the principles involved in the safe and satisfactory use of topical analgesia relate mainly to the production of analgesia without systemic reaction to the drug. In fact, absorption is so rapid that the blood concentration achieved approximates that achieved with intravenous injection. A good rule to follow is always to use the lowest possible concentration and the lowest total amount of the safest drug that will produce the desired analgesic state. Another good rule is to allow considerable time to elapse between applications of the drug. This practice allows time for development of early signs of reaction before more drug is added. It is good practice also to avoid the use of topical analgesia in areas where there has been or may be trauma. Trauma may open blood vessels and enhance absorption of the toxic agent. This is particularly likely with instillation of drugs in the urethra preceding or following intraurethral instrumentation.

Drugs commonly used for the production of topical analgesia are cocaine, tetracaine, dibucaine and lidocaine. The concentrations used are listed in Table 21-1. With respect to tetracaine and dibucaine, although these drugs are used in low concentrations they do not possess the property of vasoconstriction that characterizes cocaine. Absorption therefore is more rapid and reactions are as probable, or perhaps even more probable, than is the case with cocaine. With respect to cocaine, the addition of epinephrine will lengthen the action of cocaine by delaying its absorption. However, cocaine enhances the systemic epinephrine effect, and in patients with cardiac irregularities or with hypertension epinephrine may be excluded.

TABLE 21-1.—DETAILS OF COMMONLY USED LOCAL ANESTHETIC DRUGS

NAME	TOXICITY (RELATIVE TO PROCAINE)	CONCENTRATION (%)	MAX. SINGLE DOSE (MG)	LENGTH ACTION (HR)	OPTIMUM APPLICATION	SPECIAL PROPERTIES
Procaine	1	0.5–2	1000—Infiltration, regional, epidural 200—Spinal	1	Infiltration, regional, spinal, epidural; arrhythmias	
Lidocaine (Xylocaine)	1.25	0.5–2	750—Infiltration, regional, epidural 100—Spinal	1	As for procaine Topical	Greater diffusion Moderate topical effect
Mepivacaine (Carbocaine)	1.25	0.5–2	750—Infiltration, regional, epidural	1.5	As for procaine *except* spinal arrhythmias	Moderate vasoconstriction Longer action
Bupivacaine (Marcaine)	6	0.5–0.75	300—Infiltration, regional, epidural	2–8	Infiltration, regional, epidural	Long action Possible lower toxicity than tetracaine
Tetracaine (Pontocaine)	6	*Regional* 0.1–0.2 *Topical* 1–2	100—Infiltration, regional, epidural 20—Spinal 50—Topical	4–6	Infiltration (limited), regional, spinal, epidural (limited), topical	Long action Topical
Cocaine	4–5	*Topical* 2–10	75—Topical	2–3	Topical	Superior topical Vasoconstriction
Dibucaine (Nupercaine)	10	*Topical* 0.05–1	50—Topical 10—Spinal	4–6	Spinal, topical, regional (limited)	Good topical Long action

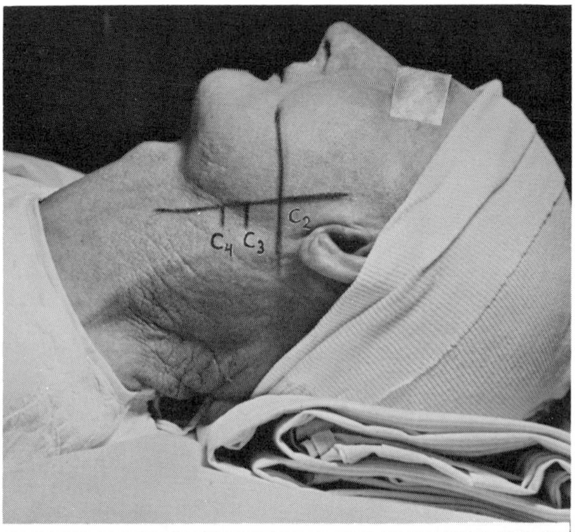

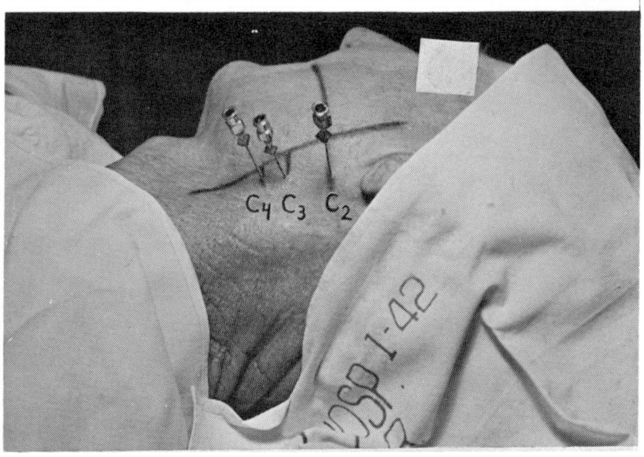

Fig. 21-6 (top).—Method of marking and position of patient's head while landmarks are being established for cervical plexus block.

Fig. 21-7 (bottom).—Position of patient's head while the needles are inserted. This also demonstrates the relative superficiality of the tips of the transverse processes, since the 5–6 cm. needles are used. In this patient, the needles are introduced slightly posterior to the line because at the level of the second and third cervical nerves the mandible is in the way.

Topical analgesia is a useful and simple technic, but it is fraught with danger because toxic drugs are used in an area in which absorption is rapid. If these hazards are kept in mind, topical analgesia can be relatively safe and satisfactory.

TECHNICS OF REGIONAL BLOCK

A number of relatively simple nerve blocks serve a useful purpose in the usual anesthetic practice. The technics for these blocks and a few of the procedures for which they may be used are discussed in the following paragraphs. The technics described are some of those compiled by Peterson during a course of study under Rovenstine and Wertheim.

Cervical Plexus Block

INDICATIONS

1. Diagnostic and therapeutic: Neuralgias in this area (which may connect with hypoglossal nerve to cause stiffness or spasm of the tongue).
2. Anesthetic: Operations on neck and scalp posterior to coronal line.

ANATOMY.—The cervical plexus comprises the anterior primary divisions of the first four cervical nerves. The first nerve is not blocked; it has no sensory branches. After emerging from the intervertebral foramina, the nerves pass behind the vertebral arteries and reach the tip of the transverse processes to lie in sulci between the anterior and posterior tubercles of the transverse processes, mostly under cover of the sternocleidomastoid muscle. They divide into superficial and deep branches, the superficial emerging along the middle of the posterior margin of the sternocleidomastoid. The tubercles lie 2 to 3 cm below the skin surface. The cervical plexus supplies sensation to a cape-like area extending from the lower edge of mandible to ear line to the spine of the scapula.

For the lateral approach, to be described, the *landmarks* include:

1. Biting surface of teeth with mouth closed.
2. Articulation of mandible with zygoma.

APPROACH (FIGS. 21-6 AND 21-7).—The patient lies supine, with his head on a small pillow to raise the occiput 10 cm off the table. The chin should be at right angles to the plane of the table (the head should not be hyperextended), the patient looking at the ceiling. With the mouth closed, a line is drawn perpendicular to the plane of the table, starting at the biting surface of the teeth. (In edentulous patients, this will have to be estimated.) Another line is drawn at right angles to the first line, starting just anterior to the articulation of the mandible with the zygoma; this line, if extended, will reach the midline near the suprasternal notch. The junction of the two lines marks the site for injection of the second cervical nerve; 2 cm distal to this juncture is the site for injection of the third cervical nerve; and 1.5 cm distal to the latter is the site for injection of the fourth cervical nerve. Block of the fifth cervical nerve is not necessary for cervical surgery.

The head is turned to the side opposite that to be blocked at an angle of about 45°, and skin wheals are raised at the three sites. The needle is then directed perpendicular to the skin until contact with the anterior tubercle of the tip of the transverse process is felt. This is usually only 2 to 3 cm from the skin surface. To check the position, the needle should be directed both cephalad and caudad. If, when this is done, no bone is encountered, the needle is in the right plane. If bone is felt both cephalad and caudad to the original point of contact, the needle is probably being directed too far posteriorly and its direction should be corrected.

After aspiration as usual, 3 ml of the appropriate solution of one's preferred local anesthetic is injected at each nerve site, the needle being in contact with the tip of the transverse process.

To facilitate more prompt onset of analgesia and to assure oneself more readily of complete skin analgesia, it is advisable to inject approximately 5 ml of anesthetic solution superficially in the angle between external jugular vein and posterior border of sternocleidomastoid muscle.

COMPLICATIONS.—The solution may enter the carotid sheath, causing compression of the vessel, if the needle is too far anterior to the tubercles. The needle may also enter the subarachnoid space, if directed too far medially. Deposition of larger amounts of anesthetic solution may result in diffusion of the solution and anesthetization of one or both recurrent laryngeal nerves, with consequent partial respiratory obstruction. This complication is apparent when the patient exhibits a "brassy" character to his voice or complains of inability to care for pharyngeal mucus and fluid.

Brachial Plexus Block

INDICATIONS

1. Diagnostic and therapeutic: Neuralgias, causalgias.
2. Anesthetic: Operations on the upper extremity up to the shoulder. For operations around the shoulder, the third and fourth cervical nerves are blocked at the time of the brachial plexus block. The intercostal humeral branch must be blocked to include the medial aspect of the humerus.

ANATOMY.—The brachial plexus is formed by the anterior primary divisions of the fifth to eighth cervical and the first dorsal spinal nerves. These nerves converge toward the upper surface of the first rib, where they emerge between the scalenus anticus and the scalenus medius muscles and pass under the midpoint of the clavicle to the apex of the axilla.

The traditional approach to the brachial plexus has been via the supraclavicular route, and this traditional approach will be outlined later. Labat, in the first edition of his text on regional anesthesia, published in 1922, described the axillary approach. Labat ascribed this approach to Hirschel. Burnham popularized this approach with the technic now to be described.

AXILLARY APPROACH.—Compared with other approaches, the advantages of this approach include (1) elimination of the dangers of pneumothorax, (2) easier location of landmarks, and (3) attainment of anesthesia at higher dermatomes because the intercostobrachial nerve is included. The last advantage is of significance in circumstances in which a tourniquet is used.

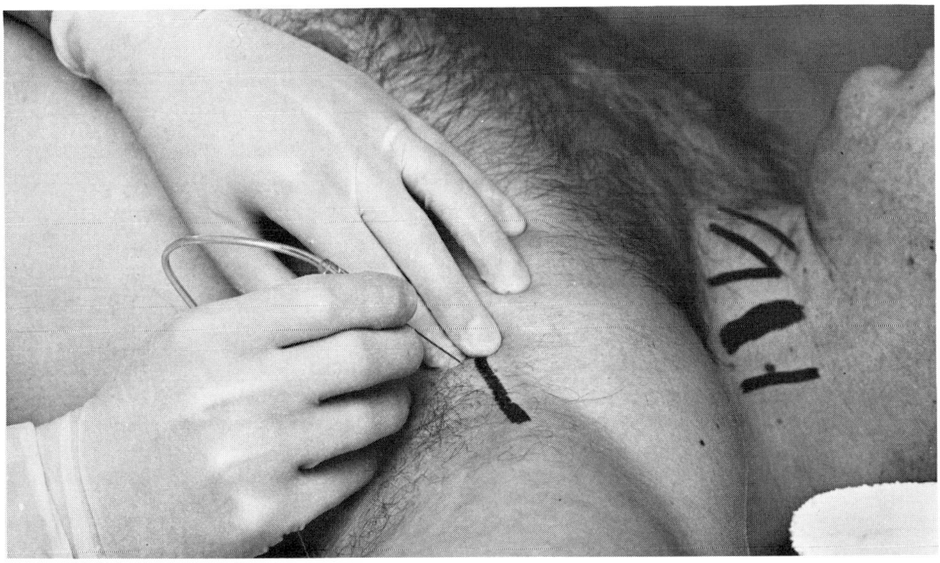

Fig. 21-8.—Axillary approach to brachial plexus block. Arm is extended at approximately 90° from body. First two fingers of left hand palpate artery, course of which is outlined by black mark. For convenience of injection and to minimize displacement of needle from point at which paresthesias are elicited, many anesthetists connect needle by tubing to syringe containing local anesthetic.

Fig. 21-9.—Interscalene approach to brachial plexus block. Medial lines depict medial and lateral aspects of sternocleidomastoid muscle. The apex of V often is at junction of posterior border of sternocleidomastoid muscle and external jugular vein. Broad mark just medial to needle indicates space between anterior and medial scalene muscles. As shown, needle is advanced in plane perpendicular to planes of neck, with head turned to opposite side.

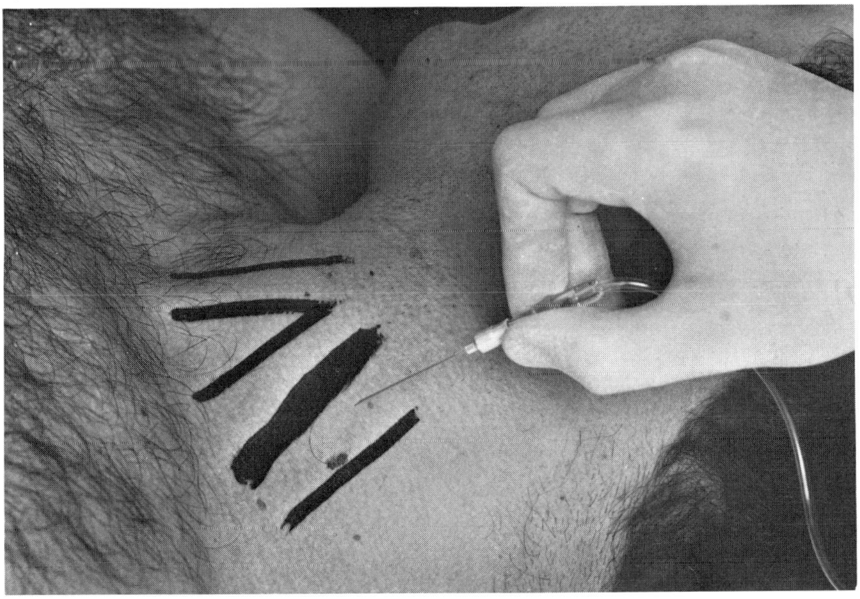

The patient lies with the arm abducted at 90°. In the axilla, the brachial artery is palpated proximal to the insertion of the pectoralis major anteriorly and the latissimus dorsi posteriorly. The artery lies in the groove beneath the coracobrachialis in the neurovascular bundle, a prolongation of the axillary fascia. As the finger of one hand palpates the artery, a needle is inserted just anterior to the vessel but in the neurovascular bundle (Fig. 21-8). As the needle penetrates the bundle a sudden release is felt, and the needle then will pulsate with the artery. Approximately 20 ml of anesthetic solution is deposited, and the needle is moved to a position posterior to the artery, where a similar amount is injected. The needle then may be advanced to contact the humerus. As the needle is slowly withdrawn, another 20 ml of solution is injected.

Paresthesias are useful in locating placement of the needle, but they are not essential.

INTERSCALENE APPROACH.—More recently, the interscalene approach used by Winnie[10] has become more popular. Both the Burnham and Winnie approaches make use of the fact that the nerves of the brachial plexus are gathered together with major vessels going to the arm in a bundle covered by fascia. The interscalene approach has the presumed advantage that the anesthetic solution is introduced closer to the origin of the nerves of the plexus; the musculocutaneous and axillary nerves, which come off high in the arm, thereby are anesthetized. Also, the approach is high enough to avoid damage to the cupula of the lung and the subclavian artery. The technic for the interscalene approach is as follows:

The level of the sixth cervical vertebra is determined by extending a line laterally from the cricoid cartilage. The line passes over Chassaignac's tubercle, the patient lying in the dorsal recumbent position and the head being turned somewhat to the opposite side. To identify the clavicular head of the sternocleidomastoid muscle, the patient raises his head. A finger placed behind the sternocleidomastoid muscle at this point lies on the anterior scalene muscle. When the finger is moved laterally on this muscle it falls into the groove between the anterior and middle scalene muscles. As the index and middle fingers impinge on this groove while astride the line drawn from the cricoid, a needle is introduced between the fingers in a direction perpendicular to the skin in all planes (Fig. 21-9). (Another useful landmark for the insertion site is the external jugular vein, which crosses the groove at this point.) The needle is advanced slowly until either paresthesias are elicited or the transverse process of the cervical vertebra is encountered. If the process is encountered without paresthesias, the needle is moved laterally in small increments until paresthesias are elicited. With the acquisition of paresthesias, 25 to 35 ml of anesthetic solution (lidocaine, procaine, mepivacaine or bupivacaine) is injected. The dose is influenced by height and age with smaller doses at the extremes of age.

Complications of the axillary and interscalene technics include intravascular injection and, with respect to the interscalene technic, injection into the intervertebral artery or entry into the subarachnoid space by reason of incorrect direction of the needle.

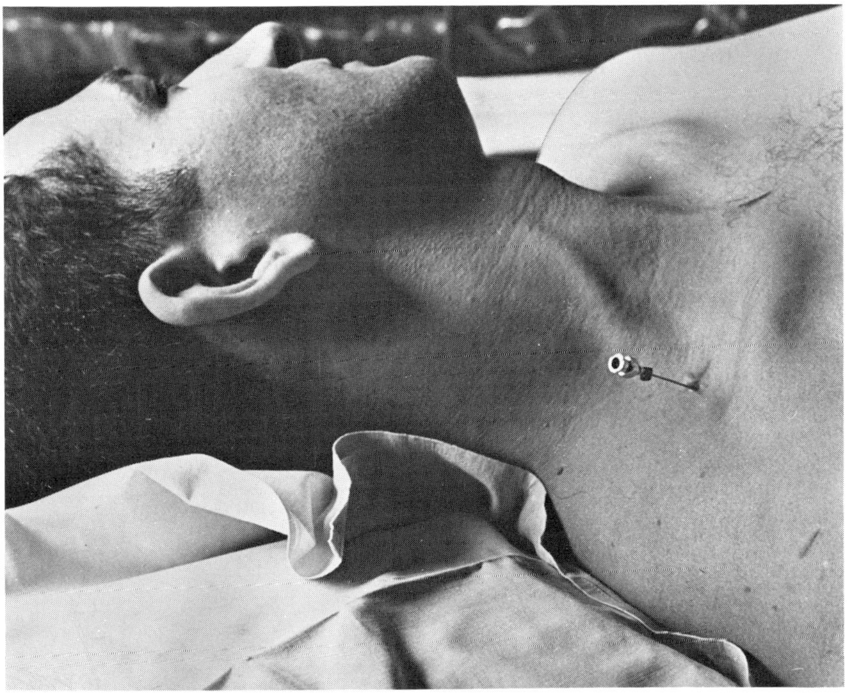

Fig. 21-10.—Supraclavicular approach to the brachial plexus block. The 5–6 cm. needle is in position on the first rib just lateral to the subclavian artery. Note how superficial the rib is. The needle is introduced at a right angle to the skin surface.

SUPRACLAVICULAR APPROACH.—The landmarks for this traditional approach include:

1. Midpoint of the clavicle.
2. Chassaignac's tubercle.
3. External jugular vein.
4. Subclavian artery.

With the patient supine and the arm alongside the body, the midpoint of the clavicle is accurately determined. Frequently, nerve cords may be palpated 1 cm above this point. A wheal is raised (Fig. 21-10). With the finger of one hand, the subclavian artery is depressed medially and caudad at an angle of about 20° in each plane. One must proceed cautiously; if paresthesias are elicited, the position of the needle must be maintained and 10 ml of anesthetic solution deposited. If paresthesias cannot be elicited, one must then make contact with the first rib, withdraw the needle 0.5 cm, and either deposit 25 ml of solution or inject 10 ml at the latter point and supplement this by 1) directing the needle for 2.5 to 3 cm toward Chassaignac's tubercle and depositing 10 ml there, and 2) directing the needle 1.5 cm below the clavicle toward the apex of the axilla and there depositing another 10 ml.

Complications.—Pneumothorax may be caused by puncture of the lung and hemothorax by puncture of large vessels. Injury to nerves may lead to motor paralysis.

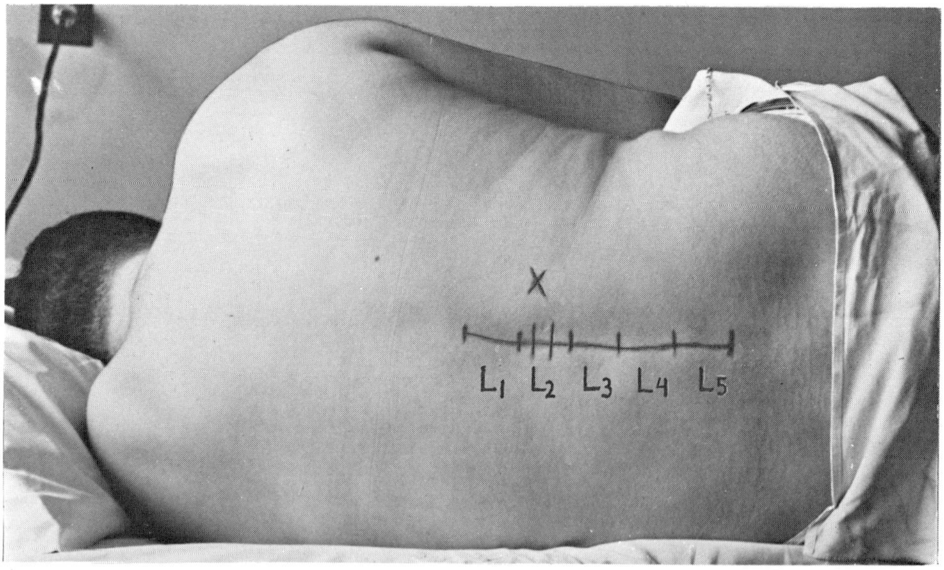

Fig. 21-11.—Marking used in locating the site of introduction of the needle for paravertebral block. The spinous process of the second lumbar vertebra is divided into thirds and the needle introduced 4–5 cm. lateral to the upper third.

Paravertebral Block—Sympathetic Ganglia in Lumbar Region

INDICATIONS

1. Diagnostic: Determination of lability of arterioles in peripheral vascular disorders and in patients with hypertension.
2. Therapeutic: Thrombophlebitis and indolent ulcers of lower extremities.

ANATOMY.—The transverse processes lie opposite their corresponding spinous processes. The important landmark is a line connecting the superior borders of the ilium and crossing either between the spinous processes of the fourth and fifth lumbar vertebrae or the fourth lumbar spinous process.

STANDARD APPROACH.—Wheals are raised 4 to 5 cm from the midline opposite the upper third of the spinous processes (Fig. 21-11). The recorder is set at 4 to 5 cm. The needle is directed perpendicularly to contact the transverse process; this is usually located at a depth of 5 cm. The needle is then directed somewhat medially and cephalad or caudad to the transverse process until it slides past the tip on its way to the body of the vertebra. The point of the 12-cm needle should rest close to the anterolateral surface of the body of the vertebra. It is useful to check the position of the needle radiographically.

LATERAL APPROACH.—With the patient supine, the midpoint between the crest of the ilium and the lower border of the rib cage at the posterior axillary line is determined. A 15-cm needle (with stilet) is directed toward the body of the vertebra and gradually redirected anteriorly until it just slides along the anterolateral surface of the vertebral body.

COMPLICATIONS.—There may be hemorrhage from rupture of vessels. It

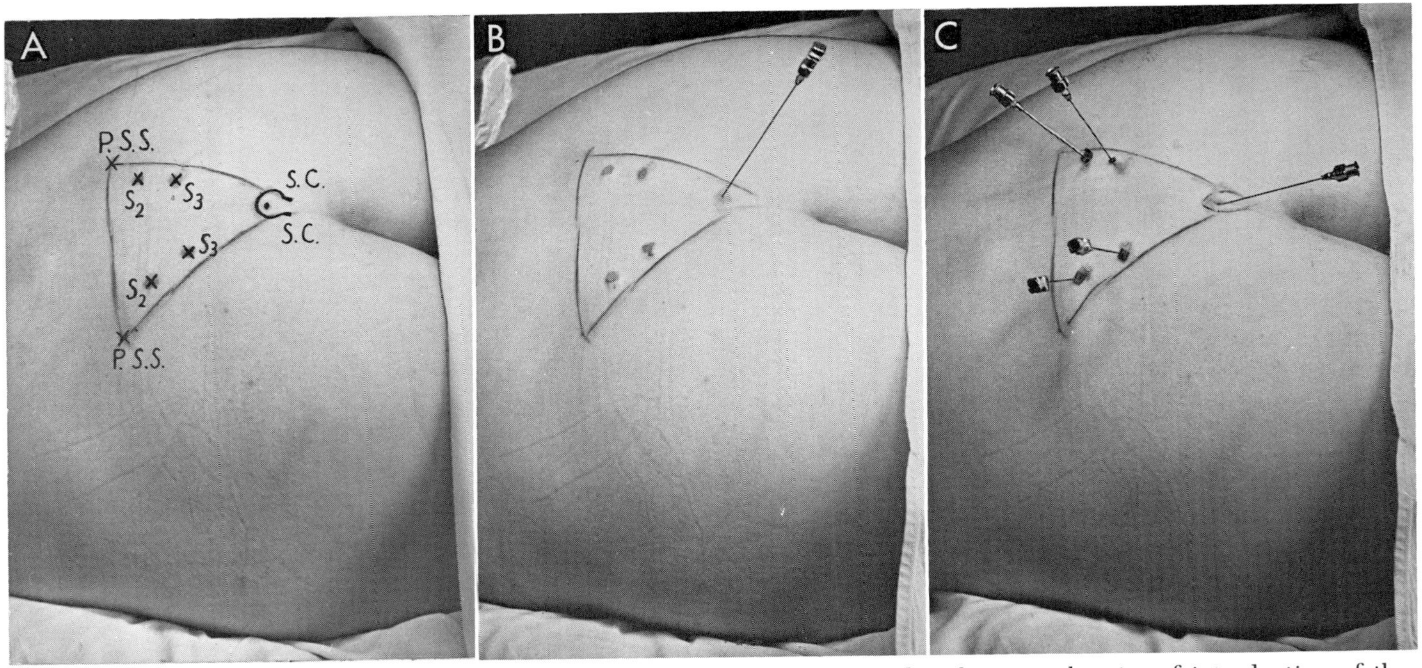

Fig. 21-12.—Procedure in transsacral and caudal block. **A**, marking used in locating the site of introduction of the needle. *P.S.S.*, the posterior superior spines; *S.C.*, the sacral cornua. The sacral hiatus is outlined by the horseshoe-shaped mark. Note the equilateral triangle. **B**, the caudal needle is introduced at a right angle to the skin surface in the most cephalad point of the hiatus. **C**, note change of angle of the caudal needle to permit it to enter the caudal canal. The sacral needles are pointed slightly caudad and medialward.

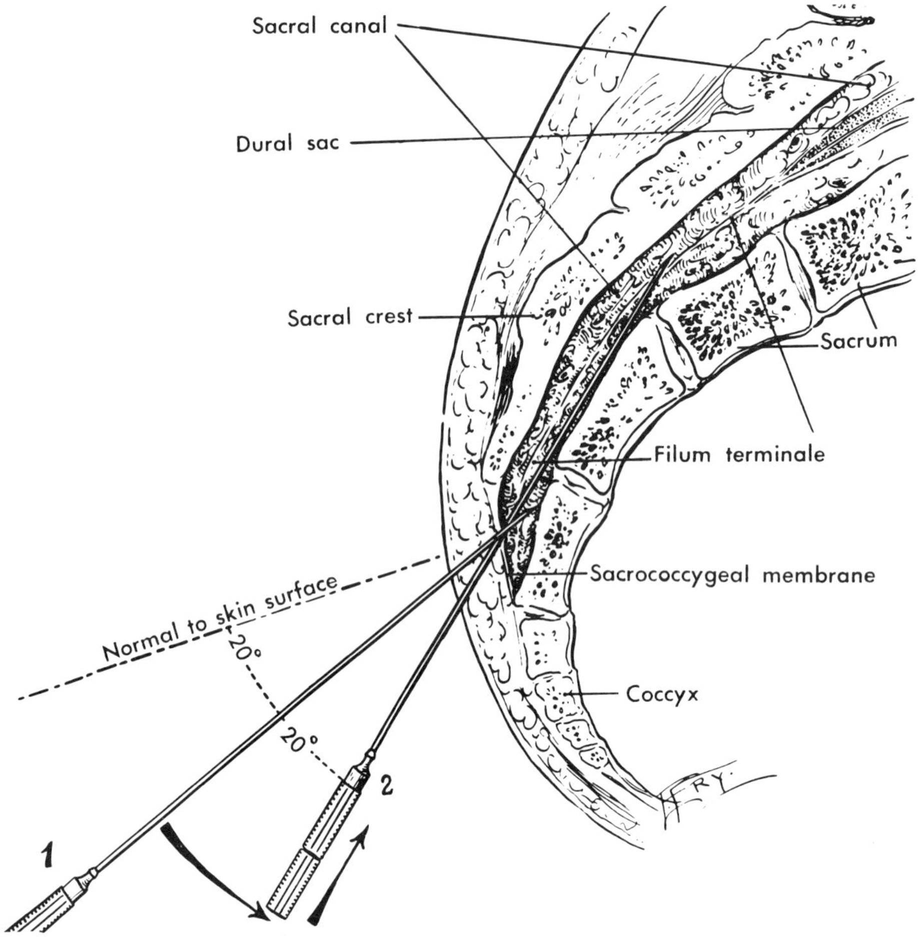

Fig. 21-13.—Relationship of needle in different positions to structures in and around the caudal hiatus and canal. (From Labat, G.: *Regional Anesthesia* [Philadelphia: W. B. Saunders Company, 1922]. Reproduced by permission.)

is possible also to inject the blocking agent accidentally into the subarachnoid space if sleeves of dura, pia mater and arachnoid extend along the somatic nerves and the rami communicantes. Many patients requiring lumbar sympathetic blocks also may be receiving anticoagulant therapy. If a patient is receiving such therapy, the block should not be done because severe bleeding in deep structures may occur.

Transsacral and Caudal Block

INDICATIONS

1. Diagnostic and therapeutic: "Sciaticas" and neuralgias.
2. Anesthetic: Operations on anus, vagina, prostate and perineum; obstetric delivery.

ANATOMY.—The first to third sacral and fourth and fifth lumbar nerves form the sacral plexus, and this plexus forms the sciatic nerve. It also innervates the musculature around the hip joint. The pudendal plexus is formed by union of anterior collateral branches of the first to fifth sacral nerves and the coccygeal nerve. The landmarks are:

1. Sacral cornua.
2. Posterior superior iliac spine.

APPROACH.—With the patient prone and supported by a pillow under the pubis, the posterior superior spines of the ilium are marked. These are defined usually as the most prominent bony eminences. The sacral cornua are then marked. These are defined by first palpating the tip of the coccyx and working the finger cephalad until the tip falls into the hiatus; then, by moving the finger lateralward, the cornu on either side can be determined. The hiatus must be located first and then the cornu. After the cornua and posterior superior spines have been located, lines are drawn between each; and if the landmarks are properly defined, an equilateral triangle will be formed (Fig. 21-12). A point 1 fingerbreadth caudad to the posterior spine and 1 cm medial to the line joining cornu and spine is marked. This point is slightly lateral and cephalad to the second sacral foramen. Another point is marked 1 fingerbreadth farther caudad on the same line for the third sacral foramen. This procedure can be repeated for the fourth and fifth sacral foramina; however, injection into these foramina is not necessary unless it is impossible to make an injection in the caudal canal.

Wheals are raised at each sacral mark and at the most cephalad point of the sacral hiatus. The spinal or caudal needle (12 cm., no. 20 gauge) is introduced perpendicular to the skin surface at the most cephalad point of the sacral hiatus and bone cephalad to this point is contacted. A no. 18 or no. 20 gauge shorter needle, such as is used for intravenous injection, may be substituted for the spinal needle. The needle is moved caudad until it falls off the bone and passes through the sacrococcygeal membrane. It is essential that the anesthetist feel the needle pass through the skin, the subcutaneous tissue and the thick membrane and space under the membrane and finally that the needle strike the bony floor of the caudal canal. The hub of the needle is then depressed, the bevel turned so that the open side is on the floor of the canal and the needle is advanced no farther than the level of the third sacral nerve (Fig. 21-13).

The 5.0- to 6.0-cm needle is then introduced through the sacral skin wheals and advanced until it comes in contact with bone. It is then withdrawn and reintroduced so that it is directed slightly caudad and medialward. It will usually enter the foramen; if it does not, the needle must be moved in a circular fashion in that area until the opening is found. One must be suspicious of a needle that is pointed cephalad because it may be resting on the top of the sacrum.

Finally, 5 ml of anesthetic solution is placed in each sacral foramen and 20 ml in the caudal canal.

The combining of injections into the second and third sacral foramina and caudal block is the most satisfactory method of producing quick and good perineal anesthesia. Furthermore, if injection into the caudal canal through the sacral hiatus is not possible, block of sacral nerves through the respective foramina makes it possible to establish sacral or caudal anesthesia. Usually there is no foramen for the fifth nerve and injection is made just lateral to the cornu.

When injecting into the caudal canal, fingertips on the sacrum will indicate the presence of a tumor from subcutaneous injection and show the

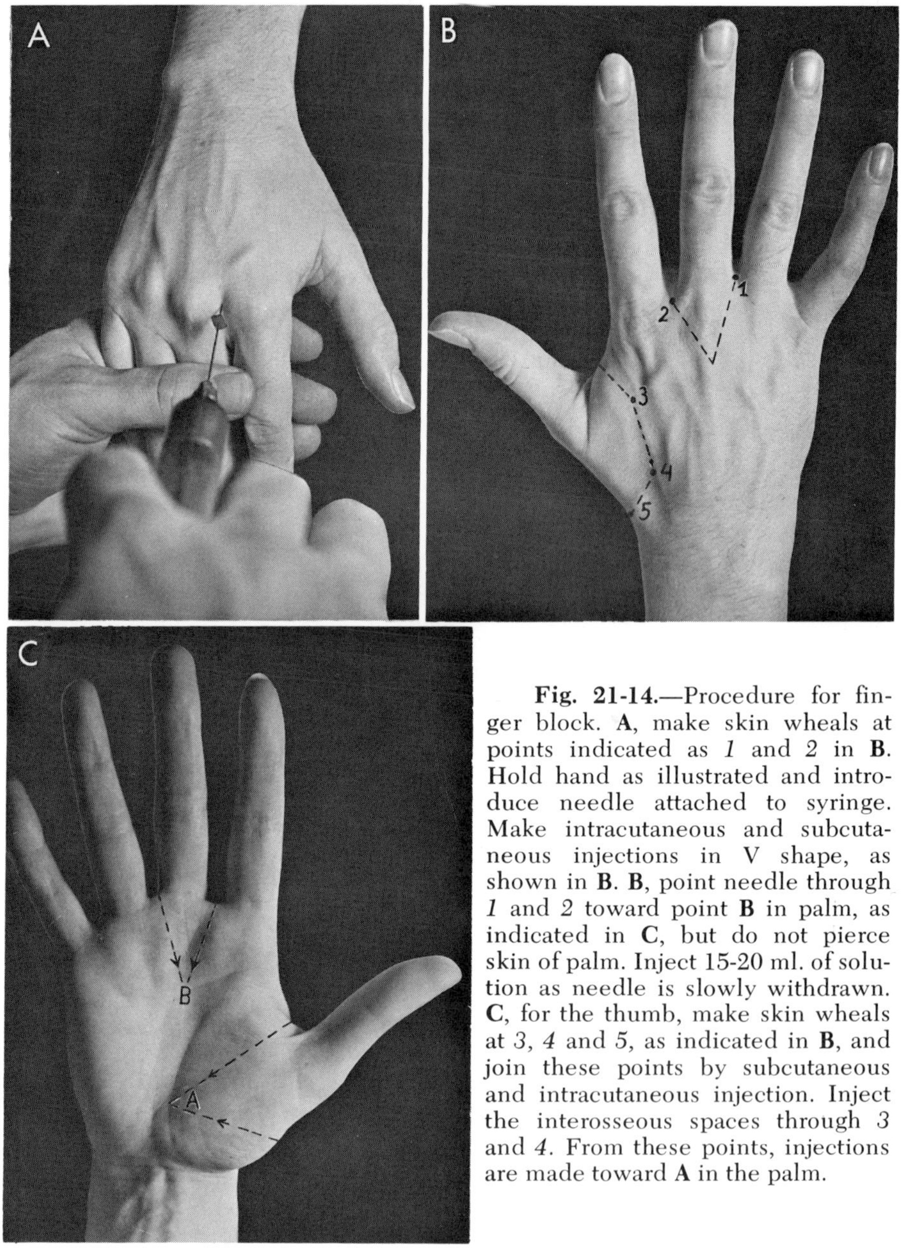

Fig. 21-14.—Procedure for finger block. **A**, make skin wheals at points indicated as *1* and *2* in **B**. Hold hand as illustrated and introduce needle attached to syringe. Make intracutaneous and subcutaneous injections in V shape, as shown in **B**. **B**, point needle through *1* and *2* toward point **B** in palm, as indicated in **C**, but do not pierce skin of palm. Inject 15-20 ml. of solution as needle is slowly withdrawn. **C**, for the thumb, make skin wheals at *3*, *4* and *5*, as indicated in **B**, and join these points by subcutaneous and intracutaneous injection. Inject the interosseous spaces through *3* and *4*. From these points, injections are made toward **A** in the palm.

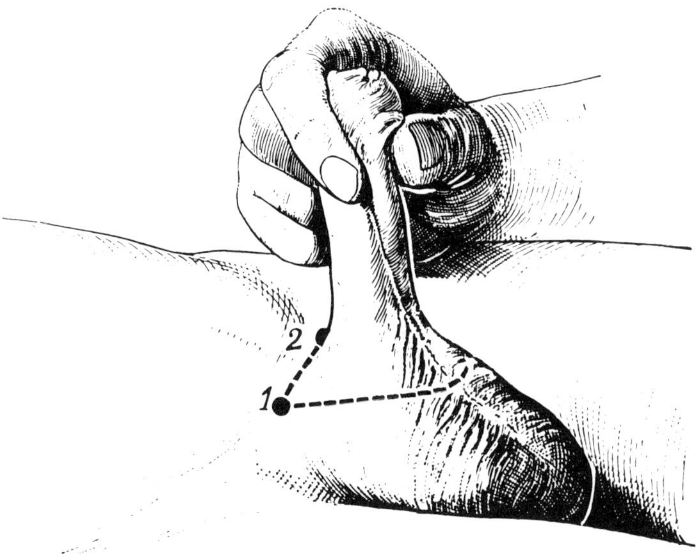

Fig. 21-15.—Field block of entire penis. *1* and *2*, pubic wheals, raised just medial to and below the pubic spine, are used for blocking dorsal nerves of the penis; the dotted lines indicate subcutaneous infiltration around the base. (From Labat, G.: *Regional Anesthesia* [Philadelphia: W. B. Saunders Company, 1922]. Reproduced by permission.)

anesthetist that he is outside the canal. An indication that the needle is properly placed is the easy flow of anesthetic solution. If it is difficult to introduce the solution the needle may not be in the caudal canal or the point may be subperiosteal.

COMPLICATIONS.—Subarachnoid injection is possible. Infection is not uncommon when the continuous needle or catheter method is employed. Infection is rare when the single-injection technic is used.

Finger Block

The procedure used in blocking the fingers can also be used in blocking the toes. This method of blocking, exemplified in Figure 21-14, is superior to the ring block of a finger or toe because it provides more complete anesthesia and is less likely to cause ischemia and subsequent necrosis.

Circumcision Block

APPROACH.—Two skin wheals are raised on each side of the base of the penis just medial to and below the pubic spine (Fig. 21-15). With the penis drawn out and held in this position, a needle attached to a syringe is introduced through each wheal and advanced deeply along the ascending ramus of the pubis as far as the corpora cavernosa; solution is injected at this point. These injections block the dorsal nerves of the penis. The needle then is withdrawn and reintroduced beneath the skin of the scrotum, where about

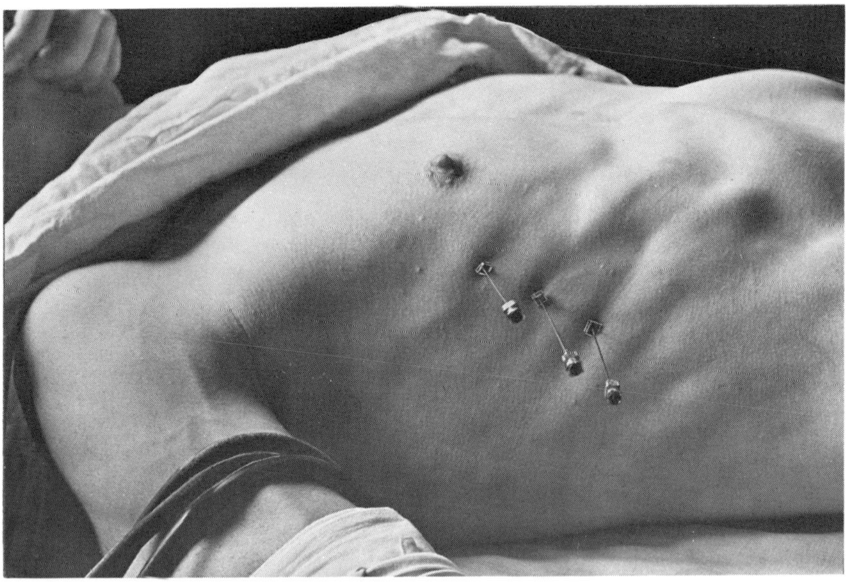

Fig. 21-16.—Placement of needles for intercostal nerve block. Note direction of the needles.

20 ml of solution is injected. It is often necessary to inject directly into the frenulum.

Intercostal Block

INDICATIONS

1. Diagnostic: Neuralgia.
2. Therapeutic: Relief of pain from fractured ribs; relief of wound pain in upper abdomen and chest; anesthesia for thoracotomy and upper abdominal surgery; and improvement of muscular relaxation in upper abdomen.

ANATOMY.—The intercostal nerves lie in the groove on the inferior surface of the rib, each being accompanied by the intercostal artery and vein.

APPROACH.—The needle is introduced perpendicular to the skin surface near the lower border of the rib in the anterior axillary or midaxillary line (Fig. 21-16). The lower border of the rib is contacted, then the needle is slipped off the lower edge and redirected cephalad and slightly medialward, seeking the groove in the inferior surface of the rib. Here, 3 to 5 ml of solution is injected.

COMPLICATIONS.—Hemorrhage from the intercostal vessels may occur. Entrance into the pleural space with varying degrees of pneumothorax is relatively frequent.

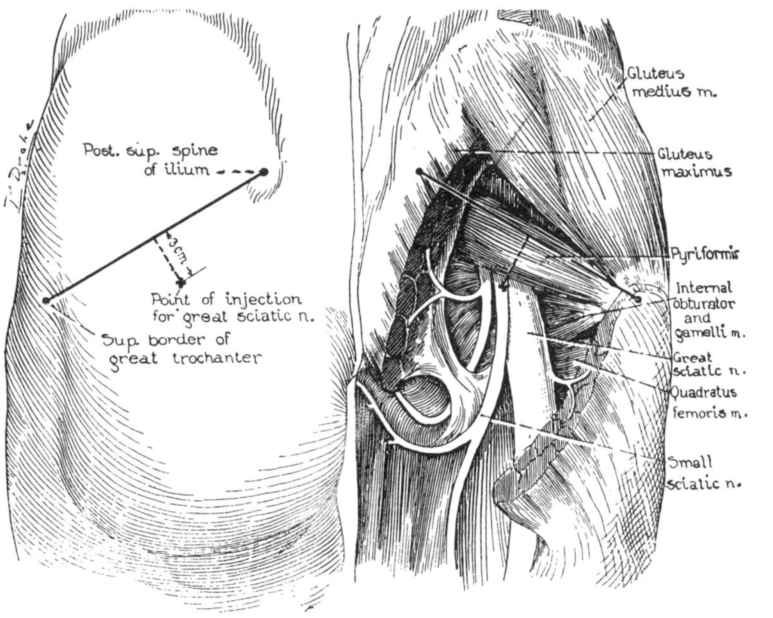

Fig. 21-17.—Great sciatic block. Superficial landmarks in relation to the deep structures. Note situation of the small sciatic nerve which is blocked at the same time as the great sciatic nerve. (From Labat, G.: *Regional Anesthesia* [Philadelphia: W. B. Saunders Company, 1922]. Reproduced by permission.)

Sciatic Block

INDICATIONS

1. Operations on the ankle and foot.
2. Sympathetic block of the lower extremity.

ANATOMY.—The great sciatic nerve leaves the pelvis through the great sacrosciatic foramen below the piriformis muscle. It turns down between the great trochanter and the tuberosity of the ischium to enter the thigh beneath the lower margin of the gluteus maximus muscle.

APPROACH.—The patient is placed in the Sims position with the side to be blocked upward and the knee on the same side brought forward (Fig. 21-17). The upper extremity of the great trochanter and the iliac spine are defined by palpation, and a straight line joining these points is marked on the skin. This line is bisected and a perpendicular line drawn down and in for a distance of 3 cm. A 10-cm needle is introduced perpendicular to the skin surface and advanced until paresthesias are elicited or until bone is contacted at a depth of 6 to 8 cm. If bone is contacted without previous paresthesias, the needle is withdrawn slightly and redirected until paresthesias are elicited. Approximately 10 to 15 ml of solution is injected.

COMPLICATIONS.—The complications from this block are minimal. Intraneural injection must be avoided. Some patients may have a profound response to the elicitation of paresthesias.

Femoral Block

INDICATION

1. Operations on the anteromedial aspect of the thigh.

ANATOMY.—The femoral nerve arises from the lumbar plexus and emerges beneath the inguinal ligament lateral to the femoral artery and vein to lie beneath the deep fascia of the thigh.

APPROACH.—The femoral artery is palpated with one finger and retracted medially. A wheal is raised just below Poupart's ligament and lateral to the artery. A 5.0- to 8.0-cm needle is advanced until it can be felt to pass through the thick fascia overlying the nerve and vessels. Approximately 10 to 15 ml of anesthetic solution is injected.

REFERENCES

1. Bromage, P. R., Burfoot, M. F., Crowell, D. E., and Truant, A. P.: Quality of epidural blockade: III, Carbonated local anesthetic solutions, Br. J. Anaesth. 39:197, 1967.
2. Bromage, P. R., and Gertel, M.: Improved brachial plexus blockade with bupivacaine hydrochloride and carbonated lidocaine, Anesthesiology 36:479, 1972.
3. Labat, G.: *Regional Anesthesia* (1st ed.; Philadelphia: W. B. Saunders Company, 1922).
4. Lundy, J. S.: *Clinical Anesthesia* (1st ed.; Philadelphia: W. B. Saunders Company, 1942).
5. Southworth, J. L., and Hingson, R. A. (eds.): Pitkin's *Conduction Anesthesia* (2d ed.; Philadelphia: J. B. Lippincott Company, 1951).
6. Adriani, J.: *Technics and Procedures of Anesthesia* (Springfield, Ill.: Charles C Thomas, Publisher, 1947).
7. Bonica, J. J.: *The Management of Pain* (Philadelphia: Lea & Febiger, 1953).
8. Moore, D. C.: *Regional Block* (1st ed.; Springfield, Ill.: Charles C Thomas, Publisher, 1953).
9. De Jong, R. H.: *Physiology and Pharmacology of Local Anesthesia* (Springfield, Ill.: Charles C Thomas, Publisher, 1970).
10. Winnie, A. P.: Interscalene brachial plexus block, Anesth. & Analg. (Cleve.) 49:455, 1970.

CHAPTER TWENTY-TWO

Spinal and Epidural Anesthesia

SPINAL ANESTHESIA

SPINAL ANESTHESIA is that state of anesthesia produced by the intrathecal injection of an appropriate local anesthetic drug. Anesthesia is confined to the area supplied by the nerve roots affected by the drug. Although only a portion of the patient is patently anesthetized, in a sense spinal anesthesia must be considered a general form of anesthesia, in that changes induced by paralysis of the nerve roots indirectly, but widely, influence homeostasis. This influence on the body as a whole is directly proportional to the number of segments that are anesthetized; that is, the higher the level of spinal anesthesia, the more profound the general effect.

It is generally believed that the interruption of transmission of nerve impulses is accomplished in a particular nerve root after it leaves the spinal cord and before it leaves the dura; the tracts of the spinal cord are not anesthetized. The degree to which nerve roots are anesthetized is, broadly, entirely dependent on the number of molecules of the drug to which they are exposed. The different modalities of sensation and the fibers controlling muscular and sympathetic tone are blocked in a relatively constant order; this is a function of the size of the various fibers within the root and the degree of their myelinization. Pain sensation disappears early; touch, kinesthetic sense and deep pressure sense disappear later and in about that order. Block of sympathetic fibers is established before the appearance of analgesia, and muscular relaxation develops shortly afterward. With low concentrations of a drug, it is entirely possible, and sometimes advantageous, to produce good analgesia and sympathetic paralysis without significant degrees of muscular paralysis (i.e., a differential spinal).

Advantages

Spinal anesthesia has several features that make it a desirable technic. It is capable of producing extreme muscular relaxation. By interruption of sympathetic pathways, it causes contraction of the small intestine, which facilitates exposure within the abdomen. Spinal anesthesia is useful when it is expedient to use electrical apparatus during surgery. It is useful also when the patient's cooperation is desired during the operative procedure and when a patient does not want to lose consciousness. A basic advantage is production of extensive anesthetic effect with minimal doses of drug.

Disadvantages

Except in continuous spinal anesthesia, the drug cannot be retrieved once it has been introduced into the subarachnoid space, and any complications that may develop must be treated symptomatically. In these respects, it is a less flexible technic than general anesthesia. There is always the likelihood of precipitate and inordinate degrees of hypotension. There are means of preventing hypotension in most patients, and there are effective means of treating it once it has developed; but one cannot guarantee that hypotension will not appear in any one patient despite adequate prophylactic measures. It is usually considered not advisable (but not absolutely contraindicated) to use spinal anesthesia for the surgical management of patients who are in surgical, traumatic or hemorrhagic shock because the peripheral vascular dilatation augments the disparity between vascular capacity and circulating volume. However, current evidence of the relative effectiveness of tissue perfusion with a relaxed, rather than a constricted, vascular bed leads one to believe that spinal anesthesia may be a reasonable choice in states of shock provided, of course, that appropriate efforts are made to restore the blood pressure by measures like transfusion and, temporarily, by the administration of vasoactive and positive inotropic cardiac drugs.

Complications During Anesthesia

HYPOTENSION.—In certain patients, it is dangerous to allow hypotension to supervene. The hypotension is due chiefly to vasodilation of peripheral arterioles as well as venous capacitance vessels in the areas from which sympathetic control has been temporarily removed, with consequent stagnation in those areas, reduced venous return and impaired cardiac output. Hypotension may be more pronounced when spinal analgesia extends above the fifth thoracic segment because of sympathetic denervation of the heart and resultant bradycardia and decreased ventricular muscle function. Hypotension appears shortly after the onset of analgesia (usually within 5 minutes) and is aggravated by alterations in the patient's position. Once the blood pressure has been stabilized either spontaneously or by use of vasopressor agents, and if extreme care is taken to prevent sudden and major changes in position, there is no repetitive fall in blood pressure due to spinal anesthesia, even though the peripheral vascular bed is still without sympathetic control for some time and beyond the period of effectiveness of the vasopressor drug. These observations lead to the belief that hypotension results from the patient's inability to rapidly adjust the dynamics of blood flow following abrupt peripheral vascular relaxation and that vasopressor agents act only to assist the patient in adapting to the alteration in blood flow and distribution. After a time (in some patients, immediately), physiologic adjustments which maintain normal blood pressure are made. If this were not true, it would be necessary to repeat the administration of vasopressor drugs throughout the duration of spinal analgesia. Changes in position, exemplified by moving the patient from the supine to the prone or lateral position or even moving the patient from operating table to the cart or bed, will cause hypotension after the blood pressure has been stabilized for a long time. A patient under spinal anesthesia, indeed any patient in whom the peripheral vascular bed may not be under complete control, should not be subjected to rough handling. Hypotension does not often occur unless there is appreciable anesthetization of the splanchnic nerves, and the incidence and degree of hypotension are much less in patients in whom the level of analgesia is below the tenth thoracic segment. The fall in blood pressure also may be augmented by paralysis of the pressor receptor mechanisms, thereby preventing reflex compensation.

Hypotension associated with spinal anesthesia results in imperfect oxygenation of the cerebral centers. Hypoxia may initiate another train of symptoms frequently noted in patients under spinal anesthesia. These are nausea and emesis, mental confusion and anxiety, air hunger and tachycardia and permanent central nervous system damage if hypoxia is prolonged.

Prophylaxis and treatment.—In most patients, hypotension can be prevented by the prophylactic intramuscular injection of a vasopressor drug approximately 10 minutes before the anticipated onset of analgesia. Drugs useful for this are ephedrine (50 mg), phenylephrine (2 mg), methoxamine (15 mg), methamphetamine (20 mg), mephenteramine (20 mg) and metaraminol (5 mg). Of these drugs, ephedrine is the most satisfactory for prophylactic use because its action is more sustained than with shorter-acting vasopressors such as metaraminol and because if spinal anesthesia is delayed in onset or impossible to achieve, the overshoot in pressure is limited. We emphasize that the prophylactic drug should be given intramuscularly and at least 10 minutes in advance of the anticipated onset of anesthesia to permit time for action. The prophylactic drug is usually unsatisfactory if given in the somewhat traditional area of the paraspinal muscles concomitant with the lumbar puncture. It is more important to administer these drugs prophylactically to the patient with hypertension than to the patient with normally low blood pressure. The patient with hypertension is less capable of compensating and may be more susceptible to thrombosis after a period of low tension. Patients with long-standing hypertension also usually have a decreased plasma volume and, as a result, the disparity between circulating volume and vascular capacity is exaggerated; vigorous hydration ("preloading") with intravenous fluids may help to prevent hypotension.

There is a tendency to treat all cases of hypotension occurring as a result of spinal anesthesia regardless of the circumstances: whether the hypotension is abrupt and profound in onset and degree or gradual in onset and minimal in degree, whether it is occurring in patients with limited circulation (coronary insufficiency, for example) or is developing in a patient with hypertension or in a patient with normotension and, finally, without regard to the fact that in many patients the blood pressure stabilizes at a reasonable and tolerable value for that patient. In this circumstance of anesthetic management, as in all others, it is important that the anesthetist keep in mind the individual patient and his problems and adjust management of the blood pressure according to the needs of the patient rather than attempting to treat the blood pressure itself. As a result, one attempts, for example, to keep the blood pressure at or near the patient's "normal" level (vigorously, if necessary) if the patient has impaired circulation (i.e., to the brain, heart, or kidney) or an abnormally high pressure. Restoration of blood pressure is also indicated if hypotension is abrupt and profound, and there is no evidence of it stabilizing. Otherwise, one often can wait to determine the rate and degree of blood pressure fall. Frequently, the pressure stabilizes by itself. A useful rule of thumb is to permit the pressure to fall to the level that one might plan to reach if deliberate hypotension were needed. The lower pressure can be tolerated well by many patients and, except in special circumstances such as angiography, there is no need to attempt to restore the blood pressure to the patient's normal tension.

There is a price to pay for the restoration of blood pressure by vasoactive drugs. One may, by so doing, cause undesirable constriction of the vascular bed and actually diminish tissue perfusion. Especially if one uses the more potent vasoconstrictors, one often encounters a "roller coaster" type of blood pressure response.

Except for prophylactic administration, the vasoactive drugs preferably should be given intravenously to ensure prompt and effective action. Subcutaneous or intramuscular injection is often ineffective in states of poor peripheral perfusion due to hypotension. The dose of ephedrine for intravenous administration is 15 mg, that of phenylephrine is 0.5 mg, that of mephenteramine is 3 mg and that of metaraminol, 0.5 mg. In our opinion, methoxamine is not indicated because of its negative inotropic effect.

Hypotension due to spinal anesthesia can be treated successfully also by giving an increased volume of intravenous solutions. The rationale is to fill up the vascular space created by the sympathetic paralysis rather than by attempting to diminish the vascular space by constriction with drugs. Often it is useful to combine use of drugs and increased fluid input. Drugs can be used for the immediate treatment of severe hypotension and fluids for the more sustained management.

Many of the symptoms associated with hypotension are due to hypoxia, and it is advisable to administer oxygen in high concentrations to patients with hypotension. This decreases the incidence of nausea and emesis and relieves mental confusion, anxiety and air hunger. In many patients in whom hypotension is only mild or moderate, administration of oxygen alone will improve the circulation.

It may be useful also to lower the patient's head. In most patients, at the time that hypotension appears, the advantage gained will offset the possible disadvantage of cephalad extension of analgesia. Raising the patient's legs is as effective, if not more so, as lowering the head.

If spinal anesthesia is high enough to block the sympathetic supply to the heart, bradycardia may occur. If this is believed to contribute to hypotension, atropine given intravenously is useful.

Many anesthetists prefer not to use vasoconstricting drugs prophylactically and to reserve their use only for treatment of hypotension when it occurs. With this approach, it is difficult to predict which patient will have a precipitate fall in pressure that may reach very low levels before therapy can be instituted. Nor is it possible to predict which patient will suffer irreparable circulatory insufficiency, such as coronary insufficiency or thrombosis in a critical vessel, with even short and not alarming periods of hypotension. It is probable that patients will suffer more from periods of profound hypotension than from a relatively insignificant hypertension due to a prophylactic vasoconstrictor.

RESPIRATORY PARALYSIS.—Another disadvantage of spinal anesthesia is the occasional production of complete intercostal and diaphragmatic paralysis. The mechanism for this loss of function is not clear. Usually, it is assumed that there is sufficient concentration of anesthetic in spinal fluid in the medullary area to cause paralysis. In many circumstances, patients feel that they are unable to breathe although they have adequate respiratory muscle function. This sense of being unable to breathe is due to loss of proprioceptive sensations associated with chest movement. Even though the patient can move his chest on command, it is often necessary to apply assistance to ventilation by mask with oxygen to relieve the patient's distress. Intercostal paralysis, with its associated decreased ventilation, may be serious in patients with deficient functional capacity. Intercostal paralysis also may be detrimental in patients placed in steep head-down positions. Fortunately, inadequate respiration associated with paralysis of intercostal muscles and diaphragm can be controlled by artificial ventilation. It is essential that the anesthetist administering spinal anesthesia be prepared to institute effective artificial respiration immediately in all patients, regardless of the anticipated height of the analgesia. This means that no spinal anesthetic should be given unless facilities for artificial ventilation are immediately available. No patient should die of spinal anesthesia because of respiratory paralysis.

NAUSEA AND EMESIS.—Nausea and emesis also may result from traction reflexes that are inadequately obtunded because the anesthetic level is too low. If the latter is the case and if the level of anesthesia cannot be raised (as it can be with continuous spinal anesthesia), it is usually necessary to induce general anesthesia to cover the deficiency in the spinal anesthesia. Indeed, many difficulties and problems result from spinal anesthesia that is too low rather than too high. Nausea and emesis often occur persistently without any obvious reason. In such circumstances, administration of oxygen may help. Drugs such as diazepam (Valium), pentobarbital and thiopental may be useful in allaying this discomfort. The combination of fentanyl and droperidol (Innovar) is effective in controlling nausea; droperidol is probably the effective agent in the combination. The antiemetics are of doubtful value. Sometimes, it is necessary to induce and maintain light levels of general anesthesia, usually with an inhalation agent. It is a common practice among some anesthetists to produce sleep in almost all patients under spinal analgesia. Nausea and emesis are said to be less severe when they do appear.

DEPRESSION OF THE COUGH REFLEX.—It has often been stated that spinal anesthesia is advantageous in patients in whom it is desirable to retain the cough reflex. This is true in part, but the fact is often overlooked that, although the patient may have his cough reflex, the ability to expel material from the tracheobronchial tree is seriously impaired by the presence of intercostal and abdominal muscle relaxation. One should not depend on retention of the cough reflex to ensure elimination of voluminous secretions in the trachea and bronchi, particularly if the spinal anesthesia is at a high level with a large intrathecal concentration of the anesthetic drug.

Suitable Drugs

A number of drugs are available for intrathecal use. Those used most commonly are procaine, lidocaine and tetracaine. Dibucaine is used occasionally if prolonged anesthesia is needed. The pharmacologic properties of these drugs have been discussed in Chapter 21.

CHOICE OF DRUG.—The selection of a drug for spinal analgesia can be made solely on a time basis. Contrary to popular opinion, the height of a spinal anesthetic is due to the volume of solution used, the position of the patient, the speed with which the solution is injected and the presence (or absence) of glucose and epinephrine; it is not due to the amount of drug used. It is the dose of drug that determines the duration of action, not height. Toxic properties of these drugs need not be considered because toxic reactions do not occur following the intrathecal use of these drugs. Small amounts are used and the absorption is so slow that toxic blood concentrations cannot develop. Features of spinal analgesia that are frequently mentioned as specific properties of certain drugs can, with the exception of duration of action, be duplicated by any of the drugs mentioned. Among these special features are height of analgesia, degrees of muscular paralysis, variations in time of onset, incidence of nausea and emesis, frequency of postanesthetic headache, postanesthetic neurologic sequelae and variations of specific gravity.

In order of increasing duration of action, the common drugs are procaine, lidocaine, tetracaine and dibucaine.

Premedication

It is usually advisable to administer a sedative-hypnotic drug and a narcotic. Most patients prefer to be somewhat sleepy during the procedure and most patients appreciate some analgesic prior to the discomfort of positioning and the lumbar puncture. It is wise not to give a dose that makes it difficult to obtain the patient's cooperation in positioning him and in determining the presence and height of spinal anesthesia.

Either of these types of drugs may be employed, of course, during the course of anesthesia to induce sleep or to minimize the discomfort of sustained position. The combination of fentanyl and droperidol (Innovar) is effective.

The Standard Technic of Spinal Anesthesia Using Procaine

Following lumbar puncture, the technic of which is described in the following section, enough cerebrospinal fluid is withdrawn to make a 5% solution with procaine crystals. After the procaine crystals have been dissolved in cerebrospinal fluid and the solution has been aspirated from the ampule, a syringe (a 5-ml glass syringe is most convenient) is attached to the spinal needle and a small amount of fluid aspirated to determine that the needle is still in the subarachnoid space. The solution is introduced rapidly if a high level of analgesia is desired and slowly if a low level is desired. A rapid rate is the injection of 1 ml of solution per 2 seconds, and a slow rate is injection of 1 ml of solution per 15 seconds. After the solution has been introduced, the needle is withdrawn and the patient placed in the supine position, the table being horizontal. The blood pressure is then determined (one must not forget to take an initial reading at the start of the entire procedure) every minute for 5 minutes, every 3 minutes for 15 minutes and every 5 minutes thereafter. Frequent observations are necessary to permit prompt treatment. The level of analgesia should be determined after about 5 minutes. The 5% solution of procaine in spinal fluid is hyperbaric and will gravitate to dependent portions of the spinal canal. If testing discloses that the level of analgesia is too low for the projected surgical procedure, some cephalad extension of analgesia can be secured within 15 minutes of injection of the drug by lowering the head of the table. After 15 minutes the level is not likely to change, and it is safe to permit extreme head-down positions if they will facilitate the surgery. If it is found that the level of analgesia is too high, it is not advisable or beneficial to elevate the head in an attempt to restrict the cephalad extension. The head-up position may cause severe hypotension.

Testing for height can be done either with a needle or with a cotton pledget with alcohol. Obviously, the pledget tests for loss of temperature sensation and the needle tests for analgesia. With either method, it is important to give the patient time to respond. Most patients are sedated, some have analgesics as premedication, and some elderly patients are confused. More precise determination of level of height of the spinal anesthetic can be made if the patient is asked to respond to each application of the testing device (i.e., sensation or no sensation, cold or not, sharp or dull). If the tester is moved continuously in a cephalad direction, the patient often responds so slowly that the tester is two or three dermatomes higher than the actual level of anesthesia.

The safe maximum dose for a single injection is ordinarily considered to be 200 mg of procaine crystals. In the average healthy middle-aged adult, this dose will produce anesthesia lasting approximately 75 minutes. Smaller doses will give anesthesia for proportionately less time. Larger doses give smaller increments of increased length of action. In other words, 200 mg will not increase the length of action by 100% over that obtained with 100 mg; actually, it increases the duration by only about 60%. Older persons and patients with debilitating diseases will experience longer anesthesia from the same doses used in the middle-aged group. Young patients will experience shorter anesthesia, presumably because the drug is absorbed and metabolized more readily. Spinal anesthesia may be used in children; in proportion to their size they require relatively large doses of procaine to effect appreciable duration of action.

VARIATIONS IN THE STANDARD TECHNIC.—*Epinephrine.*—The standard procaine technic may be varied in a number of ways. The duration of action may be increased by adding epinephrine to the solution introduced intrathecally or by the use of the continuous spinal technic. Epinephrine added to the solution to make a 1:10,000 concentration (0.1 ml of the standard 1:1,000 preparation of epinephrine is added to 1 ml of the anesthetic solution) will, on the average, increase the length of action by approximately 30%. Clinical experience and laboratory investigation indicate that no damage to nerve roots or spinal cord results from the introduction of epinephrine. The quantity used is so small and absorption of it from the cerebrospinal fluid into the blood stream is so slow that systemic effects of the epinephrine do not become evident, and the use of vasopressor drugs to control blood pressure is still necessary. Cephalad progression of the level of analgesia is hindered by the addition of epinephrine to the anesthetic solution and onset of anesthesia is slightly delayed. It is usually necessary to inject the solution rapidly, and to lower the head immediately after injection for as long as 5 minutes to produce anesthesia to the sixth thoracic segment. The delay in onset of analgesia and the slow cephalad progression can be interpreted as added safety factors.

There is a strong clinical impression that other vasoconstricting drugs such as ephedrine and phenylephrine act to prolong the anesthesia from drugs introduced intrathecally. In our experience these drugs are less effective than epinephrine.

Continuous technic.—The continuous spinal technic permits repeated injection of anesthetic drug as often as desired. Repeated injections are made possible by the introduction into the subarachnoid space of a small flexible catheter, which is left in place during the anesthetic procedure. Advantages ascribed to this technic are (1) the lack of any limitation of duration of action, (2) the use of smaller doses of the drug in the intrathecal space at any one time, (3) the presence of low effective concentrations of the drug (i.e., 2 to 5%) and (4) termination of the analgesia at will by the removal of cerebrospinal fluid. Disadvantages accrue largely from the necessity to introduce a large-bore needle, which increases the opportunity for leakage of spinal fluid and subsequent headache, and the use of a catheter, which may abrade rootlets or entrap them as it curls in the subarachnoid space.

The catheter (usually polyethylene) is introduced through a no. 15-gauge Huber-pointed Tuohy needle, after which the needle is removed. Once the catheter has passed the end of the needle, it should not be withdrawn unless the needle also is withdrawn. Failure to exercise this precaution may result in shearing off the end of the catheter within the subarachnoid or epidural space.

Glucose.—Glucose (5 or 10%) may be added to the procaine-cerebrospinal fluid solution. Either concentration of glucose is usually added in equal parts to the procaine-cerebrospinal fluid solution, and the total amount of mixture should equal that used when procaine and cerebrospinal fluid are used alone. Glucose supposedly hastens the onset of analgesia, but its principal function is to make the injected solution definitely heavier than cerebrospinal fluid so that its distribution in the spinal canal can be more accurately controlled. It is theorized—and there is some experimental evidence to support the theory—that the heavy mixture settles into the thoracic and sacral concavities of the spinal column when the patient is in the supine position and is thereby prevented from progressing farther cephalad. It is usually necessary to place the patient in the 10° head-down position to permit analgesia to spread as high as the sixth thoracic segment. When very low analgesia is desired, the solution can be injected slowly with the patient in the horizontal or sitting position. Low analgesia accomplished in this manner has been popularized as "saddle block" and used extensively in obstetric practice. A critical analysis of most of the "saddle blocks" will reveal that the analgesic area extends appreciably above the saddle region and that, in essence, this type of anesthesia is simply low spinal analgesia and subject to all the factors influencing spinal analgesia.

Hypobaricity.—Procaine solutions can be made hypobaric by dilution or by warming. Hypobaric solutions are sometimes useful when an early head-down position is desired or when the patient has to be placed in the lateral position for surgery and it seems expedient to keep the anesthetic solution in the upper side. Generally speaking, hypobaric solutions are not so easily controlled as hyperbaric solutions; and their use is always subject to the dangers of excessive cephalad distribution, with consequent unwanted medullary depression.

Differential spinal.—The degree of muscular paralysis can be varied with procaine by altering the concentration of the injected solution. Low concentrations (i.e., 2 to 3%) will produce sensory analgesia and sympathetic block with little or no appreciable motor paresis.

Use of lidocaine hydrochloride (Xylocaine).—For practical purposes, lidocaine is used in the same manner as procaine. Somewhat longer action can be anticipated for an equianesthetic dose. The dose employed ranges from 10 to 30 mg. Its presumed advantages are its common availability and its slightly longer action.

Use of tetracaine hydrochloride (Pontocaine).—For reasons that are not entirely clear (except that perhaps there is currently a tendency to longer surgical procedures), tetracaine is used more frequently than any of the other drugs for spinal anesthesia. Unfortunately, this established habit pattern mitigates against the use of the shorter-acting drugs (procaine and lidocaine) for short surgical procedures of approximately 1 hour.

Tetracaine has a much longer duration of action than procaine. The usual maximal dose for a single injection is 20 mg, and its effect will last approximately 3½ hours in the average healthy middle-aged adult. It is prepared either in the crystal (niphanoid) form or in a 1% solution. When it is injected either dissolved only in spinal fluid or from the ampule of 1% solution, its specific gravity is about that of spinal fluid; thus, its diffusion, and therefore the level of analgesia it will produce, cannot be predicted with any degree of accuracy. As a consequence, it is nearly always used with glucose. Epinephrine may be added, and it may be used in the continuous technic.

Tetracaine can also be made hypobaric by warming or diluting it. A commonly used mixture contains 10 mg of niphanoid tetracaine in 1.25 ml of cerebrospinal fluid or 1 ml of 1% tetracaine, 0.25 ml of 1:1,000 epinephrine solution and 1.5 ml of glucose (10%). The action of tetracaine is appreciably prolonged by the addition of epinephrine and in many instances use of the combination has made the continuous spinal technic unnecessary for operations of long duration. One can usually guarantee anesthesia of 2 hours' duration with the use of 10 mg of tetracaine in the healthy middle-aged adult. Another significant advantage of this combination is the ability to secure analgesia of long duration with smaller quantities of the drug. It is a most satisfactory drug if moderately long analgesia from a single injection is desired. We repeat that it is advisable when one is using epinephrine and glucose to lower the head of the patient after intrathecal injection to ensure a high enough level of anesthesia. Anesthesia usually progresses cephalad sufficiently slowly so that constant checking of the height after injection permits one to return the patient to the horizontal position after the anesthesia has reached a level one or two dermatomes below the desired level.

Use of dibucaine hydrochloride (Nupercaine).—Dibucaine has the longest duration of action of the drugs commonly used in spinal anesthesia. The most frequently employed maximum dose is 10 mg, which will provide analgesia for 3 to 4 hours in the average healthy middle-aged adult. It is prepared either in the "light," or hypobaric, solution (Jones's solution, 1:1,500) or in the heavy solution (1:200). The 1:1,500 solution is used in the manner described for hypobaric solutions of procaine and the heavy solution is used in the same manner as tetracaine. Epinephrine may be added to either solution; and either may be used in the continuous technic, although the hypobaric solution is more difficult to control by the continuous technic. Dibucaine is a satisfactory drug if analgesia of long duration is desired from a single injection.

Technic of Lumbar Puncture

Satisfactory lumbar puncture is essential to the proper use of spinal anesthesia. Certain fundamentals in the performance of a lumbar puncture facilitate its execution.

Position and choice of interspace.—The patient may be in the lateral or the sitting position. The lateral position is usual and is most satisfactory for patients who are ill or heavily sedated. The sitting position is useful when it is difficult to separate the spinous processes adequately or if a low level of analgesia is desired. With the patient in the lateral position, lumbar puncture is most easily done if the back is at right angles to the plane of the table on which the patient is lying. The back should be well flexed, but it is not necessary to force the patient into an uncomfortable or painful posture. The midline of the line of spinous processes should then be determined by palpation, and marked. The midline of the line of spinous pro-

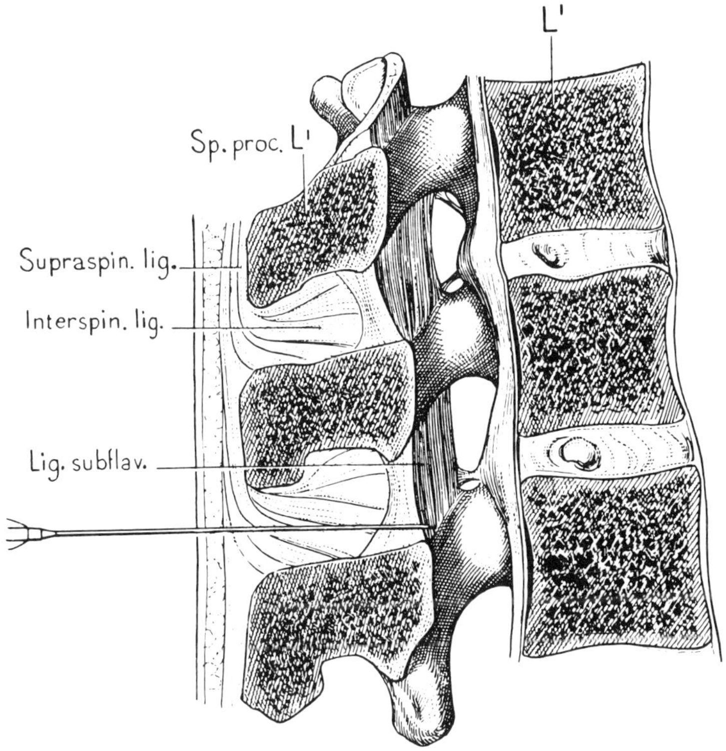

Fig. 22-1.—Sagittal section of structures through which the spinal needle passes. An appreciation of these structures and their relationships will expedite lumbar puncture. (From Labat, G.: *Regional Anesthesia* [Philadelphia: W. B. Saunders Company, 1922]. Reproduced by permission.)

cesses will not necessarily be the midline of the skin of the back, and it is important to recognize this difference when it exists. A convenient and well-defined lumbar interspace then should be located and marked. This interspace may be the second, third, fourth or fifth lumbar interspace; the second and third lumbar interspaces are usually the most convenient. With patients with pronounced lordosis it is advisable to stay out of the depression in the lumbar area and perform the puncture at higher levels. One need not be particular about the interspace selected, because the interspace selected has little to do with development of the level of analgesia. Moreover, we see little need for the traditional practice of feeling for the iliac crest. The critical element is to find and use the interspace that can be most easily defined. Assuming that the anesthetist is meticulous in placing the needle so that it is not advanced any more than enough to ensure the entry of the opening in the intrathecal space, we have no concern about introducing the needle at levels at which the spinal cord is present. One needs to remember, of course, that the higher the needle is introduced, the higher may be the level of anesthesia.

ADVANCEMENT OF NEEDLE.—After the midline of the line of the spinous processes and the interspace have been defined and marked, the needle should be introduced at right angles to the plane of the back and directed somewhat cephalad. Most patients in the lateral position do not have their back perpendicular to the plane of the table; and one of the more common errors in lumbar puncture is to have the anesthetist introduce the needle parallel to the plane of the table rather than at right angles to the plane of the patient's back. The needle should be introduced steadily and slowly through the thick and resistant ligamentum flavum until the point of the needle jumps free of the ligament. It is then advanced until it snaps through the dura into the subarachnoid space. Unfortunately, most of the needles used today, including those in the commercially packaged sterile sets, have relatively long bevels and the "snap" associated with entry into the subarachnoid space is not as apparent as it is with the shorter bevel of the Pitkin needle. After it is felt to snap through the dura, it should be advanced a little farther to ensure complete entry of the bevel of the needle into the subarachnoid space.

If the needle is in the midline of the line of spinous processes and in the interspace and if it is introduced at right angles to the plane of the back and slightly cephalad, it is almost impossible to avoid entering the subarachnoid space. An unsuccessful spinal tap, or a "dry tap," is almost always due to improper direction of the needle and is rarely due to lack of available cerebrospinal fluid. It is important that the anesthetist or any other person attempting a spinal puncture familiarize himself with the anatomy of the spinal column and the dura and its contents (Fig. 22-1). Knowledge of the areas through which the needle passes and the obstacles which it may encounter will enable the anesthetist to recognize obstructions and to alter the direction of the needle intelligently. There is no more exasperating sight to a teacher and no more unpleasant experience for the patient than to have an inexperienced and uninformed individual make repeated wild pokes with a spinal needle in random attempts to penetrate the dura.

CHOICE OF NEEDLE.—The needle used for spinal puncture prior to anesthesia should be no. 22 gauge or smaller, and approximately 9 cm long. Such a needle permits free flow of spinal fluid and does not make a large cut in the dura. The use of a 22-gauge needle makes it unnecessary to raise a skin wheal at the site of introduction of the needle. This discomfort associated with the production of the skin wheal is no less, and is often greater, than that associated with the introduction of the 22-gauge needle. However, if one anticipates or experiences a need for multiple insertions of the needle, a skin wheal is indicated. If one uses a 25-gauge needle, it is advisable to use a larger needle as an "introducer." Passing the fine needle through the larger needle diminishes the tendency of the 25-gauge needle to be misdirected by resistant structures on the way to the dura. These fine needles have been known to tie themselves into a knot and to be either impossible to remove or to break on attempts at removal. If short, larger-gauge needles are used as "introducers" or "guides" for fine lumbar puncture needles, a skin wheal of procaine (or similar drug) is indicated. There is good evidence that small-gauge needles are effective in reducing lumbar puncture headaches. In the light of this evidence, one must be prepared to defend the use of needles larger than no. 22 gauge, except in patients older than 50 years.

Once the needle has entered the dura and one is reasonably certain that the bevel is entirely inside the subarachnoid space, it is important that the needle be fixed by grasping the hub between thumb and forefinger of one hand and by resting that hand against the patient's back. If this is not done during removal of fluid and injection of solution, the needle is apt to be displaced by traction or pressure on the syringe attached to the needle.

THE LATERAL APPROACH.—In some patients in whom it is difficult to introduce the needle in the midline, a lateral approach may be used. In this circumstance, the needle is introduced at a point approximately 3 to 5 cm lateral to the midline of the spinous processes and opposite the posterior portion of the spinous process. It is angled medially and slightly cephalad so that it traverses the space between the lamina to enter the dura and intrathecal space. If bone is encountered, one must determine whether the needle is impinging on the lateral aspect of spinous process, in which case it is redirected less medially and more cephalad or caudad. Impingement may be on the lamina, in which case the needle is redirected either cephalad or caudad and perhaps more medial in an attempt to enter the interlaminal space or intervertebral foramen. As with interspinous lumbar puncture, one must be aware of the anatomy of the area in order to introduce the needle appropriately, rather than with "blind stabs."

FAILURE TO OBTAIN ANALGESIA.—Failure to obtain analgesia after an analgesic drug has been introduced into the subarachnoid space can, in 99% of instances, be ascribed to failure to introduce all or part of the analgesic solution into the subarachnoid space. The needle may be dislodged or the bevel may not lie totally within the subarachnoid space. When there is failure to obtain analgesia, it is perfectly permissible to reintroduce the needle and reinject the same or a lesser amount and concentration of analgesic solution. One should wait a sufficient length of time to assure oneself that lack of anesthesia is not due merely to a delay in onset.

In a few rare individuals, anesthesia cannot be secured even after repeated injections. In these patients, it is sometimes advantageous to use another analgesic agent. In a few of them it appears that the pH of the spinal fluid is such that precipitation of the drug as a base is not effected and the drug is incapable of inducing analgesia. In these patients, it is probable that no drug used for spinal analgesia will be suitable. In some patients, the anesthetist succeeds in introducing the needle and obtaining a flow of cerebrospinal fluid but finds it difficult or impossible to aspirate cerebrospinal fluid into the syringe. When this occurs, it is sometimes beneficial to rotate the needle because the flow is probably obstructed by a segment of pia mater or arachnoid or a dentate ligament. It is advisable to aspirate gently, because strong suction will tend only to plug the lumen of the needle more firmly. A complication of this nature is most often due to the fact that the needle is not in the absolute midline of the dural sac; and unless fluid can be obtained by one of the maneuvers just mentioned, it is good practice to remove and reinsert the needle in the midline. Failure to produce spinal anesthesia is not uncommon when free flow of fluid is not present at the time of aspiration or injection because the needle is easily displaced if it is not in the midline. If bleeding is encountered and this continues, one should avoid introducing the anesthetic drug. If the cerebrospinal fluid clears rapidly, there is no contraindication to injecting the drug. If paresthesias are encountered with introduction of the needle or the injection of the solution, it is wise to adjust the needle so that paresthesias are no longer elicited. Often it is necessary to remove and reinsert the needle either in the same space or in a different space to eliminate the paresthesias.

STERILIZATION OF AMPULES.—Ampules of crystals or solutions of anesthetic drugs used for spinal analgesia may be sterilized by autoclaving. The evidence is convincing that sterilization of ampules in antiseptic solutions is dangerous. Minute quantities of the solution may enter defective ampules and not be detected, even though colored. These strong solutions, even in minute amounts, may cause severe neurologic damage.

Postanesthetic Complications

In addition to the complications already mentioned that may occur during spinal analgesia, other postanalgesia complications occur with varying frequency.

HEADACHE.—Headache of varying degrees of intensity is a relatively common complication, the incidence being about 10% after lumbar puncture except in patients older than 50 years. Its unique characteristic is its onset or recurrence if the sitting or standing position is assumed and its complete relief in the recumbent position. It has been theorized that headache is due to leakage of spinal fluid and to chemical meningitis. To minimize the extent of the rent in the dura, 22-gauge needles or pencil-point needles are used for lumbar puncture. The incidence of headache can be lessened by the use of these needles, but one must recognize that lumbar puncture is somewhat more difficult than it is with larger needles. Contrary to common practice, it is probably advisable also to permit the patient complete freedom of movement in the postanesthetic period, even to the extent of walking if this is otherwise permissible. There is little controlled evidence to indicate that the prophylactic procedure of keeping the patient flat on his back with his head low lessens the incidence or severity of headache.

Headache usually can be relieved by mild analgesic drugs. There is good evidence to believe that hydration of the patient may result in a reduced incidence of headache and benefit the patient with a headache. This may be accomplished by any route available in the patient and the fluids need not be hypertonic. Headaches have also been treated by the intrathecal introduction of 5% glucose or by the epidural introduction of normal saline until a cerebrospinal fluid pressure that approaches normal limits is re-established. This may require as much as 20 to 30 ml of solution. There is almost always immediate relief of headache with this therapy, but in some patients headache may recur and repeated injections are indicated. Some headaches may persist for several days or several weeks. Headache after spinal anesthesia may be treated also by what is known as the epidural patch. This technic involves the withdrawal of approximately 10 ml of the patient's own blood, which is then introduced into the epidural space. It is postulated that the blood coagulates and forms a "patch" over the rent in the dura. It has proved a useful mode of therapy in headaches that persist and are refractory to the modes of therapy previously proposed.

MENINGITIS.—Aseptic or chemical meningitis may develop, but it usually subsides without specific therapy. The intensity of the patient's response to aseptic or chemical meningitis often provokes the attending physician to institute heroic, but unnecessary, therapy. This complication of spinal anesthesia is characterized by a rapid onset (i.e., hours) and the patient appears incapacitated, disoriented, and generally ill. Examination of the spinal fluid, however, reveals no cells, a somewhat ground-glass appearance of the fluid, and no growth of bacteria on culture. The return of normal appearance and function in the patient is remarkable and rapid, occurring usually within 24 hours.

Septic meningitis, on the other hand, is somewhat longer in its onset, and the patient exhibits the traditional signs and symptoms of a bacterial infection. The cerebrospinal fluid contains cells and often grows bacteria on culture. Vigorous treatment with antibiotics and chemotherapy is necessary.

OTHER NEUROLOGIC SEQUELAE.—Other neurologic sequelae, such as urinary retention, anal sphincter paralysis and paresthesias in the lower extremities, may occur. The frequency of these complications has been estimated to range from 1 in 3,000 to 1 in 20,000 cases. Some of these sequelae may be permanent, but most of them disappear in a few weeks without specific therapy. The most frequent neurologic sequela is unilateral or bilateral paralysis of the abducens nerve. This is presumed to be due to traction on the nerve from loss of spinal fluid. The etiologic factors in the production of other neurologic sequelae have never been proved.

If paresthesias are encountered on introduction of the needle into the subarachnoid space, it is advisable to adjust its position until paresthesias are no longer elicited. If adjustment in position does not eliminate the paresthesias, it is advisable to remove the needle and insert it in another interspace. If paresthesias are not present at time of injection, there is no evidence that injection of the drug results in any increase in the incidence of neurologic sequelae.

PULMONARY COMPLICATIONS.—Pulmonary complications following spinal analgesia are as common as, and in some instances more common than, those following well-conducted inhalation anesthesia. It is important that a comparison of pulmonary complications be made only in circumstances in which inhalation and spinal anesthesia are equally well administered. Comparison of the incidence of complications in situations in which spinal analgesia is administered expertly and inhalation anesthesia poorly, or vice versa, is not valid. The fact remains, and evidence is mounting, that, all other factors being equal, use of spinal analgesia will not diminish the incidence of postanesthetic pulmonary complications below that occurring following inhalation anesthesia. This is true whether or not pulmonary or upper respiratory complications are present before anesthesia is induced.

EXTRADURAL (EPIDURAL) ANALGESIA

Analgesia may be obtained by the introduction of the analgesic drug into the extradural space. The advantages cited for this technic are as follows: (1) the epidural space is limited at the foramen magnum and the analgesic solution cannot reach the medullary centers; (2) there is a tendency for the extent of the area of anesthesia to be "band like" with the center around the site of introduction of the drug so that anesthesia can be "regional"; and (3) the intrathecal space is not entered, which diminishes the contact of nerve roots and spinal cord with anesthetic drug and also eliminates headache.

The Technic of Extradural Injection

The technic consists essentially in introducing a 16- to 20-gauge spinal needle, usually the Huber-Tuohy needle, into the extradural space and introducing into this space a quantity of anesthetic solution. The caudal approach to the extradural space may be used (see Chapter 8). This is useful for the saddle type of block or low anesthesia and it is, of course, more efficient in that the solution is introduced closer to the area in which anesthesia is desired. However, the disadvantages of the caudal approach (i.e., difficulty and discomfort in placement of needle) make the lumbar approach more satisfactory, even for obstetric anesthesia.

After a skin wheal of local anesthetic has been made, the large needle is introduced through the skin and advanced until it is reasonably firmly placed and does not sag when released. At this point it may be proximal to ligamentum flavum or in the ligament. To determine entry of the needle into the extradural space, the "loss of resistance" technic is used most frequently. A syringe (in which the barrel moves freely) is attached to the needle. The syringe may contain a solution such as saline or the anesthetic solution to be used, or air, or both solution and air. Firm pressure is then applied to the end of the barrel and one notes whether or not air or solution enters the tissue. Pressure may be applied continuously or intermittently as the needle is advanced. If air or solution enters tissue but only with firm pressure, one assumes that the point of the needle is proximal to the ligamentum. The needle is then advanced cautiously in small increments with repeated firm pressure until it is evident that with very firm pressure on the end of the barrel no air or fluid enters tissue. This resistance is due to the ligament. The needle is then again advanced in small increments until there is a sudden release of air or fluid into tissue with little or no pressure on the barrel. The point of the needle is then in the epidural space. This sequence of (1) entry of air or fluid from the syringe into tissue with slight pressure on barrel, (2) no entry of air or fluid with very firm pressure and (3) sudden entry of air or fluid with no pressure is critical to establishment of the proper placement of the needle.

Less precise is the use of the fact that the epidural space has a lower pressure than the atmosphere. A drop of fluid may be placed in the hub of the needle after its engagement in the ligament. As the point enters the epidural space the fluid is sucked into the epidural space.

After one has determined that the needle is properly placed in the extradural space, anesthetic solution may be introduced. If lidocaine is used, the recommended practice is to inject 5 ml of a 1.5 or 2% solution including 1:200,000 epinephrine and then to wait 2 minutes to note the presence or absence of intrathecal analgesia. If the solution had entered the subarachnoid space, there would be the signs of spinal analgesia. If no sensory analgesia or motor paresis develops in the lower extremities or saddle area during this 2-minute period, the remainder of the anesthetic solution is injected. The volume used is generally 20 ml of 1.5 or 2% lidocaine (with epinephrine), although other drugs may be used, in concentrations that are employed for regional or infiltration anesthesia. If good muscle relaxation is essential, and especially if the patient is muscular, it is advisable to use a 2% solution. The solution is injected at a moderate rate and the patient returned to the supine position on a horizontal table.

The height of anesthesia is determined mostly by the volume of solution introduced. Gravity has a minimal effect and, as a result, lowering or raising the head of the patient has little effect on height of anesthesia. A useful clue to the volume needed to produce a desired height is the observation whether fluid returns from the needle when solution is introduced. If the fluid returns briskly, it is reasonable to assume that the epidural space is relatively small and a relatively smaller volume of fluid will be needed to achieve the desired height. If no fluid returns, the reverse may be the case and a larger volume of fluid may be needed to achieve the desired height.

CONTINUOUS TECHNIC.—The continuous technic for epidural anesthesia offers a distinct advantage in that prolonged anesthesia can be maintained without the disadvantage of introducing a large-bore needle and catheter into the subarachnoid space. The continuous technic is used in those circumstances in which anesthesia of long duration is needed. The continuous technic of epidural anesthesia often is combined with light inhalation anesthesia. In such a circumstance, inhalation anesthesia can be maintained easily with nitrous oxide with the addition of minimal doses of supplemental drugs (narcotics or barbiturates) because the epidural blocks out most sensory input. By using a 15-gauge Huber-pointed Tuohy needle, a plastic catheter may be introduced into the extradural space and left in place after removal of the needle. Small initial doses and repeated injections can then be used.

After the catheter has once passed the tip of the needle, it should never be withdrawn until the needle also is removed. Some anesthetists, when using the catheter, inject only the test dose through the needle and introduce the remainder through the catheter. Others prefer to introduce the initial anesthetizing dose through the needle before introducing the catheter. The rationale for this, which is the technic we prefer, is that the space is distended, thus facilitating the introduction of the catheter. We believe also that introducing the initial dose through the needle diminishes the chances of the catheter entering the intrathecal space or a blood vessel. Perhaps also the likelihood of diversion of the catheter into a foramen is reduced. The onset of anesthesia is delayed if one waits to introduce the bulk of solution through the catheter. Finally, if the solution is introduced through the needle, one has at least a "single shot" epidural anesthesia, and there is time to prepare for a substitute anesthesia if surgery outlasts the one-dose anesthetic. The initial "expanding" injection may be done also with saline, but we see no reason for not using the anesthetic solution.

The catheters are of plastic and of a size permitting their introduction through the usual 16-gauge Huber-pointed Tuohy needle. A catheter is usually introduced 4 to 5 cm beyond the point of the needle. Advancing it further enhances the chances of the catheter entering a blood vessel or its being diverted into a foramen. On the other hand, if a shorter segment of catheter is introduced, the catheter is more easily displaced from the epidural space by movement or positioning of the patient or inadvertent traction while the needle is being removed. After the catheter has been introduced and before injections are made through it, it is advisable to inject no more than 100 mg of lidocaine (or its equivalent) as a test dose. Catheters have been known to enter blood vessels without any evidence of blood returning through the catheter. Another method of testing is to introduce 20 mg of succinylcholine through the catheter and observe for complaints by the patient of diplopia or a sensation of relaxation or difficulty in breathing.

With the volume recommended, anesthesia usually extends from the toes to the midthoracic region. The area of anesthesia tends to be segmental and to be distributed both ways from the site of injection. The segmentalization accounts for the failure of some epidural anesthetics to be satisfactory for pelvic surgery; the solution fails to extend caudally in sufficient amount. Insufficient spread of anesthesia either cephalad or caudad has to be corrected by injecting additional amounts of anesthetic solution. The necessity, in some circumstances, of having to use relatively large volumes of anesthetic solution constitutes one of the inefficiencies of epidural anesthesia.

Repeated injections of solution are made on a time basis. With procaine or lidocaine, the anesthetic level will begin to recede within 30 to 45 minutes. As a result, it is usually advisable to reinject at 30-minute intervals. The amount then given depends to some extent on the level reached with the initial injection. For example, if the initial injection of 20 ml resulted in a level of anesthesia extending to the fourth thoracic dermatome, probably subsequent injections need amount to no more than 5 ml. If the initial injection of 20 ml resulted in a level no higher than the eighth thoracic dermatome, subsequent injections of 8 to 10 ml would be needed. It is important to reinject on a time basis because once the anesthetic level has receded to the point of discomfort to the patient or lack of relaxation for the surgeon, much more anesthetic solution is required to reestablish satisfactory anesthesia.

Sympathetic paralysis is as intense with epidural analgesia as with intrathecal analgesia. As a result, the decrease in blood pressure with equivalent heights of analgesia is about the same as it is with spinal analgesia. The onset of hypotension, however, is usually slower than with spinal anesthesia. As a result, prophylactic vasopressor is not as necessary as with spinal anesthesia. Reactions to the anesthetic drug used are possible because a relatively large volume of a relatively high concentration of the drug is introduced into an area in which absorption is good. The technic is somewhat more difficult than that of intrathecal analgesia, and the hazard of accidental subarachnoid injection of a large volume of drug is always present. If the intrathecal space is entered in the attempt at epidural anesthesia, one can either remove the needle and reinsert it at a different interspace or leave the needle in the intrathecal space and maintain a continuous spinal anesthesia. If one elects to reinsert the needle at a different interspace it is well to remember that a rent has been made in the dura and that there is a greater likelihood of the local anesthetic from the epidural space entering the intrathecal space.

Neurologic sequelae are rare, and headache is an uncommon complication. If relatively high concentrations of the drug are used for an extended period (as with continuous technic), neurologic complications are more likely to occur. Intercostal paralysis is minimal.

PART 7

Special Problems

IN THIS BOOK, we attempt to approach problems and their solutions consistently, on the basis of the fundamental factors bearing on the problems and the various solutions. We are convinced that a comprehensive basic knowledge permits the anesthetist to analyze each problem and to apply an appropriate solution in a manner that is safer and more satisfactory for each patient and each situation than trying to establish a pattern of recall and routine for each problem. In other words, we are not presenting a set of standard patterns such as, for example, anesthesia for cholecystectomy, anesthesia for pheochromocytoma and anesthesia for gastric resection. We do recognize, however, that there are some special problems that merit discussion to facilitate management of the anesthetic, and it is these problems that we present here with our suggestions as to management.

CHAPTER TWENTY-THREE

The Obstetric Patient

WE BELIEVE, on the basis of the magnitude of the overall problem created by the birth rate (in U.S.A., 2.5 million births a year) and the distressingly high incidence of complications and deaths (both maternal and infant), associated with anesthesia for delivery, that special attention should be paid to this anesthetic problem. A woman in labor frequently epitomizes the classic unprepared or improperly prepared patient from an anesthetic standpoint. One of the more prominent problems in preparation is the mother's stomach that is partially or well filled with undigested material, which, through regurgitation or vomiting, often fills the lung. This may result in acute and fatal respiratory obstruction or longer-term pulmonary congestion that often has a similar, fatal outcome. Anxiety and fear for both mother and infant are commonplace. Medication with all sorts of drugs given at all sorts of times and in all sorts of doses reflects the lack of precise and uniform knowledge about the influence of such drugs on mother and child. Obviously, also, one must take into account the impact of anesthesia on the fetus, not only in utero, but at delivery.

TRANSFER OF DRUGS ACROSS THE PLACENTAL BARRIER

It is now well established that most drugs administered to the mother cross the placenta to enter the blood stream of the fetus. All hypnotics and analgesics are relatively poorly ionized in blood and are lipid-soluble and, as a result, are capable of crossing the placental barrier easily. The rate of transfer depends, among other things, on the route of administration. Intravenous administration of a drug to the mother, for example, induces a high maternal blood concentration with a gradient between maternal and fetal blood that accentuates transfer. Intramuscular administration, on the other hand, slows the development of the high blood concentration and also probably gives time for some metabolic degradation. The rate of transfer depends also on the timing of the arrival of the drug contained in maternal blood at the uterus in relation to contractions. The decreased uterine and fetal blood flow with each contraction slows down the transfer of drug from the maternal blood.

Other factors influencing the impact on the fetus of drug given to the mother are: (1) It is easier for drugs to penetrate fetal grey matter than adult grey matter; as a result, the influence is greater, not only because the drug is concentrated (relatively speaking) in the fetal brain, but also because the fetal circulation is such that much of the circulation bypasses the liver and is distributed directly to brain. (2) The fetus has a diminished ability to detoxify drugs and, as a result, the drug tends to accumulate and reach higher concentrations. (3) There is some evidence that drugs such as barbiturates and narcotics induce a state of cellular hypoxia in the fetus in utero.

As a consequence of this evidence, five principles are advisable: (1) to limit the amount of drugs given to the mother; (2) to avoid, if possible, the development of high blood concentrations of drug in the mother, as occurs with intravenous administration; (3) to recognize that the slower development of fetal levels that occurs with intramuscular or subcutaneous administration leads to depression of the fetus approximately 2 to 3 hours after administration to the mother; (4) to consider the possibility of combined narcotic and narcotic antagonist (although in general we oppose the premixed combination of any drugs); and (5) to be conservative about the administration of barbiturates.

There seems to be no evidence that any of the newer *narcotics* are any less likely to induce depression in the fetus. Sedative-hypnotics such as diazepam (Valium) and hydroxyzine (Vistaril) given in ordinary doses (though not in the high doses associated with psychiatric therapy) seem to depress the infant minimally. This is true also of the tranquilizers such as chlordiazepoxide (Librium).

The *inhalation agents* as a group, cross the placenta easily. The speed of transfer is related to their rapid rates of diffusion, their relatively high fat solubility and their relatively low molecular weight. The degree of neonatal depression is proportional to the depth and duration of the inhalation anesthesia. *Skeletal muscle relaxants*, in general, are highly ionized and have a low fat solubility. As a result, transfer is clinically insignificant.

Contrary to well established concepts, it is now clearly demonstrated[1] that *local anesthetics* cross the placental barrier and in sufficient concentrations to affect the fetus. After injection, as in epidural or paracervical block, the local anesthetic enters the fetal blood stream within 2 to 3 minutes. The gradient between maternal arterial and umbilical venous blood is approximately 2:1. The rate of decrease of maternal and fetal concentrations of local anesthetic parallel each other which suggests that the infant is capable of breaking down (as well as redistributing) the local anesthetic. It is clear that local anesthetics cannot be used for obstetric anesthesia on the assumption that they are totally innocuous to the fetus. Reports substantiate the unfavorable impact of local anesthetic inadvertently injected into the fetal brain during delivery under paracervical, pudendal or even caudal block.

SURGERY DURING PREGNANCY

The anesthetist, surgeon, patient and patient's husband usually face surgery in the pregnant patient with apprehension because of a notion that either the anesthetic may induce birth defects or the pregnancy may be interrupted by the anesthetic or the surgical procedure. There has been little reliable documentation of the association between surgery and anesthesia and pregnancy, but a review of this problem offers reasonably reliable data that one can use to make satisfactory predictions.[2] In a review of 9073 patients, it was found that 147 (1.62%) had surgery during various stages of the pregnancy. Certain findings are of interest to the anesthetist. (1) Premature labor and delivery after surgery was correlated more with the surgical problem than with the type of anesthetic used; for example, the Shirodkar procedure was associated with a high incidence of premature delivery, whereas procedures such as appendectomy was not followed by any significant percentage of premature deliveries. (2) No particular agent or technic in anesthesia demonstrated any subsequent higher incidence of premature delivery or fetal mortality provided, of course, that the anesthetic was well managed (e.g., there was no hypoxia, no protracted hypotension or no overdose). (3) There was no greater incidence of birth defects in the patients who had surgery than in those who did not. However, the number operated and anesthetized in the first trimester were too few to provide predictive data. There is laboratory evidence that anesthetics administered in the first trimester induce birth defects, and it is therefore probably advisable to avoid, if possible, administration of anesthesia (of any type) in the first trimester.

Physiologic Changes

The anesthetist (and obstetrician) must be aware that especially during the last trimester the pregnant patient has (1) increased cardiac output; (2) increased blood volume; (3) increased oxygen consumption; (4) diminished liver function; (5) decreased vital capacity and pulmonary resistance; (6) decreased glomerular filtration rate and renal plasma flow; (7) decreased serum cholinesterase activity; and (8) the likelihood of developing the supine hypotensive syndrome of pregnancy. Each of these can, of course, be easily, promptly and effectively managed provided the anesthetist takes them into account and is prepared to deal with them. Probably one of the less readily recognized, although simple, problems is the supine hypotensive syndrome. The evidence indicates that the hypotension is a function of decreased venous return through the large vessels of the abdomen caused by compression of the gravid uterus. At any time that hypotension develops in the supine position, one should manually displace the uterus laterally, preferably to the left.

POSTPARTUM HYPERTENSION

Abrupt and severe hypertension in the postpartum period is an uncomfortable and potentially dangerous disorder. It may be due to (1) oxytocic drugs, (2) vasopressor drugs (or more particularly a combination of the two), (3) hypoxia, (4) hypervolemia and (5) toxemia of pregnancy. If conduction anesthesia such as spinal or epidural anesthesia has been used for delivery, hypertension may appear as the anesthetic wears off which permits blood vessels to constrict on the unadjusted hypervolemic state. Immediate therapy is indicated not only because of the severe headache but also because of the potential for cerebral vascular rupture. Probably one of the more effective approaches is the use of chlorpromazine (Thorazine) given intravenously in increments of 2.5 mg every minute until the blood pressure falls. Spinal or epidural anesthesia also can be reestablished.

ANESTHETIC MANAGEMENT

As in any patient requiring anesthesia, the patient about to deliver must be considered as a patient with an individual problem. All the basic principles that have been outlined earlier apply equally well to the obstetric patient. Fortunately, although the onset of the actual delivery may be precipitate, the need for anesthesia at delivery is recognized months in advance. As a result, instead of a one-time and often too brief encounter between patient and anesthetist prior to anesthesia, the anesthetist and patient can arrange for several interviews in which the anesthetist can explain the sequence of those events prior to and at the time of delivery that will influence the anesthetic or that will be influenced by the anesthetic. The anesthetist thus is well identified by the patient and a useful rapport established. The patient is not required to make a decision on a type of anesthesia in a few minutes, as in the case in most other circumstances. With cooperation of obstetrician, anesthetist and patient, it is possible to prepare for "natural delivery"; it is not essential that the anesthetist use drugs in providing pain relief. Even if delivery proceeds with the use of pain-relieving drugs, the anesthetist can certainly diminish, by educating and informing the patient, the need for drugs (such as the narcotics and barbiturates) during labor. Finally, the anesthetist can make a better evaluation of the patient's suitability for a particular type of anesthetic.

Choice of Anesthesia

Although any of the anesthetic agents and technics available may be used for anesthesia for delivery, the consensus is that conduction anesthesia probably is safer for both mother and fetus. Conduction anesthesia does not eliminate but does diminish the likelihood of depression of the fetus from placental transfer of drugs, it is adaptable to relatively long-term use in prolonged and difficult labor and it significantly diminishes (but does not eliminate) the ever-present possibility of regurgitation and vomiting and associated pulmonary obstruction and contamination.

CONDUCTION ANESTHESIA.—Conduction anesthesia seems to be the preferred approach to the anesthetic problems posed by the women about to deliver. Several technics are available for the production of conduction anesthesia. These include paracervical and pudendal block, epidural anesthesia and spinal anesthesia. Choice of technic depends on (1) the availability and qualifications of personnel, (2) the desire and preference of patient, (3) the rapidity of progress of labor, and (4) the need for relief of either (or both) uterine contraction or perineal pain. The latter factor, of course, is related to the stage of labor. In general, epidural anesthesia (either by the caudal or lumbar approach) is reserved for the longer labors and for relief of both perineal and uterine contraction pain. Paracervical block is used for relief of contraction pain, usually in the middle stages of labor. Spinal anesthesia is usually reserved for cesarean section or for anesthesia shortly before delivery; emergency needs for anesthesia also can often be fulfilled more quickly and completely (by conduction anesthesia) with spinal anesthesia. Pudendal blocks are reserved usually for the terminal phase of labor at which stage the need is relief of perineal pain, especially to facilitate episiotomy.

INHALATION ANALGESIA.—If sufficient and qualified personnel are available, analgesia produced by low concentrations of inhalation agents is a satisfactory way of managing the discomfort of the second stage of labor. Any of the inhalation agents may be used; analgesia is more effective if the agent is given continuously. If intermittent analgesia with each contraction is desired, the agents with low solubility in plasma, such as nitrous oxide, are better because an effective plasma concentration is attained more rapidly. Inhalation analgesia for the first stage of labor, although effective, has the disadvantage of requiring the direct and long-term presence of personnel to supervise or administer anesthesia. Inhalers have been devised, and are in use, to facilitate the self-administration of intermittent analgesia by inhalation agents. The agents most commonly used in inhalers are trichlorethylene (Trilene) and methoxyflurane (Penthrane). Methoxyflurane seems effective as an analgesic agent in low concentrations (even on an intermittent basis) despite its low vapor pressure and a high solubility in plasma. Its effectiveness, in spite of its physical shortcomings, may be due to the fact that the patient in need of analgesia usually hyperventilates and has a hyperactive pulmonary circulation, each of which enhance uptake. It is advisable to avoid using methoxyflurane if there is known or suspected kidney deficiency (see Chapter 14). Except for the self-hypnosis induced by the use of these inhalers, their value is doubtful and they present some hazard. The hazard derives from the fact that unexpected deeper levels of anesthesia sometimes may be produced by the concentration delivered by the inhaler, with consequent upper airway obstruction and asphyxia. Furthermore, rather than relaxing as analgesia is induced and letting the apparatus fall away from the face, some patients tighten the grip on the apparatus and airway obstruction is made worse.

Administration of inhalation anesthesia for delivery must take into account all the factors pertinent to proper management of this type of anesthesia in any circumstance. Inhalation anesthesia is currently reserved for those situations in which conduction anesthesia is not suitable. In emergency problems such as prolapse of the cord and abruptio placenta, there may be insufficient time to induce conduction anesthesia. If inhalation anesthesia is used, endotracheal intubation is usually indicated to minimize the likelihood of aspiration of stomach contents. Intubation may be done with the patient awake; if this is unsatisfactory, a "crash" induction using thiopental and succinylcholine with cricoid pressure and other measures to pre-

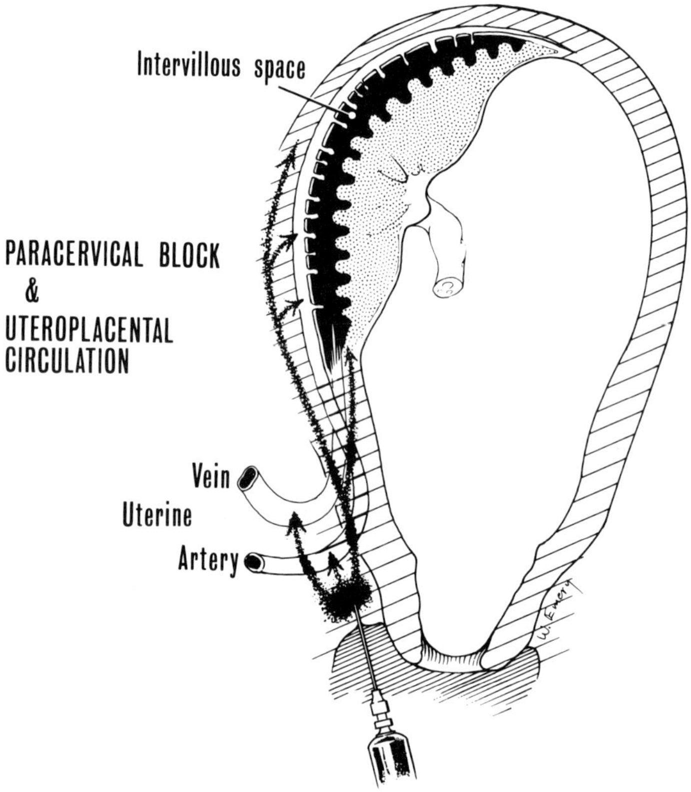

Fig. 23-1.—Absorption of local anesthetic in paracervical block. Slight deviation from optimal site for paracervical injection can introduce anesthetic agent either directly into circulation leading to placenta or into close enough relationship that significant absorption is possible. (From Asling, J. H., Shnider, S. M., Margolis, A. J., Wilkinson, G. L., and Way, E. L.: Paracervical block anesthesia in obstetrics. II. Etiology of fetal bradycardia following paracervical block anesthesia, Am. J. Obstet. & Gynecol. 107:626, 1970.)

vent regurgitation or emesis can be used. Any of the inhalation agents may be used, although there is evidence to indicate that halothane causes increased uterine bleeding.[3] Light levels of anesthesia are preferred (prior to delivery) to diminish the transfer of agent to the fetus. Light levels can be facilitated by use of relaxants.

In emergency circumstances such as placenta previa, separation of the placenta, prolapse of the cord, persistent tetanic uterine contraction, abruptio placentae and eclampsia, an inhalation agent such as cyclopropane, halothane or fluroxene may be used. These potent agents, as opposed to nitrous oxide, permit the administration of higher concentrations of oxygen, which, in emergency situations, often protects both mother and infant. Since transfer of anesthetic agent across the placental barrier is related to both dose and time, it is advisable to delay administration of the anesthetic until all possible preparations have been accomplished, such as for example, skin preparation and draping. One should avoid also excessive hyperventilation in the patient with its decreased PCO_2 and its alkalosis, which can induce fetal hypoxia and acidosis from a shift in dissociation curve and perhaps diminished blood flow to the tissue. Hypoventilation on the other hand, may induce fetal hypoxia and acidosis from hypercarbia. Induction of inhalation anesthesia may be made more comfortable for the patient by administering small (sleep) doses of thiopental; the larger doses of thiopental used for induction actually may slow the induction of subsequent inhalation anesthesia because of respiratory depression. Furthermore, larger doses of the barbiturate cross the placenta and depress the fetus.

Ether, halothane and chloroform diminish uterine contractions, even in the lighter planes of anesthesia. Cyclopropane, usually does not diminsh contractions unless higher concentrations are used. Thiopental, nitrous oxide, ethylene and muscle relaxants have no demonstrable effects on uterine contraction. Apparently, this is also true of methoxyflurane and trichlorethylene.

Paracervical and Pudendal Blocks

PARACERVICAL BLOCK.—The injection of an appropriate local anesthetic (see Chapter 21) injected circumferentially at the level of the cervix constitutes paracervical block. The technic is generally considered to be innocuous. However, investigations indicate that there is substantial uptake of the local anesthetic by the fetus with subsequent bradycardia, acidosis and fetal depression.[4] It is postulated that the local anesthetic reaches the fetus by a direct route: the systemic absorption of drug via the uterine artery (Fig. 23-1).

As a consequence, those practicing this technic must both be careful to avoid indiscriminate use of larger doses of local anesthetic than necessary and be as precise as possible in positioning of the needles.

PUDENDAL BLOCK.—In transvaginal pudendal block, the nerves to the perineum are blocked by infiltration of appropriate local anesthetic in close proximity to the pudendal nerve. The block is done simply by directing the needle, along a finger placed in the vagina, toward the ischial spine and infiltrating solution in proximity to the pudendal nerve as it branches in and about the ischial spine and Alcock's canal.

The complications associated with this block are those associated with the use of local anesthesia such as toxic reactions, possible inadvertent placement of the needle in the rectum or the injection of local anesthetic intravenously in a deeply placed vessel.

Epidural Block (Caudal or Lumbar Approach)

Epidural anesthesia is used when there is a relatively long-term need for relief of pain ensuing from both uterine contractions and the perineum. The caudal approach to epidural anesthesia, popular some years ago, is associated with technical problems of needle placement in many patients and problems of catheter placement also; hence the use of this approach to epidural anesthesia is now less popular than the lumbar approach. Moreover, use of the lumbar approach requires much less drug to effect relief of uterine contraction pain, presumably because the solution is deposited closer to the nerves supplying the uterus. The technic is the same as that used for producing epidural anesthesia by the lumbar route in other situations (see Chapter 22). In general, lower initial and repetitive doses are needed than for abdominal operative procedures. The technics, of course, require the presence of a qualified anesthetist, although the immediate attention to the patient is not as time-consuming as with analgesia by inhalation. Usually, epidural anesthesia is not initiated until there is engagement of the head of the fetus; cervical dilation should be 7 to 8 cm in the primipara and 6 to 7 cm in the multipara. If oxytocic drugs (to provoke and stimulate contractions) are used, analgesia by epidural technic may be started when the cervix is dilated 1 cm.

Spinal Block

This technic is generally used when labor has progressed to the point at which delivery is imminent and there is not time to establish epidural analgesia. It is useful also in providing anesthesia for cesarean section. The technic is identical to that described for other surgical procedures (see Chapter 22). As with epidural anesthesia for obstetric purpose, the doses of drugs required are less than in the patient who is not pregnant. For example, one usually uses 2 to 3 mg of tetracaine for vaginal delivery and 8 mg for cesarean section. This is presumably due to engorgement of the intrathecal veins and (relative flattening) of the normal spinal curves.

Complications of epidural and spinal anesthesia.—The complications are no different from those in the patient who is not pregnant. *Hypotension,* however, seems to be more frequent and more pronounced. As a consequence, it is wise to have an intravenous line in place and also to use a prophylactic vasopressor drug, preferably ephedrine. Hypotension not only has obvious disadvantages to the mother but also, as ample evidence indicates, the fetus exposed to maternal hypotension suffers significant acidosis from the inadequate placental circulation. One always must keep in mind the likelihood of compression of the vena cava and manually displace the uterus as a first step in management of the hypotension. Some obstetricians and anesthetists have been reluctant to use vasopressor drugs in the pregnant and full-term patient because some evidence suggests that the uterine vessels are constricted and blood flow to the fetus is impaired. However, recent data indicate that only those vasopressor drugs acting through the alpha receptors, such as methoxamine, phenylephrine and levarterenol, produce uterine vessel constriction. Therefore, when prophylactic or therapeutic elevation of blood pressure is needed, the intravenous use of drugs such as ephedrine (in doses of 15 to 25 mg) or dilute solutions of metaraminol (0.002%) should be considered because they produce their effect primarily through enhancement of myocardial function and do not impair uterine and placental blood flow.

Headache is also a significant problem in the younger patient (in the pregnant age group) with more resilient cerebral vessels and less fixation of dural structures. The incidence and severity of headache can be diminished significantly by the use of 25-gauge needles.

NEONATAL RESUSCITATION

It is useful for the anesthetist to be familiar with resuscitation of the newborn not only because he should understand the factors for which he is responsible and which contribute to fetal depression but also because he is often called upon, because of his expertise in resuscitation, to be responsible for infant resuscitation or to assist obstetrician and/or pediatrician.

We have outlined the various factors contributing to fetal depression, such as depression from narcotics and other depressant drugs, anesthetics (including local anesthetics), impaired circulation (e.g., hypotension, vasopressors and interruption of fetal blood supply) and hypoventilation in the mother. Assuming that these contributing factors have not been corrected either adequately or in time, one may expect delivery of a depressed infant. Monitoring by traditional methods (i.e., recording the heart rate) is mandatory, but recent technics permit more precise evaluation of the state of the fetus; these include amniotic sampling and scalp-vein sampling in utero with analysis of the blood gases and acid-base balance.

Whether or not one anticipates a depressed infant at delivery, preparation for prompt and vigorous and effective therapy is mandatory. A program of therapy is useful so that after assessing the state of the infant one may proceed logically and effectively. If depression is minimal, one may need only stimulate the infant gently by manual means (e.g., foot slapping and drying the skin with a towel), clear the pharynx of mucus, meconium and secretions and apply oxygen by funnel over the face. If there is reason to suspect narcotic depression, one may give the infant a small dose of a narcotic antagonist (1 mg nalorphine, 0.005 mg levallorphan or 0.001 mg naloxone). If one believes that the infant needs only a few inflations of the lung to initiate respiration, one may do so either by mouth-to-mouth inflation or by the application of various devices incorporating the use of oxygen.

Infants who are more severely depressed need immediate initiation of ventilation though an endotracheal catheter. Numerous devices can be attached to the endotracheal catheter; whatever device is used, one needs to ensure adequate but not overinflation of the lungs. This can be determined most effectively by observation of the chest and by listening with a stethoscope. One applies whatever pressure is needed to accomplish the inflation, recognizing that initial breaths often require higher inflation pressures. One should limit the pressure, especially at this stage, to no more than 40 cm of water. It may be beneficial also to apply end-expiratory pressure (i.e., 2 to 3 cm of water) to overcome atelectasis. If necessary, aspiration of material in the lungs and trachea is accomplished through the endotracheal catheter. One need not concern onself about the hazards of high concentrations of oxygen at this stage but, if resuscitative efforts are prolonged or continued support is necessary, one needs to decrease the inspired oxygen concentration to that which provides adequate arterial oxygen tension (i.e., 50 mm

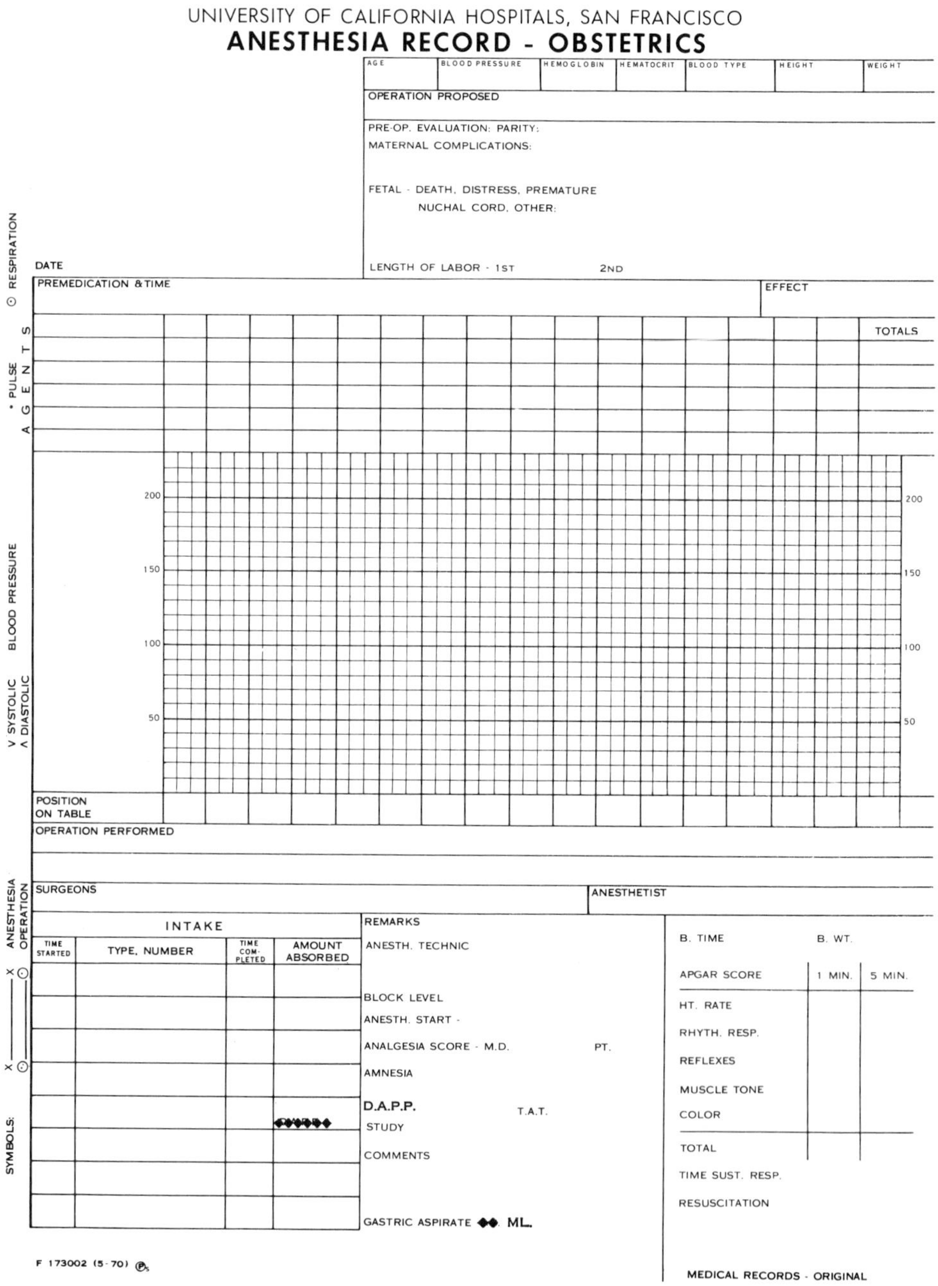
UNIVERSITY OF CALIFORNIA HOSPITALS, SAN FRANCISCO
ANESTHESIA RECORD - OBSTETRICS
AGE | BLOOD PRESSURE | HEMOGLOBIN | HEMATOCRIT | BLOOD TYPE | HEIGHT | WEIGHT
OPERATION PROPOSED
PRE-OP. EVALUATION: PARITY:
MATERNAL COMPLICATIONS:
FETAL - DEATH, DISTRESS, PREMATURE
NUCHAL CORD, OTHER:
DATE
LENGTH OF LABOR - 1ST 2ND
PREMEDICATION & TIME
EFFECT
AGENTS
TOTALS
⊙ RESPIRATION
• PULSE
V SYSTOLIC
Λ DIASTOLIC
BLOOD PRESSURE
200
150
100
50
POSITION ON TABLE
OPERATION PERFORMED
SURGEONS
ANESTHETIST
X⊙ ANESTHESIA
X⊙ OPERATION
SYMBOLS:
INTAKE
TIME STARTED | TYPE, NUMBER | TIME COMPLETED | AMOUNT ABSORBED
REMARKS
ANESTH. TECHNIC
BLOCK LEVEL
ANESTH. START -
ANALGESIA SCORE - M.D. PT.
AMNESIA
D.A.P.P. T.A.T.
STUDY
COMMENTS
GASTRIC ASPIRATE ◆◆ ML.
B. TIME B. WT.
APGAR SCORE | 1 MIN. | 5 MIN.
HT. RATE
RHYTH. RESP.
REFLEXES
MUSCLE TONE
COLOR
TOTAL
TIME SUST. RESP.
RESUSCITATION
F 173002 (5-70)
MEDICAL RECORDS - ORIGINAL

Fig. 23-2.

Hg). This can be determined most precisely by blood-gas sampling from the umbilical artery.

Because severely depressed infants usually have a substantial degree of metabolic acidosis, it is necessary to inject sodium bicarbonate. An initial dose of 5 mEq is satisfactory, but repeated administration can be determined effectively only by blood-gas analysis. Many infants also may be hypoglycemic, and glucose can be given intravenously. The immediate application of these remedial measures usually results in prompt and total recovery. Obviously those infants with congenital abnormalities of the cardiovascular and other systems and with such other disorders as Rh incompatibility must be recognized early and specific therapy initiated whenever possible.

REFERENCES

1. Shnider, S. M., and Way, E. L.: Plasma levels of Lidocaine (xylocaine) in mother and newborn following obstetrical conduction anesthesia, Anesthesiology 29:951, 1968.
2. Shnider, S. M., and Webster, G. M.: Maternal and fetal hazards of surgery during pregnancy, Am. J. Obstet. & Gynecol. 92:891, 1965.
3. Cullen, B. F., Margolis, A. J., Eger, E. I., II: Effect of anesthesia and pulmonary ventilation on blood loss during elective therapeutic abortion, Anesthesiology 32:108, 1970.
4. Asling, J. H., Shnider, S. M., Margolis, A. J., Wilkinson, G. L., and Way, E. L.: Paracervical block anesthesia in obstetrics: II. Etiology of fetal bradycardia following paracervical block anesthesia, Am. J. Obstet. & Gynecol. 107:626, 1970.

CHAPTER TWENTY-FOUR

The Infant and the Small Child

THE FUNDAMENTAL CONSIDERATIONS that we have outlined earlier apply equally well to the management of anesthesia in the pediatric patient. However, there are sufficient special considerations to merit a discussion. These special considerations include (1) tolerance to drugs, (2) temperature control, (3) anesthetic systems, (4) endotracheal intubation, (5) monitoring and (6) fluid balance.

TOLERANCE TO DRUGS

Children, including even the newborn, have a surprisingly high tolerance to depressant drugs, including anesthetics. This means that, relatively speaking, higher doses (on a weight- or age-basis) and higher induction and maintenance concentrations are required for children than for adults. To give an idea of the effect of age, Figure 7-3 gives the MAC levels for halothane at different ages.[1] This tolerance to anesthetic drugs applies also to other drugs. For example, a healthy 3-year-old child will require, for effective preanesthetic sedation, 1 to 2 mg of morphine, 25 to 50 mg of pentobarbital or equivalent doses of other sedative or narcotic drugs, or both of these latter types of drugs. Weight alone should not be the controlling factor in dosage. Although in infants and small children there is less variability in size, dose related to weight is more appropriate than in adults. Nevertheless, other factors such as the level of activity of the child and the degree of debility should be taken into account. Although many children have an aversion to needles, in general it is advisable to give the drugs intramuscularly or intravenously. Absorption of any drug from either stomach or rectum in the circumstances of stress attending trauma and anticipated anesthesia and operation is substantially delayed and generally ineffective.

A well-established custom is the administration of atropine to children in anticipation of the output of mucus and other secretions. Modern rapid induction technics, however, eliminate for practical purposes the need for inhibition of secretions. In addition to rapid induction, moderate to deep anesthesia or intubation of the trachea or both, obviate the requirement for atropine. As a result, newborn and infants up to the age of 1 year usually do not require atropine as premedication. The use of ketamine, however, provides an exception: if ketamine is used either as an induction agent or as the sole agent for anesthesia, it is advisable to use atropine for its drying effect and to forestall rapid onset of bradycardia. If problems such as bradycardia appear, atropine can be added as needed intravenously. In the child who is old enough to communicate, scopolamine in small doses (e.g., 0.1 mg at age 2 yr.) is useful in augmenting sedation and acting as a vagal blocker.

Although we have encountered no problem with the use of non-depolarizing relaxants, there is reasonable evidence to indicate that children under the age of 1 year are more susceptible to relaxants like *d*-tubocurarine. The susceptibility is supposed to be manifested by exaggerated and protracted relaxation with small doses. This susceptibility is not apparent with depolarizing drugs. However, increments of succinylcholine added to an initial dose seem to provoke bradycardia and other arrhythmias. These problems are discussed more fully in Chapter 18. Initial doses may provoke hyperthermia in susceptible children.

Not to be overlooked, of course, (as discussed in Chapter 3) is the value of establishing rapport with the youngster by visits before and after operation and by clear explanations of what is to happen. One can thus appreciably diminish the need for sedative drugs.

It often seems difficult to "settle" the management of an inhalation anesthetic and to provide anesthesia that is adequate and not repetitively light, as well as uncomplicated by laryngospasm and the secretion of large quantities of mucus, etc. In such situations, one not unusually discovers either during the procedure or at its termination that the stomach is not empty. Why a full or partially full stomach is associated with difficulty in obtaining a stable anesthetic is not known, but the association is obvious and should be suspected whenever it is difficult to establish and maintain a stable anesthetic in a child.

TEMPERATURE MEASUREMENT AND CONTROL

The measurement and control of temperature are critical elements in the proper management of infants and children during anesthesia and operation. Wide swings of temperature in either direction occur readily either because of the cold atmosphere of most operating rooms or because of the heat produced by operating-room lights or from heat retention under surgical drapes. As a result, monitoring of temperature is essential in all but the shortest of anesthetic and surgical procedures. Monitoring of the rectal temperature is probably the easiest, but it must be remembered that there is a substantial delay in the response of the rectal temperature in relation to core temperature changes. More accurate and meaningful monitoring can be done with an esophageal probe. The tympanic membrane thermistor is equally, if not more, indicative of and sensitive to core temperature.

The temperature can be controlled by the use of simple devices such as the K-pad, a small unit through which water at varying temperatures can be circulated. One must be careful not to have the water temperature in the pad above 40° C, and it is wise to check the pad temperature with a mercury thermometer placed under the pad. One must avoid placing any kind of heating device in which the temperature exceeds 40° C next to a child (or adult); severe burns have resulted from violation of this rule. Obviously, for any heating (or cooling) unit to be effective, there must be substantial body surface contact. Control of hyperthermia can be managed by cooling units or by simple measures such as ice packs in appropriate cloth containers placed in contact with the body. If the anesthetist is concerned about heat retention, a high flow or non-rebreathing system, or both, diminishes the possibility of heat retention more than does the circle system because of greater heat loss from the lungs. In the case of a child in whom the temperature is elevated at the time of anesthesia and operation, one is obligated to make continuous observations of the temperature and to be prepared to take steps to limit the elevation or to lower the temperature. A child with an existing temperature elevation may be prone to rapid development of severe hyperthermia.

ANESTHETIC SYSTEMS

In addition to temperature control, decrease of resistance to a minimum and also convenience are factors in determining the optimum anesthetic system for children, especially the newborn and small child. Maintenance of hydration is important; high-flow (non-rebreathing) systems, for example, tend to dehydrate the child.

Almost imperceptible resistances (i.e., 1 to 2 cm of water) are critical in the infant and small child, especially in those who are debilitated or in whom respiration is depressed by depressant drugs or muscle relaxants. As a result, an anesthetic system such as the Ayre's T-piece (see Chapter 11), which has no valves and depends upon high flows to prevent rebreathing of exhaled CO_2, is more suitable than the conventional circle system for the infant under 1 year of age. Most children over 1 year of age, unless debilitated, have the power to move air in the conventional circle system provided all sites of likely resistance, such as the valves, are in optimum working order. The Ayre's T-piece system may be used for children over 1 year of age. However, one must recognize that large flows of gases are needed to avoid rebreathing. The high inflow increases not only the cost, but also the opportunity for dehydration. The Ayre's T-piece is frequently modified by adding an extension to the expiratory limb to the terminus of which is attached a small (500 ml) bag. If the volume of the extension (without an attached bag) is at least half of the tidal volume, the patient inhales only the anesthetic mixture. Without the extension, the patient inhales air as well as the anesthetic mixture. Adding the bag facilitates observation of tidal exchange and intermittent positive pressure breathing. Inflow of anesthetic mixture in a system with the extension (with or without added bag) must total 2.5 times the minute volume of the infant or child to prevent rebreathing of exhaled CO_2.

The T-piece itself can be strictly in the shape of a T or it can be modified to adapt to placement of the piece with the child in different positions and also to assist in entrainment of inspired mixture.

Many non-rebreathing valves can be inserted into an anesthetic system.

These diminish the opportunity for rebreathing but, being valves, they introduce the possibility of an increased resistance in the circuit through which the child has to move air. Systems incorporating such valves are satisfactory provided care is taken to see that the valves are working properly.

Miniaturized circle systems are available for use in infants and small children. These were developed to permit observation of tidal exchange, to minimize dehydration, to conserve agents and to minimize explosion hazards. They are useful but have the unfortunate disadvantages of necessary limitation of length of the rebreathing tubes connecting canister and valves to the patient, bulk and lack of maneuverability of apparatus and possible resistance from poorly functioning directional valves.

Small pieces of apparatus are available to incorporate in non-rebreathing systems in order to minimize drying. These humidifiers ("artificial noses") help to replace moisture lost in the high flow systems. Also, available for incorporation in non-rebreathing systems are ultrasonic humidifiers to compensate for the dehydrating effect of the system.

ENDOTRACHEAL INTUBATION

Endotracheal intubation serves the same function in the pediatric patient as in the adult (see Chapter 6). The need to minimize dead space may be more critical in the infant and small child, and the anesthetist must be more precise and careful in the use of endotracheal intubation in children. The susceptibility of children to the development of laryngeal edema after laryngeal intubation has caused much debate. The debate centers around the age at which children are most susceptible; it is generally held that they are more susceptible at about the age of 5 years. Ample evidence however, indicates that all children are more susceptible to laryngeal edema than are adults. As a result, the major problem of endotracheal intubation in the child is minimizing the opportunity for laryngeal edema (or the development of subsequent papillomata). There is reasonable evidence to indicate that this can be effected by (1) taking special precautions to ensure asepsis in the technic, (2) selecting the optimum size of tube, (3) avoiding excessive movement of the tube while in place in the trachea and (4) using a tube with the least possibility for local reaction.

Asepsis is facilitated by assiduous cleaning, rinsing and packaging in containers that are opened only at the time of use. With proper and meticulous cleaning and packaging, sterilization is not indicated. If gas sterilization is used, a protracted time is needed to clear the tube and package of gas. If the tubes are to be lubricated prior to introduction, the ointment should be sterile and applied in a manner that eliminates, as much as possible, the likelihood of contamination. Many anesthetists believe that the safest and most effective lubricant is the patient's own oral secretions. Aspiration of the trachea through the endotracheal tube also should be done with a catheter that is sterile and in a manner that is as aseptic as possible.

The optimum size of the endotracheal tube is easily determined by directly observing the glottic opening and by inserting a tube with minimal

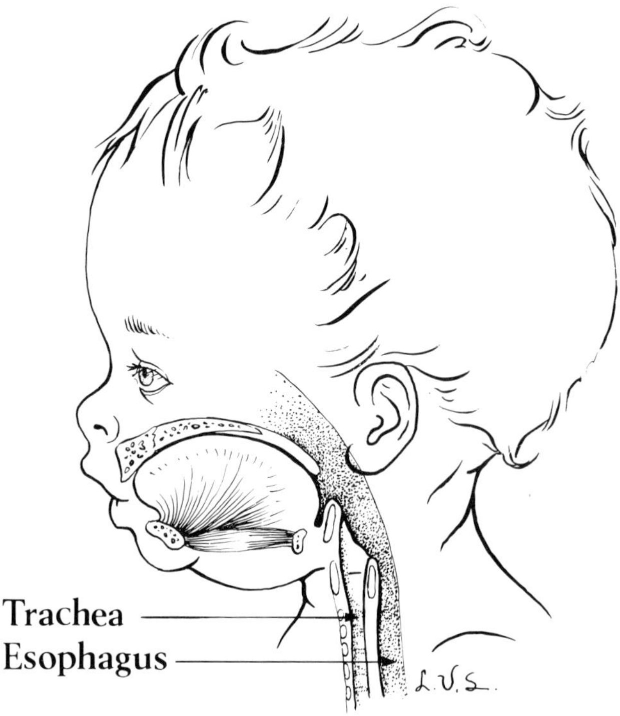

Fig. 24-1.—Differences in airway of infant and small child. Note large tongue, high-riding epiglottis and larynx, and cone shape of larynx.

resistance. In observing the glottic opening, one should remember that the upper airway (larynx and upper trachea) in the small child is cone-shaped, with the larger base at the glottic opening and the smaller dimension at the cricoid ring (Fig. 24-1). The proper size of tube, preferably uncuffed, should permit a slight leak of air about the tube when minimal pressure on the inflow of gases is applied. An inflatable cuff, even when applied closely, adds to the outside diameter of the tube and tends therefore to permit introduction only of a tube with a smaller inside diameter; moreover, the presence of a cuff leads to a tendency to inflate the cuff and thereby increase pressure on the larynx and trachea and the opportunity for ischemia. Low-pressure cuffs can be used, but their size diminishes even more the size of tube that can be introduced. With a minimal leak about an uncuffed tube, ventilation of the lungs by intermittent positive pressure is easily accomplished. Aspiration of material from the pharynx into the trachea can be prevented by having a tube with an inflatable cuff, but aspiration past a small leak with an uncuffed tube is minimal and the possibility of harm from slight aspiration must be weighed against the hazards of pressure from the inflated cuff, and the smaller size of tube permitted.

It is apparent, then, that the anesthetist should have available tubes of at least three sizes: one that he believes is the correct size, one that is smaller than this and one that is larger. If there is resistance to insertion or if there is no audible air flow (i.e., no leak) around the tube with application of positive

TABLE 24-1.—GUIDE TO SIZE AND LENGTH OF ENDOTRACHEAL TUBES IN CHILDREN

AGE	WEIGHT KG	WEIGHT LB	INT. DIAM. OF TUBE, MM	EXT. DIAM. (FRENCH)	TRACHEAL LENGTH (CORD TO CARINA), CM	LENGTH OF TUBE, CM
Neonate	1.5–3.5	3–7	2.5–3.5	11–16	4.0	10–12
1–6 mo.	3.5–6.5	7–14	4.0–4.5	16–18	4.0–4.2	12–14
6–12 mo.	6.5–9.5	14–20	4.5–5.0	18–20	4.2–4.3	14–16
2–3 yr.	12.5–14.0	27–31	5.0–5.5	20–22	4.5–5.3	16–18
4–6 yr.	16.0–22.5	35–50	5.5–6.5	24–26	5.4–5.7	18–20
7–10 yr.	24.0–36.5	55–80	6.5–7.0	26–28		20–22
10–14 yr.	45.0–50.0	100–120	7.0–7.5	28–30		22–24

pressure ventilation, the tube should be replaced by a smaller one. A useful clue as to tube size may be obtained by noting the size of the external opening of the nares. This opening and the glottic opening are of equivalent size. However, as has been mentioned, the glottic opening is larger than the opening at the cricoid level. Others estimate the size of the glottis (in adults as well as children) by making a direct correlation with the size of the ear conch. One can obtain a reasonable estimate of the proper size of tube by reference to Table 24-1.

One must be especially careful to avoid inserting the endotracheal tube too far into the trachea. One usually forgets how short the trachea is from the distal end of the larynx to the tracheal bifurcation. As a result, it is essential to auscultate the chest to assure oneself that the tube is not in either of the main bronchi, usually the right. Auscultation, however, may not reveal any evidence of endobronchial intubation. This may be revealed only by roentgenography or by a low Pa_{O_2} associated with shunting. The tube even may be endotracheal with the head in the face-up position but endobronchial with the head flexed. Another possibility is that the tube may have a relatively long bevel and also be soft, especially when warm; one then needs to remember that changes in the position of the head and neck may cause the bevel to lie against the tracheal wall and cause obstruction, usually to expiration. The tube always should be rigidly secured to avoid its being displaced or removed but particularly to avoid constant movement either with the patient's own respiration or with assisted or controlled respiration. If it is desirable to leave the tube in place after anesthesia for some time or for resuscitative or aspiration purposes, the tube may be passed through the nose. For this, however, the tube may have to be smaller than the tube selected for oral intubation, and sometimes it results in kinking of the tube at the nasopharyngeal junction. If properly secured, the orally placed tube functions better for long-term use. It seems to be generally accepted that there is less local reaction to the endotracheal tube made of plastic rather than red rubber or neoprene. One can expect, also, that the decrease in airway size that is effected by insertion of the tube (especially in the newborn and small child) will increase airway resistance substantially. The healthy child can usually compensate for this increase in resistance, but for the debilitated child or in long procedures it is often advisable to either assist the child in his respiratory efforts or to control ventilation completely.

MONITORING

The necessity for monitoring temperature in the pediatric patient has already been mentioned. Monitoring for other factors also is essential, as it is in the adult (see Chapter 5). The monitoring of blood pressure by cuff and stethoscope requires that the cuff be appropriate for the size of the child's arm in order to obtain reasonably accurate absolute values of the arterial tension. Especially useful in obtaining reliable blood pressure measurement in the infant and small child is the apparatus that makes use of the Doppler effect. Central venous pressure monitoring is also valuable in children in whom fluid balance problems already exist or may be anticipated because of the small volumes determining competence or incompetence of the circulation.

FLUID MANAGEMENT

Establishment and maintenance of fluid and blood volume is critical in the care of the child undergoing major surgery (see Chapter 20). Close and repetitive determinations must be made of blood and plasma volume, electrolytes and water shifts and losses. The anesthetist must constantly check blood and fluid loss during surgery and always keep in mind that because of the normally small blood volume and fluid requirements, small losses (in relation to losses in the adult) represent high percentage losses in the infant and small child. Thus, 10-ml loss of blood for the newborn is a critical loss. Insensible losses such as those from an open abdomen and a high-flow anesthetic system can be substantial and must be taken into account in estimating the loss and the necessary replacement.

Conduction anesthesia should not be excluded automatically in the child. Children with whom one can communicate and who are cooperative often are surprisingly receptive to conduction anesthesia. This often resolves the problem of the patient with the full stomach.

REFERENCE

1. Gregory, G. A., Eger, E. I., II, and Munson, E. S.: The relationship between age and halothane requirement in man, Anesthesiology 30:488, 1969.

CHAPTER TWENTY-FIVE

The Elderly Patient

SEVERAL FACTORS increase the number of older patients who now undergo anesthesia and surgery. These are the improved nutritional, economic and health care standards that have become available to people. Not only has the upper age limit been extended somewhat but also more people are reaching an older age. Surgical science and art also has made it possible for older patients to undergo major surgery with reliable chances for excellent recovery. Contributing to this success, of course, is better anesthetic management. The good results of anesthesia and surgery in the elderly patient can be assigned also to the likely probability that the elderly patient survives anesthesia and surgery because he has whatever it takes to reach an older age. Despite these considerations, the geriatric patient has some special problems that the anesthetist must take into account if he wishes to enhance the patient's chances for survival and optimum recovery.

RESPIRATORY DEFICIENCIES

The older patient usually has some deficiency in respiration. This may be varying degrees of impairment of gas exchange produced by such factors as emphysema, bronchiectasis, skeletal deformities, long-term smoking and decreased elasticity of lungs and rib cage. As with any patient with preexisting lung disease, preanesthetic preparation should include special efforts to improve gas exchange by respiratory exercises, aided by appliances such as those inducing intermittent positive airway pressures or artificial coughs.

CIRCULATORY DEFICIENCIES

Deficiencies in the heart and peripheral circulation may be expected also in the aged patient. These may vary from borderline cardiac compensation to decompensation that is frank and difficult to control. Other patients have the same problems but, in the aged patient, there is a basic deficiency in cardiac reserve. This is manifested often by a failure of the heart to compensate for demands of the peripheral circulation (e.g., hypovolemia, position and relaxation) by increasing the heart rate and therefore the output. Deficiencies in myocardial power account also for an inability to compensate by increasing stroke volume. The elderly patient has also a much more rigid peripheral vascular system. This may be helpful in that less hypotension may be associated with spinal anesthesia because the vessels cannot dilate. The anesthetist should become aware also of the patient's preferences for his position at rest. If he needs several pillows, this position should be maintained if at all possible; and if he cannot tolerate the head flat or below the level of the rest of the body, this should be known.

The critical problems in management of anesthesia include the selection and application of agents and technics so that there is a minimum of direct myocardial depression or exacerbation of arrhythmia. Above all, the approach to the management of anesthesia should be gradual to permit minute-to-minute assessment of the patient's responses. This means avoiding the "blitz" technic of intravenous thiopental and relaxant. Monitoring with the aid of an ECG apparatus is, of course, almost mandatory. If conduction anesthesia such as epidural or spinal anesthesia is elected, preparation should be made so that the influence on the peripheral circulation is minimal; hence, for example, the use of a prophylactic vasoconstrictor (e.g., ephedrine). There is no automatic preference for conduction anesthesia be it spinal, epidural or regional block in the aged patient. Certainly, there is no advantage to the elderly patient in forcing upon him a regional technic simply because he is old, when such a technic is unsuitable for either the operation or the patient. In such circumstances, the energy output of the patient and the unfavorable impact upon his heart and circulation may be more detrimental than well-conducted inhalation anesthesia. Close attention needs to be paid to fluid input and output in any patient, such as the elderly, with a rigid vascular system. Monitoring must be such (e.g., measurements of central venous pressure and urine volume) that frequent estimates can be made of the state of the circulating volume and the patient's response to it. Certainly, the elderly patient must not be denied fluid or blood when he needs it, but he can generally be kept somewhat on the "dry side".

DEGENERATIVE DISEASES

Attention should be paid also in the elderly patient to the likelihood of other degenerative diseases. These include mild diabetes, deficiencies in steroids, impairment of the cerebral and peripheral circulations, difficulties in bowel elimination and enlargement of the prostate gland. Appropriate corrective measures should be instituted and special attention paid to diminishing undesired consequences. For example, if the patient has impaired cerebral circulation, an effort should be made to avoid hypoxia and, especially, hypotension. If the patient has evidence of impaired circulation in the leg, measures such as leg wrapping and avoidance of pressure points should be taken. If the patient has difficulty in urination from an enlarged prostate, care should be taken to ensure bladder emptying.

In general, the geriatric patient is less able to compensate for such insults as abrupt and significant alterations in anesthetic concentration, fluid balance and electrolyte intake (especially of sodium and potassium), and severe changes in position as well as immobility. He is generally a more brittle and less adaptable individual, however hale and hearty he may appear. His tolerance to drugs is substantially diminished; we emphasize again that the dose of a drug must not be based upon weight alone or even primarily. In general, one manages the elderly patient gingerly and, if anesthesia is managed correctly, the outcome is often surprisingly successful.

CHAPTER TWENTY-SIX

The Full Stomach

ONE OF THE MORE DANGEROUS, frustrating and annoying problems in the management of anesthesia by inhalation is that of the full stomach. In order to avoid the hazards of the full stomach it is essential to be constantly aware that a stomach may not be empty. One must be alert, for example, to this possibility not only in the patient who has eaten recently but also in other patients such as those with gastric hemorrhage, acute and chronic peptic ulcer, intestinal obstruction and esophageal diverticula or long-standing low esophageal obstruction. It is essential also to recognize that the presence of an indwelling gastric tube does not ensure stomach emptying and even may facilitate regurgitation in the presence of deep anesthesia and/or muscle relaxants. Many patients surreptitiously imbibe water or solids prior to anesthesia and others simply have a long gastric emptying time. The latter is especially true in patients anticipating surgery, and evidence indicates that patients withhold stomach contents for 24 hours or more if they are anticipating surgery or if some other emotional factor is involved. This brings up, of course, the safe time limit between the ingestion of food and the induction of inhalation anesthesia. The customary interval is 4 hours, but it is readily apparent that this time limit is no guarantee of stomach emptying. Trauma, as for example, in the child with a fracture sustained after eating, often causes the stomach to stop emptying. Thus there can be no guarantee of a safe time limit.

The problem can be resolved more safely and satisfactorily by the use of conduction anesthesia. One should remember, of course, that conduction anesthesia does not eliminate the hazard of the full stomach. If, for example, the level of spinal anesthesia is fairly high, the patient may be unable to vomit effectively because of abdominal muscle relaxation. Furthermore, in order to facilitate the effectiveness of the conduction anesthesia by regional block, for example, the anesthetist may be tempted to use large doses of sedatives and these may interfere with the patient's ability to manage his own vomited material. If inhalation anesthesia must be used for any of a variety of reasons, there are technics that, if properly executed, all but eliminate the hazards of the full stomach.

One should be aware, of course, that the problem of aspiration is not the result of active vomiting alone. Relaxation of the esophageal sphincters with anesthesia or relaxants and concomitant regurgitation can be equally dangerous.

Probably the most effective measure (although not often used because of more refined measures) is to induce active emptying of the stomach by the patient through such measures as inserting a finger in the throat and administering emetics such as apomorphine orally or subcutaneously. If apomorphine is used, one needs to remember that it is also a depressant and contributes to the total depression of the patient. Another technic sometimes used to stimulate active emesis is to induce light anesthesia, preferably with an inhalation agent (rather than thiopental) to a stage at which the laryngeal and pharyngeal reflexes are still present and to provoke vomiting by stimulation of the gag reflex with a tongue blade, finger or oral airway. Failing to stimulate active emesis, one then can be reasonably certain of emptying the stomach by inserting a gastric tube, preferably a large-bore tube, and aspirating contents. Irrigation of the stomach increases the chances of emptying the stomach, but this method does not ensure the removal of chunks of food.

MANAGEMENT OF INDUCTION OF ANESTHESIA

The anesthetist often must proceed knowing that vomiting, regurgitation and aspiration may occur. The chances of such a disaster can be diminished by (1) awake intubation, (2) rapid induction, (3) the head-up position, (4) the use of esophageal balloons, (5) cricoid pressure and (6) by having large-bore and effective suction apparatus immediately available. Intubation of the trachea with the patient awake is one of the more effective and safe ways in which to avoid aspiration in the patient who is liable to vomit or regurgitate. Depending on the mental and physical state of the patient, sedation or analgesia or both, produced by drugs introduced parenterally, is useful. However, the drug dose should be just sufficient to permit retention of the patient's cooperation and, of course, his pharyngeal and laryngeal reflexes. Topical anesthetization of the nose (if nasotracheal intubation is contemplated), tongue, pharynx and larynx is often used. Anesthetization of the larynx and epiglottic area is opposed by some who argue that elimination of reflexes at those sites may reduce the possibility of the patient protecting himself from aspiration either at the time of intubation or after operation. We are inclined to use topical analgesia in a limited number of cases, if at all. In emergency circumstances, there is often insufficient time to provide topical analgesia. With or without topical analgesia, the technic for intubation is that outlined in Chapter 6 with the special need, of course, for a full explanation of the procedure to the patient (when possible) and extreme gentleness in the instrumentation. Obviously, immediate inflation of the cuff is indicated after intubation. One should be prepared in the interest of patient comfort to induce anesthesia immediately after intubation.

Rapid induction can be accomplished either by the "crash" technic of a combination of thiopental and succinylcholine or by the induction of inhalation anesthesia with high concentrations. The objective is to permit early insertion of a cuffed endotracheal tube. It is probably desirable to place the patient in the head-up position rather than the traditional head-down position because aspiration after regurgitation may be significantly diminished. The head-down position does not ensure or even diminish the likelihood of aspiration; ample evidence indicates that aspiration in positions other than the extremes of the head-down position occurs regularly even with inflated cuffs. Esophageal balloons may be effective but probably they are most effective in that their placement induces active vomiting; this may cause the esophagus to dilate around the balloon and permit material to get past the balloon. Cricoid pressure is effective in blocking the esophagus and probably is the most acceptable method of diminishing the opportunity for aspiration from regurgitation. This technic requires an assistant who defines the cricoid cartilage and, with thumb and forefinger applied anterolaterally on the cartilage, applies pressure on the cartilage in a posterior direction so that the cartilage impinges on the esophagus and occludes it. Pressure must be firm and applied just before the reflexes are lost and must be maintained until the endotracheal cuff is inflated. Properly but effectively applied cricoid pressure neither distorts anatomic relationships nor interferes with intubation.

TREATMENT OF ASPIRATION

If aspiration of stomach contents does occur, active and prompt measures are indicated. The severity of subsequent aspiration pneumonia seems to be related to the pH of the aspirated material. If it is highly acid (i.e., pH 2.0 to 2.5), as is the case with stomach contents, pneumonia (Mendelson's syndrome) is more severe and less easily controlled. In any event, one should make an effort to aspirate as much material as possible from the lung. One is tempted, of course, to irrigate the lungs in an effort not only to remove material but also to dilute it. There is some question about the effectiveness or the advisability of gavage of the lung. Gavage may succeed only in forcing the material into smaller units of the lung and it may wash out surfactant. Obviously, the better approach, if possible, is to get the patient to cough as soon as possible. Bronchoscopy, except for the removal of obstructing solid material, probably is no more effective than aspiration through an endotracheal tube. Antibiotics should be administered to cover the possible introduction of pathogens and to treat the bacterial pneumonia that may follow, or be associated with, the pathologic changes associated with aspiration. Steroids, in large doses, seem to be indicated also to diminish the violent reaction to the aspirated material. Oxygen, as needed to maintain an adequate Pa_{O_2}, should be administered.

CHAPTER TWENTY-SEVEN

Abnormal Respiratory Patterns

HICCOUGH

ABNORMAL OR IRREGULAR respiratory patterns, other than those related to depth of anesthesia that have already been described, do occur, especially during inhalation anesthesia. Hiccough is one of the common disruptions of the normal respiratory pattern. Hiccough, during anesthesia, as in the awake state, is a spasmodic contraction of the diaphragm. It differs from the jerky, gasping type respiration associated with deep anesthesia or paralysis with relaxants in that the movements are more vigorous and deeper. The relative violence interferes significantly with surgical maneuvers. As a result, it is desirable to eliminate hiccough. The causes are often obscure but there is a high correlation with disturbances such as uremia, gastric retention and surgical manipulation in the upper abdomen.

If uremia is a cause, it should obviously be corrected if possible; similarly gastric distention should be relieved, and manipulation in the celiac area eliminated. If hiccough persists or recurs every time there is any manipulation in the celiac area (e.g., during gastric resection and cholecystectomy), one may cure the disorder by infiltrating the celiac plexus with a local anesthetic. If hiccough occurs during anesthesia and the various therapeutic measures afford no relief, one may induce hyperventilation or hypoventilation. In either case, one attempts to disrupt the abnormal pattern by overriding the stimulus that presumably is transmitted through the phrenic nerve. This is what the awake patient often does when he either overventilates voluntarily or holds his breath. During anesthesia, if one fails to control hiccough, one can temporarily make conditions better for the surgeon by weakening the diaphragmatic contraction with a relaxant, but there is no evidence that the relaxant "cures" the hiccough. One of the more popular recent methods of treating hiccough has been the parenteral use of methylphenidate (Ritalin). There are a legion of remedies for hiccough, especially for the awake patient plagued with this disorder. We will neither attempt to delineate the more than 100 suggestions made nor assess their efficiency. The fact that there are hundreds of remedies, each of which is sometimes effective, strongly suggests that the etiology is unknown and there is no universally effective cure. For the occasional patient who is afflicted with persistent hiccough (i.e., for days or weeks) and becomes not only physically debilitated but also emotionally disturbed, phrenic nerve block can be tried in addition to all the other remedies. If the disorder persists, one may suspect that some patients are air-swallowers who provoke hiccough either intentionally or unintentionally.

"SOBBING" RESPIRATION

Babies or small children often cry during induction of inhalation anesthesia and carry the sobbing type of respiration into the anesthetic stage. This undesirable type of respiration may be eliminated by deepening anesthesia deliberately and then lightening it to the desired level. It may be corrected also by deliberate hyperventilation, either manually or by the introduction of CO_2. Sometimes the incorporation of added dead space, which increases the Pa_{CO_2} will correct the abnormal pattern. Preferably, one prevents this type of respiratory pattern by establishing better rapport with the patient or by giving more effective premedication.

CHEYNE-STOKES OR BIOT'S RESPIRATION

Occasionally, elderly patients develop a Cheyne-Stokes or Biot's type pattern of respiration with inhalation anesthesia. One assumes that there is then an alteration in the response of the respiratory centers to the Pa_{CO_2}, that there is a deficiency in the precise control of pH in the cerebrospinal fluid to which the respiratory centers respond, or that the anesthetic agent induces a disruption of a borderline competent or organized neurologic control. This type of respiration is not as disruptive to the surgical procedure as hiccough or the sobbing type just discussed. However, it often persists into the postanesthetic period and may be so pronounced as to seriously interfere with adequate oxygenation. One suspects that the irregularity may be more apt to occur in those elderly patients with severe emphysema or other lung deficiencies interfering with gas exchange and in which there is often an elevated Pa_{CO_2} "normally." There is evidence that these patients in the awake state have pronounced respiratory alkalosis.[1] This means that one should maintain the Pa_{CO_2} near the "normal" value for that patient by avoiding deliberate or inadvertent overventilation of the lung. If the pattern does appear, one can attempt to correct it by hypoventilation; hyperventilation rarely is successful. Although success is not predictable, one can use a respiratory stimulant parenterally to attempt to overcome the abnormal pattern. One also may add CO_2 in an effort to override the established abnormal pattern and, perhaps, to return the Pa_{CO_2} to its previous "normal," but elevated, level. Such patients must be watched carefully in the immediate postanesthetic period to prevent hypoxia during the periods of apnea and thus accentuation of the imperfect functioning of the respiratory centers. It is wise, of course, to add oxygen to the inspired atmosphere. Blood-gas analyses may reveal abnormal values that may then be corrected more objectively, provided one has the "normal" values for that patient as a reference point and does not attempt a return to values that are "normal" for the healthy patient.

CHEST RIGIDITY WITH NARCOTICS

If anesthesia is induced with a combination of narcotic and nitrous oxide, many narcotics, especially meperidine, fentanyl, phenazocine and alphaprodine, induce a state of tightness of the chest muscles. This may be so severe as to preclude ventilation, even if an endotracheal tube is in place with the cuff inflated. The tightness, the cause of which is unknown, can be relieved immediately and effectively by the administration of an antagonist such as nalorphine, levallorphan or naloxone or by succinylcholine. Morphine does not seem to be associated with chest rigidity.

REFERENCE

1. Sullivan, K. N., Manfredi, F., and Behnke, R. H.: Hippus in Cheyne-Stokes Respiration, Arch. Intern. Med. 122:116, 1968.

CHAPTER TWENTY-EIGHT

Hypothermia and Hyperthermia

GENERAL CONSIDERATIONS

VARIATIONS IN TEMPERATURE are common and sometimes may be profound and life-threatening. Knowledge of the control of temperature is therefore an important factor in anesthetic management. Furthermore, deliberate reduction of temperature is sometimes a useful means of diminishing the likelihood of unwanted brain damage in some circumstances of impaired cerebral circulation.

Maintenance of temperature at a reasonably constant level is a homeostatic function depending upon the balance between heat production and heat loss. Many factors influence heat production and heat loss, and adjustment of the body's mechanisms to compensate for the influence of these factors is accomplished by a control center in the midbrain (hypothalamus). Anesthetics and sedative/hypnotic drugs, especially the barbiturates, impair the ability of the center to respond to demands for adjustments. In addition, there may be genetically inherent aberrations in the control center that render the center unable to control elevations in temperature or provoke it to initiate severe states of hyperthermia.[1]

Heat production is a reflection of the metabolic rate of the individual patient. An increase in heat production may occur as a result of (1) the presence of endocrinopathies, such as thyrotoxicosis and pheochromocytoma, (2) an increase in muscular activity such as that occurring as a response to cold (i.e., shivering) and also struggling during induction of anesthesia, (3) the increased work of breathing associated with airway obstruction, decreased compliance (for a variety of reasons) and (4) elevated temperature from a disease process.

HYPERTHERMIA

There is some reason to suspect that once the temperature is elevated, as from disease, the tendency to further elevation is increased or accelerated; that is, a vicious cycle of heat production or reduced heat loss, or both, is initiated. Although some of the sources of increased heat production can be controlled, as is the case with muscular activity from shivering, induction excitement and increased work of breathing, the control of temperature is largely effected through control of the means of heat loss.

Heat loss occurs through radiation, evaporation and conduction. Involved in these processes is, of course, the distribution of heat to the surface by changes in the blood flow to extremities. Radiation and conduction account for 70% of the heat loss of an individual in a normal environment and evaporation of water from skin and lungs accounts for 23%. One can readily see that the circumstances of anesthesia and surgery interfere with heat loss. Drapes, hot lamps, closed anesthetic systems and warm operating rooms impair heat loss mechanisms, and drugs, especially atropine or scopolamine, interfere with evaporation because of decreased sweating.

There are a number of physiologic responses to hyperthermia at any level, but profound derangements occur if the temperature becomes elevated above 40°C (105°F). These changes include acidosis, dehydration, hypovolemia, hypotension and hypoxia (which is so severe that irreparable brain tissue damage can occur). Acidosis is induced and accentuated by both an increase in the output of CO_2 (there is an increase in metabolism of 7% with each increment in temperature of 1°F) and tissue hypoxia, which results in anaerobic metabolism with an increased output of lactic acid. Under the circumstances of anesthesia and surgery, an increased output of CO_2 is sometimes inadequately compensated for because of inability of the patient to augment his ventilation (due to drug depression or the use of relaxants, for example), the failure of the anesthetist to recognize the need for increased ventilation, or the use of malfunctioning apparatus (e.g., nonfunctioning soda lime absorber and poorly functioning valves) that inadequately removes CO_2. The Pa_{CO_2} itself may increase to such an extent that it acts as a respiratory depressant. The metabolic acidosis from increased lactic acid production may induce a lack of responsiveness to catecholamines, a decrease in myocardial contractility and cardiac output, with consequent hypotension, and impaired tissue circulation which, in turn, increases the metabolic acidosis.

Dehydration and hypovolemia occur as a result of fluid loss through the skin and lungs and may be severe. Furthermore, as the state of severe hyperthermia persists, the fluid changes in character from isotonic to hypo-osmotic with substantial changes in electrolytes. This loss of fluid contributes to hypotension.

Hypoxemia results from factors such as shunting from atelectasis, hypoventilation with a decreased intake of oxygen and also increased oxygen consumption. Tissue hypoxia, which is a critical element in the process, is caused not only by decreased input of oxygen to arterial blood but also by local circulatory changes due to acidosis.

These life-threatening changes associated with an elevation in temperature mean that the anesthetist always must be alert to temperature changes in his patient, to the many factors that influence temperature control and especially alert to potential problems in the patient with an elevated temperature prior to anesthesia and surgery. The anesthetist also must be aware of possible genetic susceptibility to malignant hyperthermia.

Prophylaxis

Being aware of the likelihood of hyperthermia, the anesthetist is obligated to take those steps that may diminish the possibility of its occurring. Close attention must be paid to ambient temperature, to the amount, nature and placing of drapes (plastic adherent drapes may accentuate heat retention), to avoidance of or use of a minimum of belladonna drugs, to the nature and efficiency of the anesthetic system and to the technic of monitoring of temperature. If a family history or any other finding makes one suspicious of the likelihood of a genetic tendency to malignant hyperthermia, one may be further alerted by increased concentrations of SGOT, CPK and LDH. Halothane, and perhaps other halogenated agents, seems to be associated with an increased incidence of severe hyperthermia; this is possibly due to some derangement of cellular metabolism. Finally, succinylcholine has been associated with muscular rigidity and hyperthermia and its use may provoke severe hyperthermia.[2] Many anesthetists believe that temperature monitoring is indicated in all patients who are anesthetized. Although rectal, oral or axillary temperatures can give useful clues as to the actual value as well as trends in the temperature, the most meaningful values are obtained from an esophageal or tympanic membrane lead. Certainly, instrumentation is available to permit routine temperature monitoring inexpensively and reliably.

Malignant Hyperthermia

Malignant hyperthermia is a special disorder of an especially lethal nature that is apparently genetically linked and provoked by the factors that have just been discussed. Alerting signs are muscle rigidity aggravated by succinylcholine, an unexplained increase in temperature often associated with halothane and, finally, a family history from the patient or from the family that indicates an unusual response during anesthesia.

If hyperthermia does occur, especially if it is of the malignant type, the treatment must be immediate and vigorous. The temperature itself must be lowered by several means depending upon the situation (e.g., whether the operation is in progress, soon to begin or terminated). If the abdomen is open, for example, cold solutions (preferably Ringer's lactate) may be placed in the abdomen. Ice packs, including the placing of ice directly on as much of the patient's body surface as possible, should be used. If shivering occurs as a result of this application, drugs such as meperidine or chlorpromazine may be useful. Increasing the flow rate in the anesthetic system may help by diminishing rebreathing. If surgery has not begun or is terminated, cooling appliances may be used. The presence and the degree of acidosis should be determined by analysis of arterial blood. The effectiveness of therapy should similarly be followed by serial blood-gas analyses; if one does not follow progress by this means, one often falls short of providing adequate corrective measures. A rough estimate of the amount of base needed is obtained from the equation,

$$\text{Base requirement} = \text{base deficit} \times 0.3 \times \text{body weight in kilograms}$$

The respiratory acidosis can be managed effectively by appropriate hyperventilation and high flows of gas. Tissue hypoxia is corrected by adequate input of oxygen (high oxygen inspired atmospheres), adequate ventilation, and prevention and elimination of shunting by "deep breaths." As in the case of metabolic acidosis, serial blood-gas analysis is indicated.

If there is evidence of increased intracranial pressure after return to normal temperature, one can administer solutions such as mannitol. If this is done, one needs to remember that hypovolemia may again occur with hypotension. Hypovolemia is probably due to large losses from the extracellular fluid space because there is evidence that the hematocrit does not often change. One must be aware that large volumes are often required. Monitoring of adequacy of fluid replacement can be facilitated by measurement of central venous pressure.

DELIBERATE HYPOTHERMIA

Deliberate hypothermia is useful when one anticipates interference with or interruption of the cerebral circulation. The hypothesis is that the tissue demand for oxygen is diminished by cooling (O_2 consumption decreases 50% at 30°C) and that tissue survival is thereby more likely. It is used most often in intracranial surgery for aneurysms. It is sometimes used during surgery for carotid endarterectomy; lately, however, surgical bypass procedures, halothane anesthesia (to improve cerebral circulation), hypocarbia (by hyperventilation) and high inspired oxygen concentrations have made hypothermia unnecessary. Hypothermia was used often at one stage of the development of technics for heart surgery but, with improvements in management of extracorporeal circulation, hypothermia is now used less frequently. There is serious doubt about the value of deliberate hypothermia in the treatment of the patient who has sustained cardiac arrest. If it is used in these circumstances, as in patients with other abrupt interruptions of cerebral circulation, the evidence is quite reliable that hypothermia is of value only if instituted immediately and maintained at approximately 30°C.

Except in the circumstances of profound hypothermia (i.e., 3 to 4°C) as used in cardiac surgery, hypothermia is induced by peripheral cooling. In profound hypothermia, the cooling is accomplished by heat exchangers interposed in the blood circuit of the extracorporeal pump. Peripheral cooling is facilitated by use of a small intravenous dose of chlorpromazine (10 to 25 mg). The hypothesis is that this drug diminishes the tendency for the surface vessels to constrict, which thereby augments the distribution of blood to the surface. Cooling can be accomplished by direct application of ice to the body surface. This may be done either by encasing the body in an ice pack or by immersing the patient in a tub of ice water. The latter method is effective for prompt cooling, but there is some objection in that the abrupt immersion may precipitate cardiac irregularities. If the tub method is used the patient should be anesthetized prior to immersion and, preferably, the patient should be placed in the water bath before the ice is introduced because this diminishes the "shock" of the immersion. Rapid cooling is easily effected by this method; a decrease in temperature to approximately the level desired occurs in the average 70-kg patient within 10 to 15 minutes. Constant temperature observation is mandatory, preferably by means of esophageal or tympanic membrane monitoring. Delay in response of the rectal temperature has resulted in significant overshoot, severe cardiac irregularities and cardiac arrest. One looks for the trend in the decrease in temperature. If the trend is reasonably linear, the patient is removed from the bath when the temperature falls to about 2°C above the desired level. Some patients have a relatively flat trend with a sudden "knee" in the curve. If the "knee" occurs, it usually presages a rapid subsequent drop, and it is wise to remove the patient soon after the "knee" appears, regardless of the actual temperature at the time.

Less rapid cooling is achieved with the use of ice packs around the body or by the use of cooling devices. These devices employ blankets in which coolant at the desired temperature is circulated. The more modern devices of this sort have reasonably automatic temperature controls for the coolant. These devices can be used also for heating. In the usual circumstance, the temperature of the coolant is set at approximately 10°C for the cooling period. As much as possible of the top and bottom blankets should be in contact with the patient. The coolant temperature remains at the cooling level until the patient's temperature comes to within 2 to 3°C of the desired level. One then begins to adjust the coolant temperature to slow down the cooling and to keep the patient's temperature at the level desired. As in the case of tub cooling, one must observe closely the trend of cooling. If the curve is linear and fairly flat, the change in coolant temperature need not take place until the temperature is within 1 to 2°C of the desired level. If the curve is linear but fairly steep, the coolant temperature should be changed when the patient's temperature gets within 2 to 3°C of the desired level. If there is a "knee" in the curve, the coolant temperature may need to be reversed at that point to avoid overshoot. Some anesthetists prefer to stop the flow of coolant rather than attempt to adjust the temperature of the coolant upward.

Except in profound hypothermia for cardiac surgery in which cardiac arrest is deliberately induced, the temperature of the patient usually is kept at approximately 30°C. Experience and laboratory evidence clearly indicate that severe cardiac irregularities and fibrillation increase significantly in incidence as the temperature falls below 29°C. Cooling by the slower methods (i.e., ice packs and blankets) often takes 3 to 4 hours and the timing of surgery and cooling must be integrated so that the optimum temperature of the patient is achieved at the time it is needed. Reversal of temperature may be accomplished as soon as there is no longer a need for a low temperature. The patient can be warmed by means of hot water bottles or by circulating warm fluid through the blankets. In either event, it is mandatory that the temperature of the warming fluids not exceed 40°C; if the temperature is above this point, severe burns may occur. If rapid warming is desired, the patient may be placed in a warm tub.

During cooling, it is necessary to prevent shivering. It is amazing how much heat is produced during shivering and therefore how effectively shivering prevents cooling. Shivering can be prevented by drugs such as meperidine or chlorpromazine. The accompanying anesthetic state in most situations in which cooling is desired helps to diminish shivering and, as long as measures are available for maintenance of ventilation (as during anesthesia), desensitizing relaxants can be used to eliminate the shivering.

The anesthetist must remember, of course, that during the cool state, the requirements of anesthetic agents are reduced and appropriate adjustments must be made in their input. Results of blood-gas analyses made during the cool state require conversion to normal temperature. Furthermore, because of peripheral vascular constriction in the cool state or the cooling process, it is sometimes difficult to obtain blood pressure measurements by the usual stethoscope and arm cuff. As a result, it is probably wise to institute an intraarterial pressure line if hypothermia is to be induced.

REFERENCES

1. Britt, B. A., Locher, W. G., and Kalow, W.: Hereditary Aspects of Malignant Hyperthermia, Can. Anaesth. Soc. J. 16:89, 1969.
2. Cody, J. R.: Muscle Rigidity Following Administration of Succinylcholine, Anesthesiology 29:159, 1968.

CHAPTER TWENTY-NINE

Deliberate Hypotension

OCCASIONALLY, it is in the best interest of the patient to deliberately induce a state of hypotension to minimize blood loss and to facilitate surgery. These occasions usually are limited to those surgical procedures in which extreme blood loss is anticipated or in which bleeding at the operative site impairs visibility sufficiently to interfere with effective and safe surgery. The latter situation is better exemplified by the intracranial aneurysm that has bled slightly, which may rupture even more seriously with hypertension and from which severe bleeding may seriously impair brain function. Situations in which severe blood loss may be expected are exemplified by surgical procedures such as pelvic exenteration, radical neck dissection, suprapubic or perineal prostatectomy and abdomino-perineal resection.

The hypothesis in support of the use of deliberate hypotension is that a decrease in the head of pressure diminishes the loss of blood from open vessels, especially veins and very small arterioles, but at the same time maintains reasonable perfusion in vital tissues because of lack of constriction of arteriolar beds with a consequent decrease in straight-line shunting through the arteriolar-capillary network. In fact, there are those who recommend arteriolar relaxation with drugs used for deliberate hypotension in order to improve tissue perfusion in states of hemorrhagic shock. This concept of lowered arterial tension with reasonable tissue perfusion, of course, eliminated the initial method of inducing deliberate hypotension; that is, the blood-letting method. Such bleeding, obviously, causes arteriolar-capillary bed constriction and shunting together with the hypotension and, in general, negates the benefits of the hypotensive technic.

METHODS OF INDUCING HYPOTENSION

Deliberate hypotension may be achieved by several methods. One of the first methods was the use of trimetaphan (Arfonad). This drug, when introduced intravenously in a 0.2% concentration (2 mg/ml), produced hypotension as a result of a direct action on peripheral vessels. The duration of action of the drug is short and, as a result, it is necessary to administer it as a continuous infusion. Constant adjustment of the rate of the infusion is necessary to control the level of hypotension. No significant adverse reactions to the drug itself have been reported. Recently, the use of sodium nitroprusside as a substitute for trimetaphan has been revived. Sodium nitroprusside produces hypotension also by a direct action on the peripheral vascular musculature. It is an exceedingly potent, short-acting hypotensive agent and it is easily reversed by slowing or discontinuing the drug. Hypotension due to either trimetaphan or sodium nitroprusside can be reversed by the usual vasopressors. Sodium nitroprusside is converted to thiocyanate but hypotension occurs with doses long before any significant degradation products are developed. It is administered in a continuous infusion. The usual concentration is achieved by placing 50 to 100 mg of nitroprusside in 1000 ml of dextrose or saline, or both. It is usually administered at a rate of 20 to 400 μg/min. Side effects include restlessness, agitation, muscle twitching, nausea and emesis. The presumed advantage of sodium nitroprusside over trimetaphan is its dependably prompt action and its easy reversibility.

Deliberate hypotension may be induced also by a combination of halothane and hyperventilation. Halothane effects hypotension by relaxation of the peripheral vasculature and by direct myocardial muscle depression. Hyperventilation adds to the technic by lowering the Pa_{CO_2} and perhaps by facilitating the input of halothane. If a constant elevated end-expiratory intrapulmonary pressure is also added, hypotension may be augmented by a decrease in venous return to the right atrium. Ordinarily, halothane does not cause hypotension unless its concentration is higher than that needed for the level of anesthesia required by the surgical procedure itself. However, the concentration required for hypotension is within the limits of tolerance of most patients. This technic with halothane has the advantages of immediate reversibility, greater stability than that of the trimetaphan or sodium nitroprusside technics and lack of any requirement for a continuous infusion of fluid. A major disadvantage for us is that the hypotension is acquired at the expense of myocardial muscle depression and perhaps some increased incidence of cardiac irregularities.

In either technic, hypotension is facilitated by placing the patient in a slight head-up position. For monitoring, the usual arm cuff and stethoscope can be used, but because anesthesia for major surgical procedures requires the attention of the anesthetist for many things, an intra-arterial pressure line is useful as a monitor. Another monitoring device is an indwelling urethral catheter with a device for measurement of urinary output; this helps one to assess the effectiveness of the hypotension and the limit to which one wants to go. One should be aware also that there may be some diminution of the need for anesthetic drugs and also that there will be significant changes in the blood flow through the lungs, which thereby slows the uptake of anesthetic agent.

The lower limit for hypotension has been established by clinical experience and limited laboratory investigation to be approximately 60 mm Hg (systolic). At such a pressure—assuming that there is no interference with perfusion through the arteriolar-capillary bed (e.g., in cases of atherosclerosis)—perfusion of the vital organs such as brain, heart and kidneys is adequate. A good indicator of kidney perfusion is the output of urine. If the patient's normal pressure is elevated, one is inclined to raise the lower limit to a minimum of 80 mm Hg or higher. Patients with abnormally high arterial tensions tolerate low systolic pressures provided there is no interference with tissue perfusion through the arteriolar-capillary bed and there is evidence of kidney perfusion by urinary output. Some anesthetists like to use the EEG as an indicator of brain tissue perfusion and to limit the level of hypotension to that pressure at which the voltage of brain waves begins to produce a flattened pattern. It is probably correct to state that if one wishes to gain for the patient the advantage of deliberate hypotension, there is no point in hedging about the degree of hypotension. For example, in a patient with a normal pressure (for him) of 160/100 mm Hg there is little value in limiting the hypotension to a systolic pressure of 120 mm Hg.

Since this technic is generally used when loss of blood is expected to be great, the anesthetist must frequently determine the blood loss and replace blood lost. Hemorrhage or fluid shifts must not be used to aid or substitute for drugs used for the deliberate hypotension. Usually it is wise also to reverse the hypotension at a time when the surgeon can observe his control of hemostasis in the state of normotension.

CHAPTER THIRTY

Emergency Resuscitation

THE NEED FOR EMERGENCY resuscitation may occur at any time and under any circumstances. In the eyes of the public, all physicians (regardless of specialty) are expected to be able to provide prompt and competent emergency resuscitation care should the need arise. The need may arise in a hospital where emergency facilities and equipment are readily obtainable or outside a hospital where one must provide emergency resuscitation without the aid of special facilities and equipment. In either situation, the requisite skills must not only be learned but also periodically renewed in order to be effective. Physicians seldom involved in emergency resuscitation must periodically rehearse its essential features to be adequately prepared to handle an emergency.

Emergency resuscitation has two distinct facets: 1) recognition of the need for such care; and 2) implementation of therapy. A working knowledge of one facet but not the other is of little value to patients at risk. Expertise in both areas is essential for the end result to be successful.

RESPIRATORY INSUFFICIENCY

Recognition

Recognition of acute respiratory insufficiency is not always easy either because there may be no obvious manifestations of respiratory inadequacy or because they may not focus on the respiratory system. For example, an overdose of a drug that depresses the central nervous system may cause hypoventilation, hypoxemia, hypercarbia and eventually death. Breathing may be very shallow and very quiet, lulling the untrained observer into a false sense of security that respiration is adequate. The eventual hypoxemia and hypercarbia may cause restlessness, tachycardia, arrhythmias, hypertension, sweating or cyanosis. Depending upon the various signs detected, the observer may conclude that the primary problem is circulatory and fail to institute respiratory therapy until cardiac arrest and apnea ensue. Respiratory insufficiency should be suspected in any patients found to be confused, disoriented or unconscious. Unexplained circulatory stimulation (tachycardia or hypertension), circulatory depression (bradycardia or hypotension) or cardiac irritability (arrhythmias) should evoke concern for respiratory adequacy. Cyanosis, often regarded as the hallmark of respiratory insufficiency, may be absent or not readily detectable. Patients with severe anemia or carbon monoxide poisoning may be severely hypoxemic but not cyanotic. Only by examination of the mucous membranes will cyanosis be readily detectable in patients with melanotic skin.

More commonly, patients with acute respiratory insufficiency have symptoms or signs that are referable to the respiratory system. If conscious, they will usually complain of difficulty in breathing. In this event, two life-threatening and rapidly fatal conditions should be considered; namely, airway obstruction and tension pneumothorax. The sites, types, symptoms and signs and the treatment for airway obstruction are detailed in Chapter 2. In the acute life-threatening situation, the signs and symptoms are exaggerated, especially those associated with upper airway obstruction and the patient "fights for air" in a manner that is obvious even to the layman.

Tension pneumothorax is characterized by labored breathing with little evidence of gas flow entering or leaving the lungs. Listening over the nose or mouth gives one the distinct impression that gas flow is rapid, though of small volume. This is in contradistinction to partial airway obstruction, in which case gas flow is slow to enter or leave the lungs. Examination of the chest may show tracheal deviation, an area of increased resonance to percussion and distant breath sounds.

Treatment

Assuming that, in the context of emergency respiratory resuscitation, therapy must be instituted within seconds or minutes at the most, the cause of the acute deficiency must be assessed immediately. Regardless of the accuracy of the diagnosis, the primary objective is to move air in and out of the lungs. If the resuscitator is in a situation in which all necessary equipment is available and he is qualified to use this equipment, he can proceed as outlined in Chapter 6. This may include the use of bag and mask, oxygen and artificial airways such as the oral and nasopharyngeal airways or tracheal tubes.

For the physician or layman to whom such equipment is not available and who has little or no experience in its use, other simpler yet quite effective means of moving air in and out of the lungs are available. If there is obvious contamination of the upper airway by fluid, vomitus, gum, dentures, chunks of food, etc., an effort should be made quickly, in a matter of seconds only, to remove this material. This can be done by using a portable suction device or by turning the patient onto his side with the head down and sweeping the mouth with one's fingers. As soon as possible (again, in a matter of seconds), efforts to move air must be made. In the absence of equipment, this can be done most effectively by mouth-to-mouth breathing. The elements of this technic are simple. The patient should be placed on his back. The resuscitator sits at the side of the patient by the patient's head and puts one arm under the neck of the patient so that the head drops back (i.e., the head is extended). Letting the head drop back (hyperextending it) relieves much of the airway obstruction due to the tongue and soft structures of the mouth and throat. The resuscitator grasps the nose of the patient with his other hand and closes it. The resuscitator then inhales deeply and blows his air into the opened mouth of the patient. While blowing he observes the chest of the patient to see if it moves. If the chest moves, air is being forced into the lungs. If the chest does not move, the resuscitator does not have his mouth tightly placed on that of the patient, the head of the patient is not sufficiently extended, the nose is not closed or there is material obstructing the upper airway. A check of all these possibilities must be made quickly. If the chest does rise, the resuscitator ceases blowing and turns his head away from that of the patient allowing the air in the lung to come out. This process is repeated 10 to 12 times each minute until it is determined that the patient either is not resuscitatable or begins breathing on his own. Do not give up quickly; it may take as long as 30 minutes with several resuscitators working in shifts before success is attained.

Artificial airways, such as the oral and nasopharyngeal airways, are of doubtful value for the inexperienced physician or layman resuscitator. Often they are improperly placed and actually worsen upper airway obstruction, or their placement in the semiconscious patient induces vomiting.

Mechanical devices for ventilation, such as the Elder valve, may be used. These, however, are ineffective unless one takes the same measures that are used for mouth-to-mouth breathing to ensure an open airway. The devices should be of a type that provide positive pressure only. One looks for chest movement as the most reliable sign of effective air movement as in mouth-to-mouth breathing.

Some recommend mouth-to-airway or mouth-to-mask methods. These are somewhat more delicate but can be ineffective because of poor placement or poor fits of airway or mask.

No mention is made of use of the traditional manual methods for ventilation, such as the Schaefer and the Sylvester, because it has been unquestionably established that these methods are much less effective (if they are effective at all) than intermittent positive-pressure ventilation.

A note of caution is necessary with respect to the care of a patient who has developed acute respiratory insufficiency. That patient must not be left unattended or unobserved for any reason. Death from respiratory insufficiency can occur extremely rapidly. Personnel capable of instituting cardiopulmonary resuscitation must be in constant attendance on this type of patient.

If tension pneumothorax is the suspected diagnosis, confirmation can be obtained by a chest roentgenogram and appropriate therapy instituted. However, signs of circulatory failure (i.e., hypotension, increased central venous pressure, tachycardia and distant heart sounds) indicate impending cardiac arrest, and delay in treatment until a chest roentgenogram can be obtained may be fatal for the patient. Instead, therapy should be begun by inserting an 18- or 19-gauge needle into the chest on the suspected side at the second intercostal space just lateral to the sternal border. If a small glass syringe is attached to the needle prior to insertion, the plunger will be forced out of the syringe barrel by the excessive pressure in the chest. This will quickly confirm the diagnosis for all observers.

CARDIOVASCULAR INSUFFICIENCY

Recognition

Circulatory insufficiency is characterized by hypotension with or without tachycardia (usually this is absent in the elderly), arrhythmias, confusion, disorientation, anxiety, sweating and cold, clammy extremities. Many of these changes are the same as those that occur in cases of acute respiratory insufficiency, which makes it difficult to determine whether the primary event is respiratory or circulatory. Because of this, treatment is directed toward both systems.

The extreme form of cardiovascular insufficiency is circulatory or cardiac arrest, which is characterized by unconsciousness and the absence of pulses in large arteries. The patient may be apneic or exhibit periodic gasping respiration. Pupillary dilation is an additional sign but one should not wait for this to occur because it may take up to 1 minute to develop and may never occur in some patients. If a patient is unconscious and a femoral or carotid artery pulsation cannot be felt, it should be assumed that the patient has sustained a cardiac arrest. One should not spend more than a few seconds attempting to detect pulses. With cardiac arrest, time is of the essence. For therapy to be successful, it must be instituted within 3 to 4 minutes after cessation of circulation.

Treatment

The treatment of circulatory insufficiency (hypotension) is directed toward improving venous return, maintaining the heart rate and cardiac contractility and then correcting the cause of the insufficiency. Tilting the patient 5 to 10° head down or elevating both lower extremities provides an immediate transfusion to the central circulation. An intravenous infusion should be started and, if the patient has bradycardia (pulse rate less than 60/min), atropine (0.2 to 0.4 mg) should be given intravenously. If the blood pressure has not returned to near normal values within a few minutes, ephedrine (25 to 50 mg) should be given intravenously. The patient also should be given oxygen to breathe. These measures will usually restore circulation to normal and allow the physician time to determine the cause of the insufficiency.

If a cardiac arrest is suspected, external cardiac compression must be started immediately. With the patient lying supine, downward compression on the lower half of the sternum compresses the heart between the sternum and the spine, which thereby forces blood out of the heart into the circulation. When sternal pressure is released, the thorax expands to its normal resting position and blood is sucked into the heart from the extrathoracic veins.

The specifics of the technic of external cardiac compression are as follows. Place the patient on a hard surface (e.g., the floor or a bed board) and position yourself either to one side or over the patient. Place the heel of one hand over the lower half of the sternum and put the heel of the other hand on top of the first hand. Compress downward about 5 cm (2 inches) and release. To minimize fatigue, keep the arms straight and use the weight of your body to compress the sternum. Repeat this action every second (i.e., at a rate of 60 per minute). In infants or children two fingers or one hand only should be used and the rate of compression should be 100 to 120 times per minute. If you are alone, quickly ventilate the lungs twice after every 15 compressions of the chest. As soon as help arrives, assign the assistant to one of the two major tasks and synchronize tasks so that the ratio of ventilation to cardiac compression is 1:5.

As additional help arrives, assign each assistant one of the following tasks:

1. Place a blood pressure cuff on an arm and determine if cardiac compression is producing a systolic beat. If no cuff is available, ask the assistant to feel for a carotid or femoral pulse with each cardiac compression.

2. Start an intravenous infusion of fluid (any type), either percutaneously using a plastic catheter or by cutdown.

3. Orotracheal or nasotracheal intubation should be performed when one trained in this technic arrives.

4. An ECG should be obtained as soon as possible to determine cardiac rhythm.

5. Start treatment for metabolic acidosis. Give sodium bicarbonate in a dose of 1 to 2 mEq/kg body weight for every 10 minutes of resuscitation time until spontaneous circulation is adequately restored.

6. Give epinephrine in a dose of 1 mg by intravenous or intracardiac injection without waiting for the electrocardiographic diagnosis of rhythm. If the heart is in asystole, epinephrine will help to start cardiac action. If the heart is in ventricular fibrillation, epinephrine will facilitate restoration of a normal circulation once defibrillation by countershock has been effected.

7. If ventricular fibrillation is detected by electrocardiography, apply electric countershock, using direct current if available. Apply generous amounts of conductive electrode paste to each of the paddles. Place one paddle just below the right clavicle and the second paddle over the apex of the heart. Apply firm pressure and ask the resuscitation team to break contact with the patient. The recommended energies are 200 watt-seconds or more for adults and 100 watt-seconds for children.

8. If multiple countershocks are unsuccessful, continue closed-chest massage and give additional sodium bicarbonate. Lidocaine should also be given in doses of 1 mg/kg and countershock repeated 1 or 2 minutes later. Lidocaine seems to be the best of the antiarrhythmic drugs for use with countershock in the treatment of intractable ventricular fibrillation. If electrocardiographic signs of cardiac irritability continue, a continuous infusion of lidocaine may be necessary.

9. If conditions permit, arterial blood should be obtained for assessment of the adequacy of oxygenation, ventilation and therapy for acidosis.

10. Vasopressors such as phenylephrine, metaraminol or norepinephrine may be of value to support the blood pressure once effective cardiac action has been restored.

Therapy should continue until physicians experienced in emergency resuscitation have had an opportunity to assess the patient's responses and to decide whether continued efforts might prove successful. Generally, if no effective cardiac action is achieved within 1 hour of expert resuscitation, further attempts are futile. If resuscitation is successful, management becomes long-term and beyond the scope of this chapter.

CHAPTER THIRTY-ONE

Electrical Hazards

WITH THE CONTINUING DECREASE in the use of flammable and explosive anesthetic agents and their total elimination in many hospitals, there is a tendency for one to be less concerned about electrical hazards. What has been overlooked or ignored is the concomitant increase in the use of electrical equipment in the operating room, including such items as the electrosurgical unit, the electrical or otherwise heated direct cautery, temperature controlling devices, extracorporeal circulation apparatus, mobile suction apparatus (as for therapeutic abortion) and numerous monitoring devices incorporating electrical circuits. From the standpoint of patient morbidity and mortality, we are willing to venture that the combined use of electrical devices mentioned introduces a greater hazard to the patient than that of injury from explosion or fire; furthermore, the incidence of harm to patients is distinctly lower with the commonsense use of explosive agents than halogenated agents at all well administered. That is, fewer patients will be injured by explosion than, for example, hepatic damage, and cardiac and circulatory depression.

We outline in this chapter the steps necessary to avoid explosions from flammable agents. Unfortunately, some hospitals, in an effort to save money and in a misguided lack of concern over such hazards with the limited use of explosive agents, are not taking the steps necessary to avoid injury to patients and operating room personnel.

THE POTENTIAL FOR HAZARD

Commonly used electrical systems involve a "hot" lead and a "neutral" or ground lead. Household types of electrical devices often use only two-conductor-line cords and plugs rather than a three-wire system, which adds an additional ground path via a third wire. All is well with this type of installation in the absence of an open ground lead (broken wire) or a "short" (e.g., imperfect insulation or "hot" lead in contact with shell of the device). In either circumstance grounding occurs through all available paths. The greatest current flows through the path of least resistance. In the common household accident this occurs in the bathroom, grounding taking place through the person's body to a metal bathtub drain or other plumbing fixture that is connected to ground. Fortunately, in household use two pieces of electrical equipment are rarely used at the same time with the person's body being interposed or connected to both units. The built-in hazard of the two-wire system when two electrical devices are used simultaneously is that one has a fifty-fifty chance of plugging in the devices to the wall outlet in such a way that both units have the same lead attached to the "hot" lead. In such a circumstance, if a ground connection within one apparatus is disconnected, ground will be sought by the current through the other device. If the person's body happens to be interposed, the current passes through the body on the way to ground. When the plugs are in the opposite relationship, an excessively high leakage current may flow from one instrument case through a patient to the other case, which is grounded even when there is no break in the wiring or other defect present.

As a result, it is essential in patient care areas to use a three-wire system that maintains grounding of the apparatus if the usual ground lead is broken or if contact is made with the shell of the apparatus by the "hot" lead. This latter defect in an instrument will result in a blown fuse instead of the primary ground path going through the body.

Isolation Circuit

In order to insure more certainly against hazards from undesired grounding in the operating room where many paths to ground are available to a patient, it is wise to isolate the operating room electrical circuit from the main hospital circuit. This is done by installation of an isolation transformer, which provides a circuit that is independent and isolated from the hospital circuit and ground; this is why isolated electrical systems are also referred to as "ungrounded" electrical systems. Such a system is a complete circuit within itself; grounding to an external ground does not take place even with a fault, except to trigger an alarm through the "line isolation monitor." An electrical shock hazard through accidental grounding only takes place when a second fault occurs before the first one is corrected. Unfortunately, hospitals have neglected to install or have deliberately avoided installation of the isolation circuit because of the erroneous notion that elimination of explosive agents has solved all of the problems. In fact, the costs to hospitals of proper electrical systems in the operating room area have not been lessened by the elimination of explosive agents. Explosive and flammable agents are used less, or their use has been eliminated, because of the presence and use of electrical equipment that is not properly designed to exclude entry of explosive atmospheres into the apparatus in which sparks may be generated or which are of heavy construction with close-fitting connections. These will contain a fire if it occurs and flame cannot spread through a very small opening, hence the name "explosion proof."

Conductive Flooring

Conductive flooring is needed to dissipate static electricity whenever flammable anesthetics are used. This floor must be carefully maintained to insure that it is 25,000 ohms above true ground. This is to minimize electrical shock hazards. If flammable anesthetics are never used there is no need for a conductive floor. This will be discussed more fully later.

Electrical Burns

Current deliberately passed through a human body, as in the case of the electrosurgical unit, causes heating where the area of electrode contact is small. This principle is made use of in the electrosurgical unit when the small tip of the instrument (active electrode) is brought in contact with the tissue for use as a knife or for cauterization. A ground plate (indifferent electrode) with a broad surface is used at the current outlet site or return path to prevent concentration of the current (with heating) and associated unintended burning of tissues. Obviously, it is necessary therefore to be certain that the ground plate contact with the body is not limited to a small area; the mere placement of the broad electrode does not always insure a broad area of contact. A disruption in the ground plate or its connecting wire will lead to a burn at some other small area contact with ground.

This mechanism often operates with the use of ECG leads, and when needle electrodes are used this danger is significantly increased. Even the currently popular small disc type of leads permits burning when the ground plate and its connections fail to work.

It is apparent then that a very important factor in the safe use of electrical equipment, especially when more than one unit is in use on the same patient, is the ensurance that grounding is taking place through the proper channels. It is important to see that the opportunity for accidental grounding through the patient is minimized by use of the third-wire ground, high quality instruments and, in the operating room, an isolated electrical system.

EXPLOSION HAZARDS

Ignition of flammable or explosive anesthetic agents is a potential danger that accompanies the use of these agents. Fortunately—despite careless handling of these agents—the incidence of fires and explosions is extremely low. One must be aware, however, of the likelihood of ignition whenever these agents are used; one must develop a consciousness of explosions in the same way that a surgeon develops a consciousness of sepsis and the need for asepsis. It is possible to avoid fire and explosion by always applying certain fundamental principles and a rigid discipline concerning safety in daily practice.

TABLE 31-1.—LIMITS OF INFLAMMABILITY (IN PERCENTAGE)

	AIR	OXYGEN
Ethylene	2.75	to 79.9
Cyclopropane	2.40	to 63.1
Divinyl Ether	4.00	to 14.8
Ethyl Ether	1.70	to 83.5
Fluroxene	4.00	—

Table 31-1 provides details of inflammability in air or oxygen of the flammable gases and liquids. The prophylactic measures to be outlined are developed on the basis of these physical properties and associated factors.

Factors Necessary to Explosions

Three factors are essential to each explosion: (1) a flammable material, (2) an ignition source and (3) an oxygen supply. One other factor is often present—a lack of common sense (which also may be reclassified as carelessness or inattention to details).

Materials and Concentrations

The flammable materials used in anesthetic practice are the gases, ethylene and cyclopropane, and the volatile liquids, ethyl ether, divinyl ether, ethyl chloride and fluroxene. Inhalation agents that are nonflammable in anesthetic concentrations are nitrous oxide, chloroform, trichlorethylene, halothane, methoxyflurane, isoflurane and enflurane. Cyclopropane, as well as the other flammable agents, may be used in a closed system; and even in the presence of a gross leak, it is difficult to develop explosive concentrations at any appreciable distance from the machine. A hazard exists with static electricity when attaching and detaching the external circuit from the patient. Ethyl ether, divinyl ether and ethyl chloride are heavier than air and gravitate to the floor when released into the atmosphere. It is difficult to produce flammable concentrations of these agents in areas distant from the mask or machine unless there is gross spilling in a small room with minimal ventilation. Table 31-1 shows that all of these agents are flammable within the range needed for anesthesia. Fortunately, fluroxene usually is flammable only when given in the concentration needed for induction. Fluroxene should be used with caution in the presence of ignition sources and not at all if ignition sources are close to an output of the vapor.

Oxygen to support the combustion may come from the oxygen added to the anesthetic mixture, from the air or from nitrous oxide. There is an increase in range of explosiveness and rate of propagation of flame when oxygen is added to the explosive or flammable agents. The accelerated rate of propagation of the flame in an oxygen atmosphere is the factor that is most dangerous to the patient because it facilitates the entrance of flame into the lung.

Ignition Sources

Ignition may originate in electrical equipment or static discharge. Electrical equipment, including switches, should be explosion-proof whenever possible, and electrical circuits should be designed as isolation circuits. If it is at all possible, all electrical equipment should be kept off the floor and switches, outlet boxes, etc., should be placed at least 5 feet (150 cm) above the floor. The best means for avoiding ignition from electrical equipment is to avoid the use of explosive agents whenever equipment such as electro-surgical units, electric saws and x-ray machines are to be used.

Static discharges are the most difficult ignition sources to eliminate or suppress. Static is developed by friction, and a spark occurs when one object with a high potential discharges to another object with a low potential.

A few examples of the potentials that can be developed in an operating room are as follows:

1,000–2,000 volts: a nurse walking 20 feet on a tile floor;
2,000–3,000 volts: scuffing of feet on a tile floor;
4,000 volts: draping the patient on an operating table;
50,000 volts: an anesthetist sliding on a stool cushioned with rubber.

Woolen or synthetic fibre blankets are potent sources of static and should be eliminated from areas where explosive agents are used. The making and breaking of contact with rubber to metal or metal to metal connections are common sources of static discharge.

PREVENTION OF STATIC PRODUCTION AND DISCHARGE.—Production of static should be lessened by ensuring that the humidity in the operating room exceeds 55%. This permits the slow discharge of potentials without spark. If air conditioning is in use, one must be careful that washing of the air is not so efficient that all small dust particles are removed, because the dust particles also transmit potentials and prevent the development of high potentials.

All metallic and otherwise conductive equipment, including tables and other furniture, must be grounded to make less likely the development of high potentials relative to other pieces of equipment or persons. If one piece of equipment or a person is not grounded, the discharge of the static load from such an object will be facilitated by contact with the grounded equipment and sparking will occur. It is essential to install a proper conductive floor that includes an area outside of the door so that high potentials will drain off before persons entering can come into contact with the grounded equipment. A conductive floor should be maintained so that the resistance to ground remains greater than 25,000 ohms and any reading between special weighted electrodes 3 feet apart does not exceed 1 million ohms.

Another method of establishing equipotentials between objects and for disposition of static charges is the use of wet towels. Towels should be placed from the machine to the floor, from the operating table to the floor and from the patient around a nonconducting table mattress to the metal of the table. Particularly in rooms with poorly conductive floors, the anesthetist should stand on a wet sheet or towel. The towels should be spread out to increase the area permitting discharge of the static.

The anesthetic tubing and mask should be made of conductive rubber and tested periodically to ensure that stretching and use has not destroyed the conductivity. Nonmetallic parts of gas machines and operating room tables should be conductive. This includes tires, mattresses, tubing, etc. Overcrowding of operating rooms should be avoided, not only from the standpoint of increased ignition source but also from that of an increased possibility for contamination of the operative site.

Only approved conductive shoes or shoe covers should be allowed in flammable anesthetizing areas. Nonconductive soles or shoes, and wool, silk and nylon outer clothing (except for stockings) should not be permitted in the operating room when flammable agents are being used. Shoes with protruding nails or with metal heel or toe plates should not be permitted because of the mechanical development of sparks.

Thus, fires and explosions can be kept at an absolute minimum by careful and proper use of electrical equipment, by maintaining humidity in the operating room above 55%, by keeping the potential equal between patient, operating table, anesthetist, gas machine and floor and by eliminating wool blankets, rubber-soled shoes, and wool, silk or nylon outer clothing. There is no device that can substitute for the constant alertness and consciousness of the anesthetist of the hazards associated with the use of explosive agents.

SUMMARY

It is a curious paradox that even when the opportunity and the indications exist for the use of a flammable agent such as cyclopropane, the current generation of anesthetists seems to be much more afraid of a very, very low incidence of explosion than of the hypotension, cardiac irregularities, hepatotoxicity, hypoventilation and other complications regularly associated with the use of an agent such as halothane. Perhaps much of the reason for their selection lies in the fact that most surgeons today demand the use of the electrosurgical unit in nearly every case. Finally, we know of no anesthetists who have developed hepatitis (or other sensitivities) to cyclopropane or ether.

REFERENCE

1. Standard for Use of Inhalation Anesthetics. N.F.P.A. Bulletin 56A, 1973. National Fire Protection Association, 60 Batterymarch Street, Boston, Massachusetts.

Index

B

D